Sex and People

Kenneth L. Jones
Louis W. Shainberg
Curtis O. Byer

Mt. San Antonio College

Harper & Row, Publishers

New York, Hagerstown, San Francisco, London

Sex and People

Sponsoring Editor: Joe Ingram
Project Editor: David Nickol
Designer: Howard S. Leiderman
Production Supervisor: Will C. Jomarrón
Photo Researcher: Myra Schachne
Compositor: The Clarinda Company
Printer: The Murray Printing Company
Binder: Halliday Lithograph Corporation
Art Studio: Danmark & Michaels Inc.

Photographs: *Figures 5.1, 6.2, and 6.3, Lester Bergman and Associates; Figure 13.11 courtesy Parke, Davis & Co.; Figure 14.3 courtesy Nicholas Fiumara, M.D.; Figure 14.6 (top) courtesy U.S. Public Health Service, Communicable Disease Center, Atlanta, Georgia; Figure 14.6 (bottom) courtesy Sidney Olansky, M.D.; Figure 14.11, Lester Bergman and Associates.*

Library of Congress Cataloging in Publication Data

Jones, Kenneth Lamar, Date–
Sex and people.

Bibliography: p.
Includes index.
1. Sex instruction for youth. I. Shainberg, Louis W., joint author. II. Byer, Curtis O., joint author III. Title.
HQ35.2.J65   301.41'8'055   76-43981
ISBN 0-06-043434-1

Contents

Preface

We are quite pleased with the way in which the college human sexuality course has grown and matured since our first text for this course was published in 1969. At that time, few colleges even offered such a course, and where it was offered, instructors were often uncertain as to the direction their course should take. Today, excellent courses are being presented in a great many institutions.

The experience of many instructors over these few years has led them to conclude that the most effective course in human sexuality contains a balance of biological, psychological, and sociological material. Few sexual experiences can be fully understood without drawing upon all of these disciplines. We feel that *Sex and People* offers a good balance of the cultural, emotional, and physical aspects of human sexuality and can serve as a basis for interesting classroom discussion in all of these areas.

We believe that a human sexuality course should do more than just present facts. While a sound factual basis is important, we see additional goals as including the development of positive attitudes toward sexuality, a sense of sexual ethics, increased ease and confidence in communicating sexual ideas and feelings, and a strengthened sense of personal sexual adequacy. We have written *Sex and People* to help achieve these goals.

We want to thank Mary Fairfax, R.N., for her contribution of materials for Chapters 1, 2, and 16 and for suggesting the title of the book.

K. L. J.
L. W. S.
C. O. B.

Sex and People

Sex and Society

1

Society and the Individual

Society's primary function is supposed to be the promotion of the welfare of its members and the provision of an atmosphere in which its members, whether many or few, can live in relative concord and agreement. Thus the population allows itself to be bound together by certain common standards, customs, values, mores, and laws, thereby conveying a degree of security to individual members. When these standards are no longer held to be valid, society is acted upon by its members so that changes will be initiated. As changes are effected, the society and its population are eventually brought into equilibrium again. Individuals and societies cannot act independently of each other; however, each has a dynamic force, and both must work at interacting cooperatively.

Sexuality has always held a prominent position in human affairs and its expression is largely determined by societal expectations. Such expectations greatly influence the individual's development as a sexual being. At various points in our lives, each of us has had either more or less self-determination in the realm of sexual attitudes and sexual behavior. But at some point, society places limitations beyond which negative consequences are meted out. Our society is apparently gravely concerned about the adequacy of the traditional value system in meeting the needs of contemporary people. While there is a lesser degree of sexual inhibition now than there used to be, and many heated controversies are challenging traditional mores, we don't view the situation as being appropriately termed a "sexual revolution." The old attitudes are not being totally altered, and there is no evidence that such changes are coming about with any extraordinary swiftness. Just as biological life forms evolve gradually and with some orderliness, societies must also evolve in order to adapt to the changing cultural milieus with which individuals are obliged to cope. Adaptation is paramount to survival, whether it be at the biological or the societal level. Some segments of our very pluralistic society view such changes with alarm, fearing rampant sexual exploitation or even societal collapse. Neither is likely to happen. The current questioning and possible rejection of outdated norms seems to reflect a genuine attempt to establish a more sensible, more humanitarian sexual morality. The new morality leans toward an individual's responsibility to self as well as to others, and a system whereby public attitudes and private behavior are in harmony.

A society experiencing change in its sexual standards places a heavy burden on the individual. Sexual matters used to be hidden under a smooth surface, and underneath there was a somewhat uniform set of regulations regarding sexual behavior. The roles played by each gender are established by society rather than by individuals themselves. Morality is hardly more than a prefabricated arrangement of do's and don'ts that in the past relied greatly on such negative controls as fear and guilt for their enforcement. While these guidelines were often riddled with hypocrisy, they did exert a stabilizing influence on people. Since the sexual climate has become freer, more demands are made on people to work out for themselves a set of standards that will serve as a basis for personal sexual fulfillment while meeting the broader regulations of the society and community.

The changing standards reflect greater concern over the persons involved in a sexual relationship than in the socially defined desirability of the sexual behavior itself. Sexual behavior is judged in accordance with its emotional impact on the partners. The new freedom places moral integrity on an individual level; standards are considered relevant only insofar as a person is committed to them. Individuals are increasingly taking the responsibility of judging the desirability of sexual actions according to their expectations of the positive or negative emotional consequences that will result from them. Determination to proceed or withdraw from intimacy has come to depend on questions like these: Has the relationship contributed to increased or decreased self-esteem in both partners? Has the relationship resulted in loss of either partner's individuality? Are both partners motivated by the same things? Has it increased or decreased either partner's personal growth? Has the relationship led to feelings of guilt, hostility, jealousy, or has it increased the ability of the partners to find satisfaction and appreciation with each other? These questions are more meaningful to many people today than the older guidelines, which said simply: Thou shalt not.

The future status of human sexuality ultimately depends on how well prepared we are to experiment with new values and standards and how judiciously we carry out such experiments. These experiments are not unlike scientific experiments, in which hypotheses are tested for validity. Indeed, we are in an era of testing social hypotheses and either qualifying or disqualifying them on the basis of our personal feelings, as well as the emotional responses of others. This is not an easy road to travel. Anything that will help us avoid missteps should therefore be well understood. We need to have accurate knowledge of our biologic sexual potential and a basic understanding of the way various learned cultural influences give rise to almost infinite variation in sexual behavior. It is also of great importance that the individual be able to distinguish between what is factual and what is an attitudinal opinion. Attitudes can come to be accepted as truths. On the other hand, a legitimate fact does not vary, no matter how many or how few people are in possession of it. Truths are not subject to deviation on the basis of individual perception. A firm grasp on the basic facts of human sexuality will be of enormous help in emotional feelings that arise from the transgression of a learned sexual attitude. Guilt, fear, hostility, anxiety, and anger need not become roots of permanent psychosexual damage if they are dealt with logically.

It is also useful to establish some uniform meanings to such broad concepts as human sexuality, sexual roles, norms, dysfunction, variation, and deviation. This does not mean that everyone is obliged to have the same perceptions and attitudes, only that we must establish enough related meaning so that communication does not become confused and nonsensical. Verbal communication on sexual matters is further complicated by lack of experience in using sexual terminology. Words like coitus, penis, orgasm, and masturbation frequently cause embarrassment, guilt, or vague states of anxiety. As children many of us were punished for using "dirty" words, and our questions about sex were evaded. The genitals were often not called by their true names, but by euphemisms. In short, sex topics were mostly taboo, so there was little opportunity to learn the language and hardly any chance to use it in the course of daily conversation. Many sexual subjects are just beginning to be open for discussion, especially in mixed company. Therefore, it is hardly realistic to expect everyone to react neutrally when sex is discussed in a roomful of strangers.

A knowledge of the origin of some traditional standards gives us new insights into the reasons that certain traditional values and customs had significance in past centuries, although today they have little if any meaning at all. Consider the idea that sex can be labeled good only when it is engaged in specifically for reproduction. This idea had a great deal more relevance when human populations were small and a high birth rate was necessary to compensate for deaths. Today's population is already testing the limits of the earth's ability to support it, and we run the risk of reproducing ourselves to extinction. In this context, an individual might look upon sexual intercourse as being destructive when it is engaged in for reproductive purposes. Words like marriage, masculinity, and femininity are also in states of transition; they need redefining if they are to conform with present realities. For instance, if one were to define marriage in terms of its traditional meaning, it would probably be worded something like "a legal and religious contract whereby a man and woman agree to live together, love each other, and remain forever faithful to each other until death." It sounds rather idealistic in the face of today's prevalent serial monogomy. In examining the history of sexual morality, we can see where our society falls on the sexual continuum and will realize that periods of permissiveness and restrictiveness fluctuate with regularity. We can also see that we are unique neither in desiring change nor in any of the forms of sexual behavior in which we engage. Traditions established today will also be subject to renovation in future generations.

Human Sexuality: What and Where?

Human sexuality represents a series of complex interactions between mind and body and is manifested as an indivisible component of the entire personality. The sociocultural environment responds differently to the male than it does to the female. It acts upon the biological sexual potential by providing characteristic learning experiences in the form of all relationships between the individual, other persons, and the environment. While sexuality reflects attitudes, beliefs, values, and a repertoire of sexual behaviors, patterns are gained from experience beyond the self. The self alters all of these through unique perceptual differences. Nonsexual aspects of personality influence overt and covert sexual elements, just as the sexual components of the personality influence the nonsexual.

In an attempt to appreciate the multidimensional quality of human sexuality, it seems appropriate to make a few comparisons between human and other animal sexuality. Sex among other animals is primarily oriented toward reproduction. Even the more complex sexual behavior patterns, such as courtship rituals, have as a direct goal the mating of a male and female which will result in perpetuation of the species. In humans, sex plays many roles independent of its reproductive function. Even during periods of extreme sexual suppression, when the prevailing morality has condemned nonreproductive coitus, history reveals that sex for fun has always been prevalent. Among most animals, sexual contact occurs only during the female's estrus period, or "heat." At other times sexual advances are likely to be met with indifference or resistance. In contrast, humans are amenable if not enthusiastic to sex at any time, regardless of the female's fertility status. The higher primates do exhibit more flexibility in their sexual behavior, but there is still a strong relationship between sex and reproduction.

Another basic difference between humans and other animals lies in the almost infinite number of ways humans have dealt with their sexuality. What is completely normal to a person in one culture may seem bizarre or even inhuman to someone from another culture. In animals such diverse sexual behavior is not seen. Different populations of the same species demonstrate almost identical sexual patterns. In most animals the main association between males and females relates to reproduction and care of the young. Humans deliberately seek out relationships with members of the opposite sex for purposes other than erotic sex, such as friendship, cooperation at work, or advice. It is very important for humans to be perceived favorably by the opposite sex. In marriage, sex is but one of many expectations. Often we attempt to win recognition for our sexual attractiveness, but without any intent to engage in sex, as when we flirt or tease. People frequently use their sexuality to attract attention because they want someone to notice them in other respects. Unfortunately, sexuality is also used as a tool in manipulation of other persons. In any case, sexuality influences many parts of the human personality.

Attempts are increasingly being made to explain human sexual behavior comprehensively. While at present none of these explanations are conclusive enough to be accepted as theory, the search for new data is providing fresh insights into the problems as well as stimuli to seek out additional avenues of investigation. Mounting resources give us much reason to be optimistic about our prospects in our search for an understanding of human sexuality. The main approaches thus far traveled have sought explanation through application of biological factors, assorted sociopsychological elements, and learning principles. Inasmuch as everything is still conjecture, we can simply state that quite likely in the final analysis elements from each channel will be found necessary for theory validation. Although we cannot go into the details of each proposed theory, it is still possible and appropriate to draw knowledge from them which is relevant and applicable to individuals in their search for an understanding of their own sexuality.

At one extreme, human sexuality is seen as a purely biological instinct, universally inherent in all humans. According to this belief, even if an individual were devoid of past sexual experience and had been told nothing about it, sexual behavior would become manifest sometime near the onset of physical maturity. Since no such experience-free persons exist, our past histories are rationalized as merely limiting the explicit sexual activity we have engaged in, but are not considered to have any effect on the basic development of masculinity or femininity or on the instinctive sex drive. Obviously, no concrete evidence can be put forth disproving such a simplistic notion, but the data that are available do not support it. For example, in cases of sexual ambiguity, when parents have brought up a child as a girl, say, but subsequent testing has revealed that the child is actually a boy, attempts to establish a new gender identification—to help the child to perceive himself as a boy—have largely been unsuccessful. Greater success is achieved through altering the visible sexual apparatus to coincide with the adopted or learned sex role. Cases such as these discredit the concept of a purely biological gender identification; learning in some manner must account for perception and acceptance of gender affiliation.

Thus sexuality is not simply a product of biologic maturation, but is essentially dependent on learning in one manner or another. At birth all persons possess certain biologic sexual potentials as well as certain differences, and it must be stressed that the differences are greater among individuals than between the sexes. The extent to which such potentials are developed or denied is relative to the quality of learning that incorporates one's sexuality into overall personality structure.

The most influential sources of informal sexual training include the home and family members, peer groups, and the social environment, such as advertising, movies, television, and the like. The phrase "sex education" has been deliberately avoided here because it implies a more formal learning approach with specific criteria and such goals as those found within school sex education programs. While the kind of sex instruction that is given in the classroom is of great importance, within our culture it is relatively new. Until recently people have learned their sexual rules and permissible sexual behavior on a more informal basis, usually quite inadvertently. Sex education will be discussed later on. For now let us look at some of the ways in which sexuality is taught informally and how these encounters influence a developing sexual self-concept.

Parents

Parents or other significant persons in a child's life act as the first and perhaps the most influential mediators of sexuality training. Parenting and its duties are not simple under any circumstances. In our sex-repressed culture, however, it has been particularly difficult for parents to become consciously involved and aware of their responsibility to assist their children in sexual development. To a large extent, what has been learned through parents has been only incidental to the entire child-rearing process. With or without intention, parents cannot avoid being basic models of female and male roles, various intimacies between the sexes, and intangibles such as attitudes, beliefs, and values. Children imitate these models and eventually adopt observed behaviors as their own.

Sex is a pleasurable pursuit, and when sexual needs cannot be adequately met, the result is frustration. Parents are a great threat to an individual's sexual adjustment when they act as either severe inhibitors or punishers of sexual behavior—most of which is nowhere near an erotic level during the early years. Punishment sets up an internal competition between pleasure and inhibition. In any case, sexual activity is not likely to cease despite anticipated negative consequences. Even though attitudes may conflict with the attainment of sexual pleasure, such standards are usually transgressed, resulting in psychosexual problems ranging from minor feelings of guilt or anxiety to total sexual incompetence.

Rudimentary sexual behavior is evidenced early in infancy. Male infants are capable of erection almost upon birth, and females of vaginal lubrication upon genital stimulation. These phenomena are not perceived in the erotic sense, as being preliminary to coitus. When the mothering person feels a revulsion toward such involuntary responses, as frequently occurs during diapering, her reaction is picked up by an infant.

That such sensations are pleasurable is evidenced by the way some cultures employ genital stimulation as a method of comforting irritable infants. The infant begins to explore hands, feet, face, and at some point stumbles upon the genitalia and finds that it feels good when these parts are touched. It is not likely that playing with any part of the body except the sex organs will elicit a negative parental response. When these and similar activities are consistently interfered with, in due time the genitalia come to be perceived as unclean, thus lowering total self-esteem. Inhibited, sexually anxious parents are provided with ample opportunity to restrict sexual growth. For instance, when children learn to dress and bathe, unreasonable expectations of modesty or the use of substitute words for penis, vagina, breasts, and so on also diminishes the acceptance of these areas. Many parents fail to cope with or satisfy normal sex curiosity, either by avoiding questions, giving unrealistic information, or punishing children who are mutually exploring each other's sexual apparatus. Detailed explanations of sexual physiology and elaborate descriptions of coital technique are not necessary, but in homes with healthy sexual atmospheres questions are answered promptly and information is factual and appropriate to the chronological age as well as emotional maturity of the child. There is no one big day when parents spell out the "facts of life" because the child is big enough for sex. Rather, there is a natural and gradual unfolding of information that distinguishes purely orgasmic sex from a cohesive sexuality in which relationships are as important as the sex act itself.

Interactions between parents also constitute an avenue of sexual tutoring. Affection openly displayed is a lesson in sensuousness: The child learns that close tactile contact, even though not overtly sexual, is a source of self-esteem, enhanced by the fact that it involves the awareness of another person's needs. If sensuousness is not learned in childhood, its lack often presents problems in establishing loving or caring adult relationships because the individual does not know how to get close to another person without feeling uncomfortable. As a result the cared-for person is made to feel more like an object, perhaps even a sexual object, than an appreciated multidimensional human being.

The manner in which parents act out their respective masculine/feminine roles has lasting effects on an individual's future role portrayal. Because a small child's world is so circumscribed, sex roles of family members are likely to form the basis of generalizations about all males and females. If either parent is not satisfied with his masculinity or her femininity, this dissatisfaction can affect the sexual adjustment of the child. When roles are rigidly defined by society, individuals will desperately try to conform. They will view males as dominant, competitive, successful in business, athletically adept, in control of emotions, devoid of tenderness, and very sexually oriented, if that is the pattern that is rewarded by the society. They will see females as submissive, subservient, dependent, virtuous, emotional but passionless, tender, and noncompetitive. In reality, neither sex has exclusive rights to any basic human characteristic. Independence, self-confidence, tenderness, competitiveness, and passion are neither male nor female, only human. Enough flexibility and tolerance should exist in the home so that all of its children can assume roles compatible with their unique personalities. Much of what we see as extremely masculine or feminine behavior is merely an attempt to compensate for imagined failure in some aspect of role expectation. Traditional barriers between what is appropriately male and female are breaking down, and with them the double standard is beginning to crumble. Concerned parents should endeavor to behave in such a way that male and female roles are seen as complementary rather than antagonistic. Parents do a grave disservice to their children and to themselves as well when they turn their home into a battleground in which one of them is always superior while the other is always dominated and inferior.

Parents tend to present their own attitudes, beliefs, and values as absolute truths, leaving little room for otherwise acceptable alternatives or tolerance toward people with different views. Attitudes, we believe, should be related in such a way that alternatives are also offered. For example, a parent may say, "I feel this is the right way to act because it has worked for me. But this might not be comfortable for you, so here are a few alternatives." With greater resources, the individual is better prepared to adapt to almost any sexual or nonsexual situation without having self-concepts disturbed. When differences between values and actual behavior are small, psychological problems rarely arise. Extension of attitudes beyond those of the home enables parents to discuss pros and cons of issues important to young people, rather than acting as dictators issuing orders. Parental orders in the sexual sphere are often based on fear or guilt—fear of pregnancy or disease, the belief that sexual intercourse outside of marriage is sinful, the fear that masturbation leads to the insane asylum or the penitentiary. These are standards, so to speak, but where is the morality? Once parents allow children more latitude in forming their own values, they will be able to spend less time with discipline. Consequently they can concentrate on the development of character that is a basis for choosing wise sexual behavior.

The Peer Group

After parents, friends are the most common sources of information on sex. They may be the *only* source of information if parents have totally avoided the subject. At best, the information gleaned from peers is secondhand, and it has usually been passed along from several other friends or older siblings. Much of what is learned from peers is not reliable and is full of misconceptions that will only lead to further confusion of the sexually naive individual. Another danger inherent in such sex gossip is that it is more explicitly sex-oriented than value-oriented. Discussions are rarely on a factual physiological basis and almost never involve psychological implications. Sexuality as it relates to the total personality and is integrated with nonsexual aspects of the individual's life finds little place in these exchanges of information. The principal focus is on intercourse: Have you done it? How do you do it? How far did you go? How does it feel? If members of the group have had intercourse, their experience may be a source of prestige. Thus, in order to gain greater identification with peers, some people who don't feel they are ready for the intimacy of intercourse will go ahead in spite of inner conflict, for the sole purpose of gaining status and acceptance from friends. While such experimenting will not necessarily have a negative influence on future and more mature relationships, guilt and fears of pregnancy, of getting caught, or of contracting disease can be sustained for many years, without cause.

For every negative aspect, a positive one can usually be found, and such may be the case here. Peer groups may have a beneficial effect on individuals whose sexual attitudes, as gained from the home, have been excessively restrictive or overly permissive. Friends are usually very accepting and trustful of each other. Thus young people can find acceptance of their sexual feelings from their friends when such feelings must be denied at home. In a way, permission is given to engage in a degree of sexual behavior that is condemned in the home. In this manner inhibitions may be overcome, and if development of character also continues, realization of satisfactory sexuality can be achieved despite previous negative influences.

Cultural Mediation

The cultural environment, including movies, television, magazines, newspapers, billboards, public controversy, and so on, exert indeterminable influence upon preadult sexual maturation. It is also one of the least manageable areas of learning because exposure is unavoidable. Commercialism has put dramatic emphasis on the portrayal of sex without regard to personal relationships. It is sad that sex is so often used as an advertising gimmick—purchase the product and increase your sex appeal; fly Nancy on one airline or do it the French way on another. Some of this is changing, but role portrayal in the cultural milieu has been rigidly sexist. Both women and men have been maligned by stereotyping, and this has perpetuated the polarity of the sexes. How many self-concepts have been traumatized by failure to conform with some idealized image?

Old traditions lurk everywhere because sex in the current cultural environment is still being segregated from the more "wholesome" aspects of life. We may hope that the younger generations, having the benefit of a more temperate sexual climate, will get a basic grounding in sexuality through informed, responsive parents and adequate school sex education programs, thereby reducing the importance of impressions received from the cultural media.

Sexual Maturity

In a discussion of sexual maturity, distinctions must immediately be drawn among the various aspects of maturity: biological, social, and emotional. Most conspicuously, the physiological changes accompanying puberty represent sexual maturity, but usually only insofar as reproductive capacity is concerned. Early adolescence is a period of intense self-awareness in which the struggle for independence and identity takes precedence over sensitivity to others. Behavior is characteristically impulsive and rationalizations bear heavily on decisions. Very few individuals reach a level of emotional maturity commensurate with their biological status at this stage. Therefore, it is necessary to look elsewhere for a more meaningful definition of sexual maturity.

Traditionally, sexual maturity has also been related to meeting certain societal criteria. For instance, eighteen years is a common legal age of maturity, both sexual and nonsexual. Other implied prerequisites include completion of formal education and economic stability; until recently even marriage was an expressed standard. Because there was little acceptance of the "sex for fun" attitude and because sex, marriage, and children came pretty much as a package deal, the liberties associated with maturity had to be closely guarded. Today many people do not complete their educations until their late twenties. Economic soundness likewise is delayed, and the proclivity for marriage has waned, especially in the procreative sense. Sexual desires and satisfaction cannot realistically be suppressed for so many years. In addition, sexual maturity cannot be determined by age. Many individuals remain emotionally adolescent despite advanced chronological age or social status. As such they are likely to have sexual adjustment problems, with which their partners may also be burdened.

Emotional stability is perhaps the most reliable measure of sexual maturity and usually increases the quality of the sexual relationship itself. The value of interaction between sexual partners cannot be underestimated. Sex also fulfills the nonsexual need to be physically and emotionally close to another person. If orgasmic relief were the only objective of sex, it could just as easily be satisfied through masturbation. As the level of emotional maturity rises, the potential meaningfulness of sexual intercourse increases. Personal fulfillment and self-esteem are increased, and the pleasure given and received reinforces sexual competency and communication. Such intimacy, however, requires the confidence that self-integrity will not be injured. The truly sexually mature individual realizes that a certain vulnerability exists for both partners; therefore, deliberate thought is given to sexual actions.

There are no limits on the amount of emotional maturity that can be developed. On the other hand, it is possible for a person to be emotionally prepared for one type of relationship but not another. Different kinds of sexual commitment demand varying degrees of emotional stamina. Thus a brief liaison wherein both individuals voluntarily share little more than the pleasure of sex is not likely to cause as much emotional stress and adjustment as would a marriage relationship, which requires constant nurturing. Also the nature of the sexual behavior—marital, nonmarital, extramarital—tends to place the interacting parties in a position of greater or lesser precariousness. The mature person is aware of the amount of anxiety he or she can withstand and avoids sexual encounters that would be overwhelming.

In order that sex be maximally rewarding and satisfying, under whatever circumstances, there are some guidelines that we feel should be followed. If these conditions are met, the persons concerned should feel free to act upon their mutual decisions without having to secure additional approval. There should exist a basic emotional readiness so that sexual behavior will not result in excessive guilt or prove an impediment to other life goals. Sexual maturity means that sexual behavior will be based upon knowledge of available alternatives, objectivity in evaluating the advantages and disadvantages of such behavior, and anticipation and acceptance of possible consequences. Most important, a conscious effort will be made to protect the psychological integrity of the other party as well as one's own. Practical considerations like contraception and the possibility of sexually transmitted disease should always be taken care of before initiation of sexual activity. This means that motives must be examined and mutually shared; expectations of the relationship and of each other should be understood and accepted. Honesty must be matched with openness. Both are essential elements in a rewarding sexual interaction. Finally, sexually mature persons always have an attitude of respect for their partners, caring about their general welfare. Without this respect, self-esteem is lowered by giving so fully of oneself to a person deemed unworthy to receive it.

Autonomy and Motives

Where does one look for standards or codes of sexual conduct that are neither restrictive to the point of sexual inhibition or dysfunction nor so liberal that sex becomes exploitive, decreases self-esteem, or results in lack of ability to achieve a deep psychological intimacy? You will find neither justification nor condemnation of any mode of sexual behavior here. Part of maturity, sexual or otherwise, is being able to work out standards of behavior consistent with personal beliefs. Presumably adults are autonomous—independent and self-governing—and are therefore responsible for and capable of defining their own sexual morality. By virtue of such autonomy, it is necessary for individuals to sort out and identify personal motives for sexual involvement. Care should be taken not to rationalize behavior or to pretend certain motives exist when in fact they do not.

Every behavior has an underlying motive for being acted out, and usually we are drawn toward those experiences that satisfy either physical or emotional needs. Intercourse is not necessarily engaged in for reasons of a sexual nature. Indeed, quite often the motives are hardly related to the sexual experience itself.*

Sexual Motives

The basic drive toward the pleasures derived from arousal, orgasm, and relief of physical tension constitutes a direct sexual motive. This type of involvement demands a minimal expenditure of self; thus the risk of psychological trauma is not overly great. On the other hand, such a relationship offers little in the way of emotional satisfaction. The healthiness of psychosexual adjustment would have to be questioned when superficial relationships become a pattern. Yet, on an occasional or sporadic basis, sexual satisfaction alone maybe a realistic motive and may be quite valid, if both partners agree and accept the predominantly physical nature of such involvement. It is certainly better to admit to oneself and one's partner just how limited commitment is or will be than to try to find nonexistent "higher" motives. The honesty and mutuality of motive, even though emotional attachment is lacking, demonstrates concern and may generate much tenderness because no one is being manipulated. One must question, however, just how honest it is possible to be when physical sex is the only motive. Total honesty regarding lack of commitment is rarely seen except between prostitute and customer.

Other sexual motives, although not directly related to orgasmic release itself, are the need for tactile stimulation (touching), security,

*See *Medical Aspects of Human Sexuality,* August 1975, pp. 32–41, and September 1975, pp. 8–31.

warmth, trust, and being close to someone (intimacy). Again, these desires need not be accompanied by overwhelming affection. Usually, however, people do not have intercourse with persons they dislike or view as being unattractive. Unless an individual has problems in establishing a nonsexual interest in others, it is almost inevitable that motives will extend beyond pure physical desire.

Reproduction is occasionally a motive for sex. Sometimes it is used in an effort to trap someone into marriage. Obviously this motive can have disastrous consequences and is indicative of immaturity. It is also an often-used rationalization for the pleasures of sex. The more recent trend is to validate sex with love; but when the sexual motive has been fulfilled, only too often love fades and is replaced by feelings of amazement that one could ever have been in love with that person. It is difficult to distinguish between infatuation and love. Frequently sexual intimacy serves to define feelings. The relationship may be strengthened by it so that true commitment grows and replaces original physical motivation. Or the relationship may disintegrate rapidly, indicating that real love never existed.

Nonsexual Motives

Nonsexual motives for intercourse can be very complex and quite frequently are indicative of psychological problems. It is difficult for individuals to recognize neurotic behavior in themselves. Often they identify motives falsely or avoid personal confrontation altogether. In such cases honesty between the interacting persons suffers greatly; one party is commonly the subject of exploitation, and both partners may be psychologically hurt.

Younger persons are especially vulnerable to being pressured into sexual relations by the attitudes of their friends and a desire to conform to the group's standards. When doubt exists or personal standards are overridden, however, anxiety, guilt, and even depression frequently result. There can also be a loss of faith in one's ability to make decisions.

Sexual activity is often motivated by the desire to be loved. Thus the sexual giving of oneself may be seen as a means of obtaining love and acceptance that were denied in childhood. It is not likely that such desires will be met, and the feeling that one is unlovable is reinforced. A similar motive is the desire to overcome feelings of loneliness, the purchase of companionship in exchange for sex.

Feelings of inferiority or doubts about masculinity or femininity are often combated through frequent and superficial sexual conquests. Total satisfaction is rarely achieved, however, and blame is placed on the innocent party. Numerous short-lived relationships can also be motivated by hostility toward the opposite sex. In these situations the sought-after party is usually dropped suddenly after sexual seduction.

When independence has not been adequately established, sex can be used as a means of identifying with traits one would like to see emerge within one's own personality structure. Such associations are likely to hinder subsequent development of independence and self-reliance.

Sex is also used as a means of comforting another person. In this case, an individual may fulfill some desire to act in a mothering or fathering capacity. On the other hand, offering oneself sexually may be the only way a person knows how to feel comfortable in extending consolation.

Compensation for favors or an out-of-duty motivation is not uncommon. In fact, these motivations frequently replace loving interpersonal sexuality in marriages that have lost significance with respect to intimacy, growth, and meaningfulness.

Sex Education

Sex education is of particular importance to the development of mature sexuality. There exists a legitimate need for formal sex education even at the elementary-grade level. Whereas human sexuality courses are quite well established in college curriculums, there is still a substantial lag in the establishment of adequate sex education programs below this level. Mainly this has been due to community or parental disapproval plus a lack of qualified teachers. The lack of sex education has been so great that many college-level human sexuality courses appear to be of a remedial nature. So much time has to be spent in explaining basic anatomy and physiology, or in correcting fundamental misconceptions, that exploration of the deeper meanings of interpersonal relationships often has to be sacrificed.

Increasingly more people are going to counselors, psychologists, and physicians in search of help for such sexual dysfunctions as impotence, unresponsiveness, and premature ejaculation. Many of the problems experienced by these people as adults could have been prevented had they received adequate sex education during childhood. Much of the guilt-fear-incompetence syndrome is a product of having been taught by misinformed parents that sex is shameful or that parts of the body that are sexually responsive are unclean. If effective sex education were initiated at grade-school level and continued throughout high school, we could anticipate that children would at least grow up without turning red when the words penis and vagina are mentioned. Using correct names (although not necessarily scientific names) for parts of the body helps to build the necessary vocabulary for communicating sexual ideas, and desensitizes the individual to the vulgar use of sexual words as epithets.

Basic biological sex courses would make it easier for young people to understand the prevention of sexually transmitted disease and the importance of early cure, and the necessity of choosing either contraception, pregnancy, or celibacy. It is to be hoped that in the not-too-distant future such information will be part of a broader *education for sexuality* introduced in a nonjudgmental and humanistic manner.

The greatest obstacles to sex education have been lack of public support and hostility to such programs. When sex education has been introduced, it has been difficult to make decisions as to suitable subject matter—how much and how soon. There is much concern about the manner in which sex should be taught. Should it be presented from a strictly biological standpoint, or should the course involve discussions of attitudes, values, and contemporary issues? In our opinion, sex education is frequently presented in a far too factual, dehumanized, mechanistic manner. It may not be so easy to teach concepts like caring, tolerance, and sexual decision making as it is to teach physiological sex, but this is the area of real need, in which students are going to be most helped in their quest for maximum sexual fulfillment and happiness. Many individuals reading this book will be involved as voters and parents in the formal sex-instruction controversy, and we hope to persuade you here that sex is a valid classroom subject.

Reasons for Sex Education

The home can be an excellent place for sex education, since the setting provides a living example of sexuality and spans the many years of growing up. At present, however, it is not realistic to rely completely on parents for such education, because so few have either the knowledge or the objectivity needed for this task. At the same time, there is a dire shortage of professionals qualified to deal with sexuality and its related problems. Scientific research in the area of human sexuality has greatly expanded our knowledge, but thus far the dissemination of this information has been extremely limited. Some people have proposed that parents be required to take sex education classes so that they can instruct their own children. If such a thing were possible, however, what assurance would there be that parents would feel comfortable enough to pass on this learning to their children?

One of the most cogent arguments for formal sex education is that sex, from a reproductive standpoint, is becoming less a matter of personal consequence and more a matter of societal concern. Every child born puts more stress on our total resources, and the luxury of limitless reproduction is no longer considered socially acceptable. There is a need to let many people know that there is such a thing as sex for joy and that reproduction is not the desired outcome of every act of intercourse. It is not enough that individuals be aware of contraceptive methods and the availability of abortion clinics. The lasting and really adhered-to concepts are those learned during childhood, and these should include the value of the quality of life as opposed to quantity, and the development of healthy self-images. If sex is taught only from the standpoint of reproduction, a tremendous opportunity has been lost to put forth the idea that sex is good in itself, but that if it is used indiscriminately it may create many problems for both the individual and the society.

There is yet another reason why formal sex education is essential. In years gone by, individuals had only a few "respectable" alternatives to choose from insofar as sexual behavior or sexual life style were concerned. Now we are freer to choose from many alternatives without fear of social condemnation. Unless children learn tolerance and adaptability, they are likely to encounter many problems that could be avoided in the world beyond their homes or communities. If nothing else, they will be bombarded with sex in every area of the cultural milieu, so that in one way or another sex education will be obtained, but with much confusion and without constructive purpose. With effective formal sex education, children are guaranteed at least a minimum of what they need to know if their sexual decisions are to be made wisely and knowledgeably.

Finally, when we speak of sex education it must be remembered that sexuality covers much, much more than various coital techniques, sexually transmitted disease, masturbation, and so on. While it is important to have a knowledge of these things, it is really more important that we understand the relationships between men and women, and that we value ourselves and respect others as well. In other words, sexuality is an integral part of the whole being—and this is the essence of what we believe sex education should be. Well-adjusted persons rarely have sexual problems because they see themselves as good and are self-accepting. Emotions influence sexual functioning by controlling physiological factors. So it is not enough merely to teach reproductive physiology. It is our feeling that formal sex education, perhaps more broadly defined as *humanity education,* should be considered as natural and desirable a subject as math or history.

Historical and Cultural Perspectives

2

Societies universally attempt to regulate sexual behavior. Beyond this broad generalization, however, the capacity for variation in sexual practices and the meanings attached to them seem almost infinite. We become so inundated with present sexual notions that it is easy to lose sight of important historical considerations that, despite a gap of centuries, are still affecting our lives and sexual morality. Many sexual standards currently being challenged are attitudes and beliefs far removed from contemporary society, and actually originated almost two thousand years ago (McCown, 1958).

Usually one's own cultural background is used as a basis of comparison, since most of us view our own sexual activities as natural and those of other cultures as peculiar. Often we judge people negatively if their codes differ from our own. Intolerance develops rapidly, and any custom that we don't understand tends to be labeled abnormal and treated with suspicion. Interestingly, we sometimes tolerate differences exhibited by others but are incapable of accepting the same variation in ourselves.

No sexual pattern can be universally stereotyped as normal or natural. We can say that, with the exception of the incest taboo humans are *naturally* incredibly various in their approaches to sexuality. The utmost imagination has been exercised in the creation of distinctive sexual cultures, and this is quite a feat considering that the number of physically possible variations is quite limited. Factors like gender orientation, male and female roles, and standards of sexual behavior have been approached from every conceivable viewpoint, and have been combined and recombined in almost countless ways. Seemingly identical sexual acts can have totally different meanings: One culture may find an act completely appropriate, another may attach religious significance to it, and others may perceive the same act as utterly deplorable. Many intracultural sexual variations also exist, particularly in complex modern societies like the United States, with heterogeneous populations.

Sexuality is such a dynamic force that it is an integral part of society as a whole. Even cultures that rigorously suppress sexual expression reveal the strength of their sexuality through the very restraints designed to mask it. Humans have portrayed their sexual activities in every known medium, making it a favored subject of art, literature, mythology, religion, and law.

Any overall view of human sexuality requires some knowledge of past as well as current sexual behavior, including cross-cultural perspectives. This chapter describes some of the historical events that bear on today's sexual scenario, and presents a small and very incomplete glimpse of contrasting sexual patterns in other cultures. We believe that knowledge about dimensions of sexuality lying beyond our own immediate experience serves to enhance tolerance of all sexual attitudes. It also helps us gain perspective on the continuing shifts between restrictiveness and permissiveness. Our society has made unusually rapid progress in liberalizing its sexual climate. However, there are still many unanswered questions as to how much personal sexual freedom we want or should have. When values and attitudes change rapidly, people are put under stress and the whole system is vulnerable. We could find ourselves right back in an era of sexual repression, perhaps worse than ever. If realistic, human-oriented sexual standards are to be worked out, we need to use every resource available, including all that history and other societies have to show us, so that decisions may not be made blindly.

Primitive Men and Women

Family bonds have apparently always been important in human cultures. All available evidence indicates that human beings have always formed themselves into societies and into families within those societies. The families were organized differently than ours, of course, but kinship was always recognized and was in fact the basis of primitive society. Primitive kinship systems were much more elaborate than ours, indicating that the family, in whatever way it was organized, was much more central to their lives than it is to ours.

Early anthropologists held a different concept of primitive human life, believing that people were nomadic, with the two sexes wandering about independently of each other. Mating was seen as taking place at random, when male and female paths happened to cross. No lasting pair-bonds were thought to occur; after mating, the man and woman were assumed to have wandered off separately. The father was seen as assuming no responsibility for the survival of his children. However, much anthropological evidence has accumulated in support of a much different concept of primitive life. For example, in 1976 Richard Leakey reported the discovery in Africa of the remains of what appears to be a family group of an adult male and female and three children who died together, probably in a flash flood. The site is subject to flash floods today and has been for as far back as evidence gives witness. The human remains have been dated by the carbon-14 method as 5 million years old.

The prolonged infancy and dependency of the young human consumed much of the mother's time and energy. In turn, during this period of child-care, the mother must have required the protection and probably the food-gathering assistance of a mate. Without this, the species would not have survived. In nature, all female and infant primates need and receive the protection of dominant males. It seems likely that this was true of early humans as well as the other primates. Of course, under today's conditions women can successfully raise children without male assistance, but this was apparently not the case for early people.

Beyond these generalizations, little can be said with authority concerning the sexual habits of early humans.

The only universal sexual restriction is the incest taboo. There is no definite agreement on its origin, but some theorists have speculated that it may have arisen from a need for mutual trust among people so that males could cooperate without becoming involved in disputes over sisters and mothers. Other theorists believe the incest taboo is innate, and point to the fact that our cousins the chimpanzees avoid mating with their parents and siblings. Certainly none of us has ever been specifically instructed that we must not have coitus with our parents or our siblings, yet it is very rare for any of us even to consider the matter. In any case, it is extremely doubtful that early peoples recognized the genetic risks of inbreeding. The only known exceptions to the incest taboo serve to validate its universality: Some societies, such as the ancient Egyptian, required their kings to marry their sisters. Members of royal families are always exempt from most of the restrictions imposed on commoners. Breaking the taboo was a sign of divinity. Had there been no incest taboo, there would have been no divine command that the royal heirs marry their sisters. It is also frequently pointed out that among the Hebrews before the time of Moses, brothers and sisters were permitted to marry if they had the same father, though not if they shared the same mother. But the Hebrews, and their descendents the modern Jews, have never permitted paternity to establish membership in their society. The son of a Hebrew man and a gentile woman was not a Hebrew; the son of a Hebrew woman and a gentile man *was* a Hebrew. Clearly paternity carried little weight. Half-siblings who shared only their father were not considered to be brother and sister at all.

We can only speculate that male dominance sprang from physical superiority and from the restrictions placed upon women by motherhood. The prolonged infancy of human offspring required the protection of some dominant male, just as the offspring of other primates receive the protection of the strongest males of the troop. That male was usually, but not always, the mother's mate. In some societies the man who protected the young and had authority over them was the mother's brother, while her mate protected the children of his sister. But in all known societies at least formal authority has rested in some male who is presumed to have the strength and the freedom of movement necessary to protect the young and the women who are responsible for their care. As men began to expand their knowledge and control over the territories where they lived with the tools and weapons they fashioned, women remained in bondage to their physical bodies and maternal functions.

Objects relating to fertility have been found by anthropologists among all primitive and nomadic peoples. It seems that people have always taken the survival of the species seriously. Even the most primitive art depicts male and female genitalia. Also, at the foundation of most religions there can be discerned an identification with sex, fertility, and the powers of nature. The Old Testament is full of admonitions relating to sexual matters, and contains constant reminders to the Hebrews to "be fruitful and multiply."

Early Cultural Influences

Despite the broad range of sexual attitudes and behavior within our culture, there exists a definite sexual climate that can be attributed to influences of Judeo-Christian traditions, flavorings of seventeenth-century Puritan ethics, and remnants of the Victorian era. Inasmuch as many of the early converts to Christanity were of Roman and Greek heritage, these cultures have also contributed to our potpourri of "modern" sexual customs. The following is a brief sketch of some historical events that have influenced our view of sexuality and major trends of thought toward sexual matters at various periods in the past (Lewinsohn, 1958).

Early Judaism

The early Hebrews did not separate the person into two entities, the physical and spiritual. Immortality was believed to be obtained through continuation of family lineage rather than some spiritual afterlife. The rules in regard to sexual behavior mainly emphasized the importance of marriage and family lineage. Procreation was seen as a primary obligation and nonreproductive sex was strongly discouraged. The God of the Old Testament promised Abraham that his descendents would be as numerous as the stars in the heavens. Unmarried persons were at best pitied, and for a man to remain single voluntarily was considered immoral. Men also had a responsibility to carry on the family name because it was believed that the "seed" (semen) carried the substance of life. Women came to be considered merely receptables in which the seeds grew and were nurtured until birth. Were a man to die without having a child by his wife, it was his brother's duty to impregnate the widow. The first son born was considered an offspring of the dead man and the child was given his name. The family line, however, could still be passed down only through a Hebrew woman, for if a Hebrew man impregnated a gentile woman, the child was considered to belong to her clan. A man was therefore free to have sexual relations with a gentile woman, father her child, and leave without feeling responsibility for either of them.

There existed a double standard among Hebrew men and women, inasmuch as a married man was not totally restricted to sex with his wife but the wife was limited to sexual activity with her husband. For purposes of inheritance and biological immortality, it was important for the man to know that the children his wife begot were really his own.

Marriage was a serious undertaking, and men were encouraged to select mates cautiously. A Hebrew man was forbidden to marry a woman until he had seen her—just the opposite of the injunctions of Oriental cultures. What our culture calls the honeymoon, which usually lasts for only a few days or weeks, was a very important part of newlywed life. After the marriage ceremony, the husband was not allowed to be involved in business affairs or war for a period of one year so that he could devote full time to his new wife and adjustment to married life.

Women were respected as wives and mothers but men generally had authority over their wives, their children, and their property, and they alone might initiate divorce. A woman could not divorce her husband, but he could dissolve the marriage on practically any grounds. Barenness was considered good cause for divorce, and if the husband of a barren woman did not dissolve the marriage, he was encouraged to produce children with concubines. In comparison with other societies at that time, however, Hebrew women were treated fairly and with respect. Hebrew girls were expected to remain chaste until marriage, and their fathers had more than a moral stake in their daughters' virginity, because they could demand more money for a marriage contracted with a virgin. In fact, the father could claim compensation from a man who robbed his daughter of her virginity. Engaged persons were regarded as married with respect to intercourse, and children were considered illegitimate only if they resulted from acts of adultery (sexual infidelity of a married person) or incest.

Sexual behavior was quite strictly regulated by law, and penalities ranged from ridicule to death. Adultery, incest, homosexual acts, and bestiality (sexual acts with animals) were forbidden. Male homosexuality was taboo mainly because it was nonreproductive, but also because it was associated with religious practices of other tribes that worshiped different gods. Male homosexual activity was punished by stoning to death; female homosexual acts were not so severely punished. A Hebrew prostitute was stoned to death, but gentile prostitutes were accepted. The adultery laws applied to women who were unfaithful to their husbands, not to the husbands themselves. Masturbation was also forbidden for males, because it was considered wasteful spillage of seed and the death of countless unborn Hebrews. Female masturbation seems not to have been considered worthy of notice.

Some of the other attitudes that we have accepted from Jewish tradition include the belief that menstruating women are unclean and sexual relations during this period are taboo. Although all children were loved and cared for in the Jewish family, boys were preferred to girls as offspring. We have also quite totally accepted the Jewish tradition of male circumcision, which the Jews actually adopted from the Egyptians. Our culture, like that of the early Jews, also tends to honor women in their roles as wives and mothers. Our society still tends to discourage women from competing in business or other activities outside the home. It is significant that even though sexual activity was governed by specific Jewish laws and moral standards, sex itself was considered good. It was not until the advent of Christianity that sex became widely associated with negative attitudes, many of which still persist.

Early Greek and Roman Civilizations

Both Greek and Roman sexual morality had a more secular basis than the hebrew. While the Jews were primarily concerned with procreation and wasting as little seed as possible, the Greeks were interested in limiting population growth for economic reasons. Within both Greek and Roman cultures, infanticide and abortion were legal. In the face of an anticipated food shortage, the Greeks often resorted to female infanticide, although males were not always spared either.

Early Greeks held a bisexual view of the world. According to Greek mythology, the first human-like creatures were hermaphrodites—both male and female. No pressures were placed upon men or women to assume a particular sexual orientation. Homosexual unions between males were not only common but socially acceptable. In fact, the bond between older cultured men and their youthful male companions was considered a more pure form of love than that between a man and woman. Few Greeks were exclusively homosexual, however. The mature men who delighted in their boy lovers were married men with families. Female homosexuality was not unknown among Greek women, but it appears to have been more prevalent in Roman culture. In any event, we have come to call female homosexuality "lesbianism," a word that is derived from Lesbos, an island where the Greek poetess Sappho headed a school for girls. According to the story, Sappho fell in love with one of her pupils, and when the love she sought was never returned, she threw herself into the sea.

Marriage in both classical cultures was outwardly monogamous (exclusive union between one man and one woman), as was Jewish marriage. Jewish women on the whole were accorded more freedom and respect than either Greek or Roman women. In the Greek culture, the roles of women were well defined. Female roles were divided into three basic categories that gave rise to three distinct classes of women, each performing a specific function. First there were the wives, whose function hardly went beyond that of providing their husbands with legitimate offspring. The wives rarely provided companionship to their husbands, and were not included in their husbands' social activities. About the only thing a Greek wife could claim was the permanent right to her dowry. For practical reasons the home was monogamous, but usually men had as many lovers (male and female) as they could afford. In addition, women were under almost complete domination by their husbands. Wives could be ordered to have abortions, or could be arrested for aborting themselves without their husbands' consent. Even after a wife had her husband's child, she could not protect that child's life. Until the husband chose to recognize the infant in a ceremony that took place about ten days after birth, it was legal for the infant to be killed.

Another class of women were the *hetaerae*. From the standpoint of freedom, these women were in the best situation, because they were well educated and sought after by men for both their mental and their physical charms. They were expected to provide intellectual and social companionship as well as sexual favors. The third class of women were those hired specifically for entertainment or sexual gratification. They were known by two names. What we would call prostitutes were known as *pornae*. Slaves or hired women who would entertain gatherings of men at parties were *auletrides*.

Roman sexual practices were more brutal than those of the Greeks. Infants and young children were often used to satisfy sexual needs. Animals were trained to perform all types of sexual acts with humans. Captured humans were frequently subjected to animal assault for the amusement of spectators at the Colosseum. The early sexual restrictiveness of Christianity may have been in part a response to the sexual excesses and cruelty of the Romans.

Oriental philosophies gradually found their way into Greek civilization and influenced not only Greek culture but also Judaism and Christianity. Essentially, dualism emerged and people began to see themselves as possessing both a physical and a spiritual self. Immortality was no longer a biological legacy, but rather a function of the spiritual self after death. Concern for spiritual needs was gaining ascendancy over those related to the physical body. This ascetic trend in Greece ran counter to another force called hedonism. While most people at that time were hedonists, seeking pleasure as the chief good in life, asceticism was attracting many followers, and the two forces became sources of friction and upheaval. Christianity originated in this time of turbulent transition.

Christianity

Jesus was a Palestinian Jew. Hedonism was still prevalent in this region, and he was brought up in the old tradition of naturalism. Although evidence of Jesus' views on the subject of sex is only fragmentary, we do know that he did not condemn sexual pleasure as such. But he was concerned about the welfare of sexually indiscriminate persons—prostitutes and adulterers. His teachings never denounced women as evil, as many of his later followers did. Jesus was presumed celibate, but he made no demands for sexual abstinence on the part of others. According to the New Testament, Jesus once attended a marriage ceremony, and when the host ran out of wine, Jesus changed some water into fine wine. Had Jesus taken a negative view of marriage and its implied sexuality, he probably would have chosen another type of festivity at which to perform a miracle. Regarding divorce, he supported stricter laws than the Jews traditionally had, but divorce was not condemned. Jesus was apparently against the double standard, especially with reference to adultery—he believed it should be forbidden for both men and women. Forgiveness for any human error played a substantial role in his philosophy, and he often forgave people for their "sins of the flesh." The bulk of what we call the Christian sexual ethic is based not on the teachings of Christ, but on those (almost exclusively men) who were to follow him.

Paul was one of the first followers of Christ to speak out on sexual behavior. He taught that chastity and celibacy were superior to marriage. But if sexual urgencies could not be smothered, he did concede that marriage would be better than fornication (illicit sexual intercourse by unmarried persons).

The church's attitude toward women placed them in a position of inferiority, and eventually women were blamed for almost every tragedy that has befallen humans. Wives were admonished to be subject to husbands and to remain silent in church affairs. In the fourth century St. Jerome wrote that the only justification for marriage was that it produced more virgins.

By the Middle Ages (between A.D. 500 and 1500), women had lost almost all their rights. Sometime during this period married women even ceased to have legal existence. So it was rather surprising when the Council of Macon in the sixteenth century decided that women do possess immortal souls—*by a margin of one vote.* The council also declared that women would become sexless at the final resurrection so that heaven would not have to be subjected to the feminine gender. The burden of original sin also fell upon women, and they were made responsible for the condition of human mortality. The pain of childbirth was considered part of the price women must pay for tempting men into sin.

Around the latter part of the fourth century, St. Augustine was converted to Christianity. He was in his thirties at the time and had already led a life of sexual adventure to the point of excess. According to his writings, he was involved in a constant struggle to control his sexual nature. Before his conversion he was engaged to be married, had fathered a child by a former mistress, and had a succession of love affairs throughout the years. His writings associate guilt rather than pleasure with sex. While he acknowledged the necessity of sex for reproduction, he argued that the sex act itself carries the guilt of original sin, which is passed on to each new generation. Sex was rationalized only for the purpose of having children and was to be performed with as little physical reward as possible. After a life of sexual transgressions, which he described in his autobiographical *Confessions,* he ardently went about preaching the virtues of chastity to others. He thus bequeathed his own guilts to millions of Christians for generations to follow.

By the eighth century the church had devised a set of strict rules governing sinful acts, including those of a sexual nature. The only coital position that could be assumed without committing a sin was that of the man above. Presumably other positions might be more enjoyable, and sex was not supposed to be fun. Couples were to abstain from intercourse on specified occasions that amounted to some five months of the year.

Originally the church did not have jurisdiction over marriage and divorce; these matters were governed by civil authority. About the twelfth century, however, the church took over responsibility in these areas and declared that marriage could not be dissolved except under unusual and rare circumstances. Even then, weddings were celebrated outside the church, not in it. In the fourteenth century Chaucer's Wife of Barh boasts that she has married five husbands "at the church door" — not counting, she says, "other company in youth." One suspects that many men and women managed to have a pretty good time, just as they always have.

St. Thomas Aquinas (thirteenth century) spelled out the position of the Roman Catholic church on just about all matters pertaining to sex and morality. In his *Summa Theologica,* nocturnal emissions (wet dreams) were condemned as mortal sins. Sex outside marriage was condemned because of the possibility of conceiving a child that would have but one parent. And chastity and virginity were idealized and glorified to the extent that celibate persons were said to be envied rather than pitied.

During the Reformation, which is marked by the establishment of the Protestant faiths, Martin Luther and John Calvin attacked the prevailing notions of chastity and celibacy. The status of marriage was elevated, and the stigma of sin was formally removed from marital intercourse. Both reformers accepted sex as an honorable act within marriage. Luther was of the opinion that marriage was not a strictly religious affair, and felt that it should fall under the jurisdiction of civil rather than religious authorities. He set an example by marrying at home rather than in a church. The Reformation was characteristically a period of challenge between established beliefs and new ones just emerging.

The Renaissance was characterized by many fluctuations between strict and permissive sexual morality. The revival of open interest in sex was expressed in the art and literature of this period. At any given time, however, sexual standards depended largely on the behavior of the pope who headed the Catholic church.

Puritanism (1620–1800)

Puritanism grew largely in response to early Protestant reformers' desire to break with the Church of England, which they saw as too political and still too closely tied to Catholic doctrines. They desired to return to the fundamental teachings of the Old Testament as they conceived them. After many years of persecution, they brought their convictions to the New World during the seventeenth and eighteenth centuries. Not only were they concerned about the weak nature of humans; they were also confronted with the stark realities of life in a new and threatening environment. Maintenance of the family unit was necessary for survival, and thus many of the sex-related restrictions were enforced to uphold family stability.

Contrary to popular belief, the Puritans were not antisexual people; they were actually quite realistic and open about sex. The Puritans were primarily concerned with self-discipline and felt the need for constant self-examination. The strict dress codes and restrictions on enjoyable pastimes were aimed at limiting stimulation of the senses but not necessarily at suppressing sexual thoughts. Such rigidity was part of their whole attitude toward self-discipline and hard work.

The sexual regulations were primarily aimed at maintaining the integrity of the family unit. Within marriage the sex act was considered good and natural, and there were few regulations regarding marital sex. Men were obligated to have intercourse with their wives, and failure to do so was a punishable offense. The avoidance of pleasure in the New World, including sexual pleasure, did not peak until the Victorian era.

Sexual transgressions were commonly revealed at public confessions held at church meetings. If the penalities for sexual misconduct were unduly severe, people would surely have been less willing to tell of their indiscretions. All extramarital sex was frowned upon, but it must have been ultimately forgivable, because some of our most famous American forefathers were involved in sexual escapades that would be considered scandalous even by today's standards.

Alexander Hamilton, for instance, while Secretary of the Treasury, was accused of misappropriation of funds. His explanation was simple: His financial dealings with a minor government official were not in any way corrupt; he merely had given money to a Mr. Reynolds in exchange for the favors of Mrs. Reynolds. Benjamin Franklin never married the woman who was known as his wife. Thomas Jefferson is believed to have fathered half a dozen children by a slave at his Monticello home. When Grover Cleveland was running for the presidency on the Democratic ticket in 1884, he was charged by the Republicans with having fathered an illegitimate child some years before. He readily admitted that he had had an affair with Maria Halpin, and that he had assumed responsibility for their child. Despite his sexual indiscretion, he won the election.

There was little sexual equality during this period. Women were subject to more critical reprisal than men when they violated a sexual code. And they were valued primarily on the basis of what they could produce, be it babies or farm produce or textiles. It would be a long time before they would be considered important as individuals. The husband was the head of the family; wives were confined to homes and to duties related to the family, if their husbands could afford to let them remain "idle." It was not considered proper for women to make themselves conspicuous socially. Among the poor, women have always worked. Women's place is in the home only if husbands can afford to keep them there.

The Victorian Era

Chronologically, the Victorian era spanned the reign of the English queen Alexandria Victoria (1837–1901). Attitudes characteristic of this period, however, were not strictly confined within these dates, nor to England. Since England was a very powerful nation, its ideas influenced many other countries, especially those where English was spoken.

The sexual ethics of this era contrasted with those of the Puritan period in two main ways. First, the restrictions of the Puritans were based upon religious convictions, whereas those of the Victorians were founded upon a more secular morality revolving around an emerging interest in science and the development of intellectual character. Evidently the Victorians assumed that sex interfered with achievement. The sexual nature of humans therefore had to be controlled so that higher aims could be realized. Second, whereas the Puritans were primarily interested in curtailing sexual activity outside marriage, the Victorian era is associated with attempts to restrict sexual behavior within marriage as well.

The semen theory was a pivotal theme in Victorian values. Semen (fluid produced by male reproductive organs, containing sperm) was thought to be a substance essential to a man's well-being and health. Wasting semen was considered dangerous, whether it was spilled into one's wife, another woman, or a dark closet. The people were highly conscious of saving and reinvesting capital. It was wrong to waste money on pleasure when it could be reinvested to bring even greater wealth. Sex was looked upon as a form of indiscriminate spending; the process of ejaculation (ejection of seminal fluid) was actually called "spending."

Women were likewise encouraged to save their sexual "assests" until matrimony. Those wasting their virginity prior to marriage often lost the opportunity to marry at all. According to Victorian thinking, it should not have been too difficult for females to save their respectability, since women were believed to be devoid of sexual desires. Men imposed their "animal instincts" upon gentle women who were obligated to put up with sexual intercourse. Under no circumstances were women supposed to encourage it or show pleasure while being "used."

Victorian women often brought breach-of-promise suits against men who had promised marriage but for one reason or another did not fulfill their end of the bargain. Such legal actions were valid during this era because women lost varying degrees of marriageability upon engagement, even though sexual assets had not been relinquished.

The prudery of the Victorians often teetered on the brink of absurdity. Women's legs were treated as if they did not exist. Anything even suggestive of the fact that legs were a part of the anatomy was objectionable. Sometimes piano and table legs would be hidden inside frilly coverings. Art museums conducted separate tours for men and women, so as not to cause embarrassment when paintings of nudes were seen. Doctors frequently could not examine female patients except by noting places they pointed out on a dummy. It was indecent for women to undress and allow physicians to touch their bodies. Masturbation was considered pathological for both sexes, and cages were manufactured that could be fitted over the genitals at night. Some devices had spikes sticking out of them for added protection. It is not too surprising that a large portion of the population did not adhere to such rigid standards. Even though publicly ascribing to these attitudes, in private life the rich and the poor tended to behave pretty much as they always have. It was in the rising middle class that Victorian attitudes were frequently translated into behavior.

The inhibitions built up during the Victorian era went "unspent" until around World War I. Changes started earlier in the century were speeded up by the war environment. In times of stress people behave differently than they normally do. Middle-class women as well as those of the "underclasses" were called upon to fill the jobs of absent men, and economic independence spurred them on toward greater equality. Too, during the war married men and women discovered other sexual partners, and by the time it ended some 300,000 couples had been divorced in the United States alone. Thus the Victorian era was finally laid to rest.

Cross-Cultural Contrasts

Sexual patterns of various cultures and societies can be compared from many aspects. By looking at certain sexual behaviors such as masturbation and homosexual orientation, one can readily see that different cultures approach these behaviors in quite different ways. Many cross-cultural studies have been done, and on the basis of their findings cultures have been ranged along a continuum from most restrictive to most permissive. This kind of comparison, of course, depends on our own subjective attitudes as to what is restrictive and permissive. Many of the contrasts presented here are admittedly brief and may leave you with questions as to why people would ever do these things. The main intention is not to draw full-scale pictures but rather to acquaint you with the extent of variability in adjusting to human sexuality and to point out that there are extremely few innate or "natural" attitudes.

Sexual Behaviors and Gender Orientations

Masturbation is found in almost all cultures, although it is generally considered more acceptable behavior for children than for adults. Some cultures try to stop or prevent this activity completely, while others encourage it or even provide youngsters with instruction as to how it should be done.

Among the Kwoma of New Guinea, if a little boy is caught with an erect penis he is likely to get it beaten with a stick. Eventually youngsters even learn to urinate without touching their genitals. The Lesu of New Ireland have a specific approved masturbation technique for adults. When a woman is sexually aroused she sits down and bends her right leg so that heel touches the genitalia. The men and women freely talk about this activity, and very young girls are observed doing it. In the Philippines some mothers soothe irritable babies by stroking their genitals.

Cultures vary in their attitudes about premarital sex, from the extreme of total prevention to the opposite extreme where it is considered an absolute necessity. Among some Indian tribes in the United States—Cheyenne, Papago, Arapaho—boys and girls are segregated at all times during childhood, thus eliminating almost entirely the possibility of premarital intercourse. The Hopi Indians segregate boys and girls between the ages of ten and twenty, and wherever the girls go, an older woman goes along. Among the Wapisiana of South America there is no such thing as premarital sex, because their definition of marriage is cohabitation; thus if two people have intercourse, they are by that fact married.

In many cultures prohibitions against premarital sex are removed prior to marriage, usually when the young people reach a certain stage of maturity. The attainment of such mature status is often marked by some ritual. Among the Chagga of Tanzania, if an uninitiated boy is caught having sexual intercourse, both he and his partner are staked to the ground.

In contrast, the Lepcha of India believe that girls must have intercourse in order to reach maturity. By the time most girls are eleven or twelve years old, they are having sexual intercourse regularly. The sex life of a Trobriand Island girl begins between the ages of six and eight, and of a boy between ten and twelve. The children receive explicit instruction as to what is done. They are free to engage in sexual behavior with full parental approval. Their sex play includes masturbation, oral stimulation of the genitals of the same and the opposite sex, and heterosexual intercourse. Marriage, however, is not entered into until sexual intimacy has been established for a considerable period of time. Both partners are urged to wait until they are sure of their affection for one another.

The Toda of India allow women to have several husbands and several lovers as well. They do not have a word for adultery. In some tribes of western Africa, women of the ruling families can have as many lovers as they please, but are not allowed to degrade themselves by marrying.

Homosexual Activity

In the contemporary world, forty-nine of seventy-six societies studied by Clellan Ford and Frank Beach (1951) considered homosexual activities to be normal and acceptable for at least certain members of the community. Among the Siwans of Africa, all men and boys have anal intercourse, and indeed they are considered peculiar if they do not. Men lend their sons to each other and openly discuss their male lovers as well as their women. The Keraki of New Guinea require males to have homosexual experience as part of their puberty rites. Each boy is initiated into anal intercourse by an older man. After about one year of acting as the passive partner, the boy spends the remainder of bachelorhood having anal intercourse with newly initiated boys. This activity is believed necessary for a boy to become a man. Aranda women of Australia find it quite normal and acceptable to stimulate each other by touching each other's clitoris.

Our culture has rigidly defined gender identifications and assigns to each sex rather specific activities, dress, and roles. Individuals do not cross the gender barrier often in our society because the action is likely to call forth social disapproval. Not all cultures see male and female roles as totally exclusive. Along the Alaskan coast, the Konang used to raise a certain number of boys to assume female roles in all activities. When they reached adulthood, important men of the tribe would marry them. These male "wives" were believed to possess magical powers. The Mohave

Indians also had a special class of men who dressed and functioned like women. Some would even mimic pregnancy and menstruation. They married men who were allowed to have female wives as well. In such families, the male "wife" held a very respected position. The men of the Pilaga Indian tribe of the Argentine Gran Chaco outnumber the women. Here the women have the advantage and get their choice of sexual partners as well as husbands. Upon marriage, a man moves in with the family of the wife in her village.

Whereas we picture married people as living together in one residence, the men and women of Marind Anim (New Guinea) live separately even after marriage. Wives sleep in the women's house and men in their own. Domestic and social life take place mostly outdoors, in the space between the houses. Sexual intercourse takes place outdoors in the forest, not in either house.

Sexuality: An Integrated Part of Society

Let us look now at sexual behavior within the context of the general cultural life styles of two little-known island societies and of a few modern societies with which most of us are familiar.

The Marquesans of Polynesia Sexually, the Marquesans are probably more sophisticated than the people of any Western culture. In 1962 Robert Suggs wrote about them in his book *Hidden Worlds of Polynesia,* and in 1972 anthropologist W. Menard published an article about them. Over the span of ten years, it does not appear that the intrusion of Westerners has significantly altered the unique and beautiful sexual abandon of these people. Missionaries have exerted some influence, however. Sexual acts that once supported group solidarity are becoming sources of friction and guilt for those who have absorbed the sexual negativism of Christianity.

Marquesan children are given sex instruction early in life. Infant boys have their genitals massaged to promote sexual development. Mothers teach daughters about intercourse and methods of contraception. Long before puberty (when the ability to reproduce is first reached), girls are shown how to enlarge the clitoris by manual stimulation. Vaginal responsiveness is supposedly heightened through the use of carved phalli (dildoes). Medical examinations are said to confirm the effectiveness of such preparation, and have shown that Marquesan women do indeed possess more highly developed, responsive internal and external genitalia.

Both sexes begin masturbating in infancy, like all children everywhere, but here they are not discouraged. By six children are often found involved in playful homosexual acts. Until the circumcision rite at twelve to fourteen years, it is not felt proper for boys to engage in heterosexual acts. Boys are gradually introduced to heterosexual intercourse by carefully selected older, experienced girls. Girls begin adult sexual activity before boys and frequently have sexual intercourse before menarche (first menstrual period).

Even though it is considered normal for adolescents to engage in coitus regularly and with a variety of partners, complete openness is not permitted by parents. Total parental approval is withheld with the intention of preventing early marriage and subsequent broken union later on. When a couple is caught, the girl's father puts on a frightening display of anger, and threatens to kill both offenders. The daughter and even her mother traditionally receive harsh beatings, but the offending boy is likely to receive nothing but a few discouraging words. All in all, these incidents are viewed as community entertainment, and topics of gossip.

Marquesans have a form of behavior similar to what we call gang-banging, but such activity is socially accepted and girls willingly spend a night having sex with several boys. Thus behavior considered pathological by Western standards is seen as normal here, and in fact exceptional performances are admired.

Girls often bear one or more children before marriage. All children are adored by and belong to the whole community. Paternity is of no concern. Marriage ceremonies involve the participation of the oldest able citizens, and missionaries have not had much success in getting couples to marry in Christian ceremonies.

Recognition is given to people who cater to the sexual needs of persons who deviate from usual sexual norms. Women who freely choose to be prostitutes are called *vehine mako.* They play an important role in Marquesan society by providing sexual outlets for young men without sex partners, for older married men, and for foreigners. Married women and young marriageable girls are protected from unwanted sexual attention, and social equilibrium is preserved. Males having an exclusive homosexual orientation are rare, but those who do are known as *mahu.* Often they are also transvestites and specialize in "women's work," such as dressmaking or laundering. Married people freely engage in extramarital sex. Extending sexual hospitality to visitors and mate swapping are both socially sanctioned behaviors.

A Folk Community in Ireland In 1971 John Messenger published an account of Inis Beag, an island community off the coast of Ireland, which demonstrates an unusual degree of sexual repression. The community has maintained its stability for some two hundred years. Most islanders are devout Roman Catholics, but they also cling to many pagan beliefs of ancient Celtic origin, such as belief in magic, spirits, and witches.

Children are brought up without any reference to sex either in the home or outside of it. Most people learn about sex only after they marry. Boys and girls are segregated both in school and in church. Dating or courtship customs do not exist, and, according to Messenger, premarital intercourse is virtually unknown.

Marriages are usually contracted for economic reasons, and late marriages are the rule. The average age for men to marry is thirty-six, and for women twenty-five. Love is of little concern, and the sexes rarely mingle socially even after marriage.

Women are quite ignorant of the biological significance of menstruation and menopause. Menarche is usually a traumatic experience for girls because they do not receive any preparation for it. They believe that menopause (end of reproductive ability) can cause "madness." Women have been known to take to their beds at the beginning of menopause and to stay there till they die. Men have equally erroneous ideas. They think that coitus is physically debilitating and that women are dangerous during menstruation and for many months after childbirth.

Sexual intercourse is kept as pleasure-free as possible. Men make all sexual advances, and employ little foreplay. The only position used is that of the man above, and usually neither partner completely undresses. Messenger found no evidence of female orgasm.

Sexual repression is learned early in the home, and is later supported by sermons at church and in the classrooms. Sex is never discussed in the presence of children, and masturbation, mutual body observation, or even the use of sex-related words is subject to disapproval and frequently severe punishment. After late infancy mothers limit physical contact with their babies, and affection is thereafter shown only verbally. Because of the sexual connotations, breast feeding is rare. Even though the islanders are surrounded by water, none of them learn to swim because such an activity would require them to shed some clothing. Medical treatment is also avoided for the same reason. Bodily hygiene is, as you would expect, very poor. Only babies have their whole bodies washed; all others limit bathing to face and extremities.

Sweden In the past, fruitful marriages were very important to the Swedes, and pregnancy before marriage was good assurance of such fertility. If a couple dated for some time and no pregnancy resulted, both partners were free to seek other sexual companions with whom they might be more successful. This tradition and modern circumstance, including economic stability, have continued to social acceptability of premarital sex. It is estimated that about 98 percent of married Swedes have had premarital intercourse.

Early marriages are not encouraged and long engagements are

common. Although contraceptives and instruction in their use are widely available, births out of wedlock still account for approximately 10 percent of all births. They do not call these children "illegitimate," however, and unmarried mothers and their children are not socially stigmatized. Sex is considered an important part of life whether persons are married or not.

Sex education as a regular part of schooling was introduced in 1940. In 1956 it became compulsory for all children from the age of seven. One of the main objectives of the sex-education program is to promote understanding of the physiology and anatomy of sex, so that ignorance won't interfere with the development of harmonious interpersonal relationships. Sex education also focuses on how closely sex life is linked with total personality, social relationships, and society as a whole. Swedish students are taught that sexual attentions should never be forced on others, that men and women have equal rights and responsibilities, and that sexual minorities are to be respected. The use of contraceptives is encouraged unless parenthood is desired by both partners.

Switzerland The Swiss have a patriarchal society that is very male-oriented. Men dominate in Swiss society, women are submissive to their husbands' wishes, and children are firmly disciplined. Men pride themselves on knowing how to control "their" women.

Women were not conceded the right to vote or hold federal office until 1971. Despite gains in the status of women, marriage is still male-dominated. When a women marries, her husband takes claim to whatever money she may have. Married women cannot buy property or incur debts without their husbands' consent. In the business world women still do not hold high positions, and in the jobs they do hold they receive about 25 percent less pay than a man who performs the same work.

The USSR Through education, the Soviet government attempts to structure sexual attitudes that are in the interest of certain political aims. Sex in general is deemphasized and is associated almost exclusively with marriage. In line with Soviet educational aims, children are taught that personal happiness can be achieved only in family love and that sex is appropriate only within marriage. The image of a good Soviet citizen is equated with that of a stable married person. Sexual repressiveness, however, has not always been a Soviet theme.

After the overthrow of the czarist state during World War I, marriage and its religious associations were rejected as being representative of bourgeois ideals. During the first few decades of Soviet government, economic life was tightly controlled but the citizens' sex lives were their own concern. The new government abolished traditional marriage and replaced it with civil registration. Divorce could be obtained merely by going to the registrar. The only requirement was that both parties consent. Marxists really did not take a position on sexual values, and agreed only that marriage in bourgeois society had been corrupted by capitalist influences. They believed that the abolition of private property would stop women from being exploited by marriages for money, and from being used as domestic slaves.

In 1927 divorce was made easier than it had been and husbands and wives could get divorced without the consent of the other partner. The liberal system was abused and family tragedies led to public reaction. More importantly, however, short-term marriages did not bring the state as many children as it had hoped for. Policy makers wanted many people for the new generation, and marriage for life seemed to be the best method of obtaining them. Up until 1936, legislation actually facilitated sexual license. Free sexual cohabitation was on the same level as marriage. But in 1936 new laws were passed which reversed the liberal ones and divorces were no longer easily arranged—the biggest deterrent being a progressive tax on each action. In 1917, after the revolution, abortion was legalized so that women could have more freedom to work. Later, abortion was outlawed except for medical reasons. It was stated that abortions were dangerous to health, sexual enjoyment, and future fertility. In 1955, however, abortion again became legal.

Today children's time is systematically filled with schoolwork and physical training. Actually such activities play a substantial role in the Soviet sex-education program. There is little time available for the usual impulses of the young.

Conclusion

We cannot overemphasize the diversity people have shown with respect to integrating sexual behavior with all other dimensions of social interaction and interdependency. Whatever basic sexual nature we possess becomes thoroughly affected by cultural learning. Who are we to judge one way or another as being most "normal" or "natural" when our true naturalness was probably relinquished millions of years ago in favor of community life? If any given populace maintains a sociosexual structure capable of fulfilling the needs of both individual members and the group as a whole, then it is successful; beyond this our evaluations become a matter of personal prejudice.

Glandular Control of Sexual Physiology

3

Human sexuality is greatly influenced by the actions of various glands. Glands are classified into two groups according to the way their products are secreted and distributed. *Exocrine glands* secrete their materials into ducts leading to specific areas where the products are used. *Endocrine glands* have no ducts and secrete almost directly into the bloodstream. The term "endocrine gland" is used synonymously with "hormone secreting gland" because the materials secreted are *hormones.*

The Neuro-Endocrine System

The body contains two communication systems: the nervous system, with its great network of nerves throughout the body, and the hormones, which are blood-borne messengers regulating all cellular functions of the body. Hormones are chemical substances synthesized by a specific gland, secreted into the bloodstream, and carried to another part of the body where their chemical control activities are exerted. Hormones serve to control and integrate body functions.

Despite the many ways hormones differ from each other, several general characteristics and principles apply to virtually all of them. Although hormones are distributed throughout the body by the bloodstream, only specific organs and cells are capable of responding to specific hormones. These organs are known as *target organs.* Hormones are not secreted at constant rates. Their rates are increased or decreased by a *negative-feedback mechanism* in which the target organ of the hormone releases another hormone in response; this hormone "feeds back" to the initial endocrine gland controlling the secretion of the original hormone. Such a self-limiting system of controls is highly effective in damping hormonal response—limiting extremes of hormonal activity. As shown in Figure 3.1, follicle-stimualting hormone (FSH) and luteinizing hormone (LH), which is often called interstitial-cell-stimulating hormone (ICSH) in males, flow into the bloodstream and act upon the ovaries of the female or the testes of the male. They cause the release of estrogen and progesterone (female sex hormones) in the female, and testosterone (male sex hormone) in the male. These hormones then flow back to regulate the subsequent release of the FSH and LH (or ISCH).

Different hormones are often very similar in chemical structure, and slight differences may produce great alterations of physiological activity. For example, as shown in Figure 3.2, the chemical structure of the male sex hormone, testosterone, and the female sex hormone, progesterone, are extremely similar, yet they perform very distinct functions. Also, there is often a *series* of chemicals being secreted by endocrine glands, all of which show the same or similar actions. Consequently, the

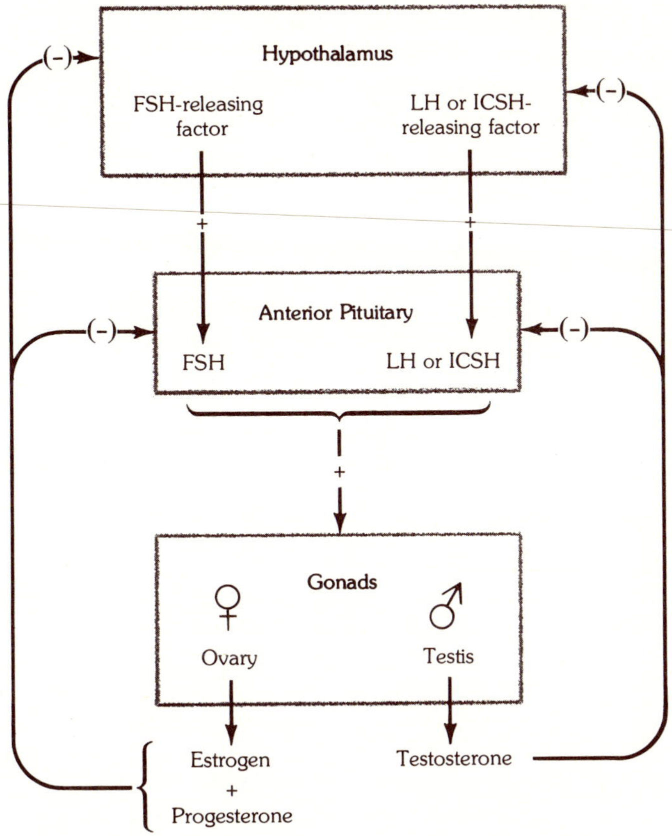

FIGURE 3.1 Negative feedback of target-organ hormones

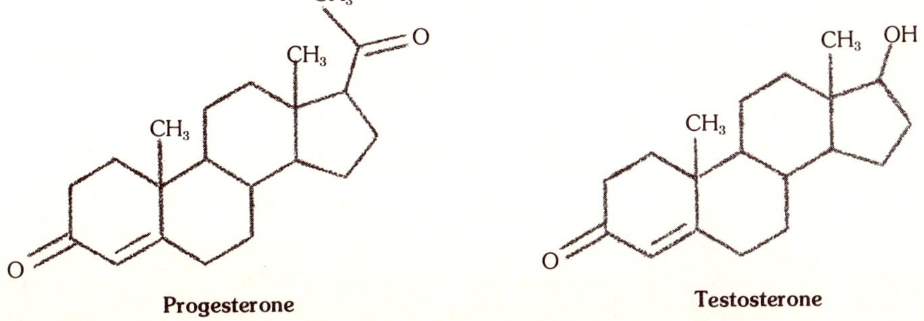

FIGURE 3.2 Chemical structure of testosterone and progesterone

complete series is given one name and referred to as a *single* hormone. Another significant term is *trophic*. Any hormone that affects another hormonal gland is termed a trophic hormone. The hormones that affect the *gonads* (ovaries of the female and testes of the male) are termed *gonadotropins*. The major human gonadotropins that we shall refer to most frequently are FSH and LH (or ICSH).

Physiological Sexuality and the Brain

There are three primary divisions of the brain: the *brainstem*, the *cerebellum*, and the *cerebrum* (Figure 3.3). The brainstem is literally the stalk of the brain. All nerve fibers that relay signals between the body and the

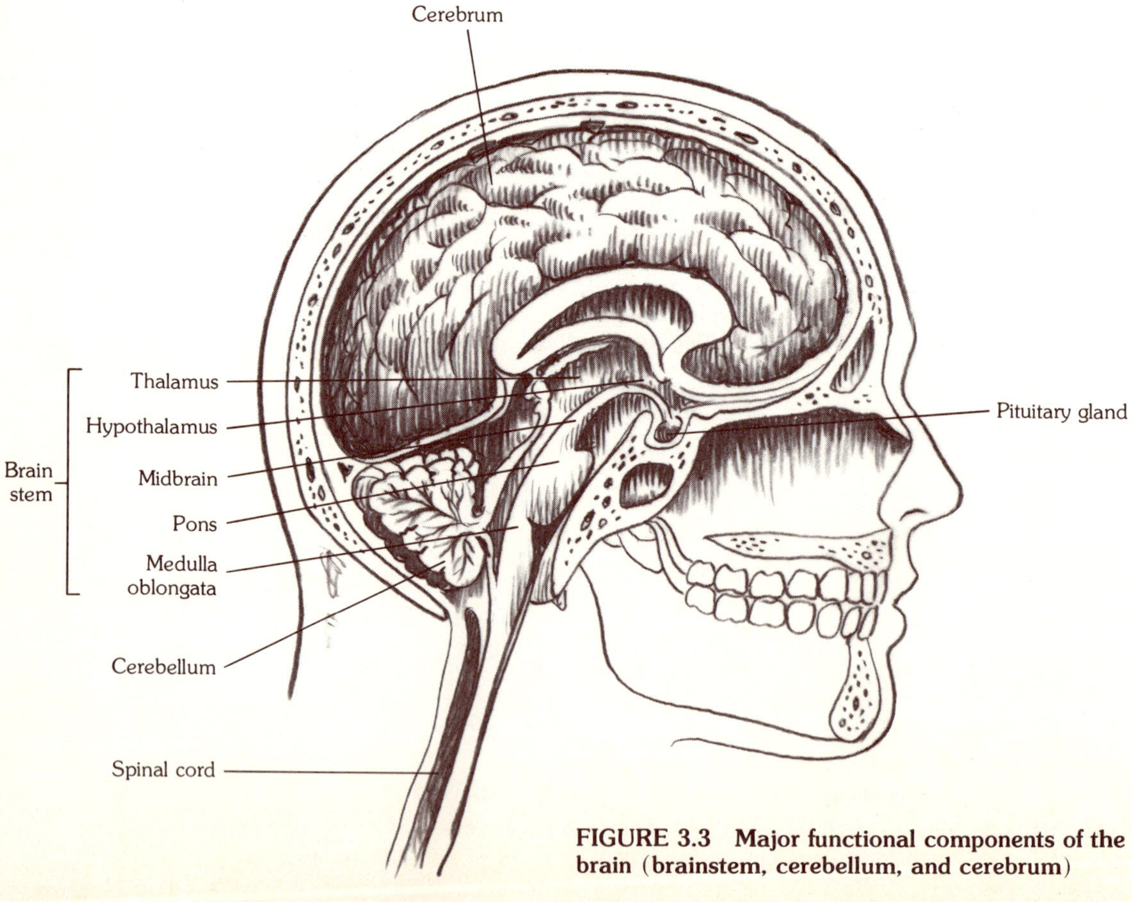

FIGURE 3.3 Major functional components of the brain (brainstem, cerebellum, and cerebrum)

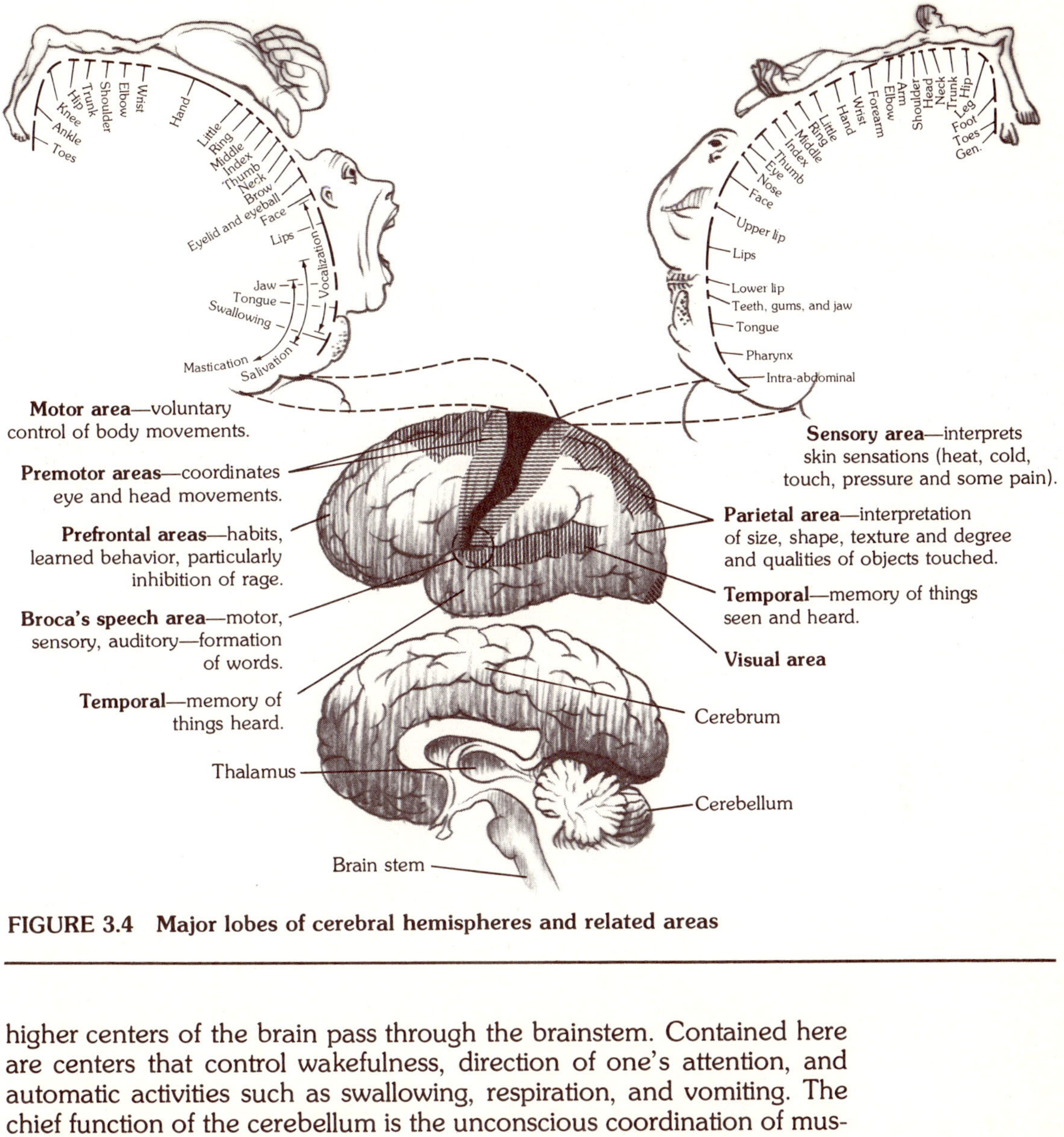

FIGURE 3.4 Major lobes of cerebral hemispheres and related areas

higher centers of the brain pass through the brainstem. Contained here are centers that control wakefulness, direction of one's attention, and automatic activities such as swallowing, respiration, and vomiting. The chief function of the cerebellum is the unconscious coordination of muscle movements. The remainder of the brain is the cerebrum or areas closely related to the functioning of the cerebrum. All other functions of the brain are associated with these structures.

The major lobes of the cerebrum (Figure 3.4) record and control all higher functions of human behavior, learning, and recognition of sensual stimuli. Deep within the cerebrum lies the *thalamus,* a conducting and integrating center for all sensory stimuli (except smell) entering the cerebrum, and the *hypothalamus,* which lies below the thalamus and directly above the hypophysis (pituitary) endocrine gland (Figure 3.5).

The hypothalamus is especially important to us because it is responsible for integrating many basic behavioral patterns that are correlated with the automatic functions, hormones, and reactions of the body to its environment. It is associated with the expression of one's emotions. Behavior is experienced as rewarding and pleasurable when some areas of the hypothalamus are stimulated, and unpleasant and punishing when other areas are stimulated. The hypothalamus seems to be the single most important internal control center of the brain.

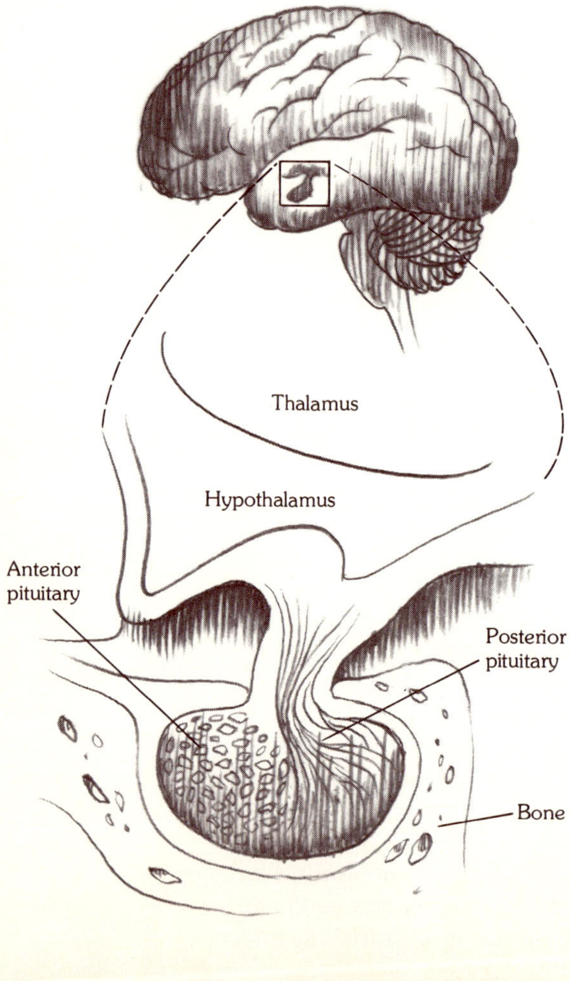

FIGURE 3.5 Relationship between the thalamus and hypothalamus of the brain, and the hypophysis (pituitary gland)

Hypophysis (Pituitary Gland)

The hypophysis, or pituitary gland, is an endocrine gland, suspended from the lower surface of the brain. It lies in a pocket of bone just below the hypothalamus (Figure 3.5). The *posterior lobe,* or *neurohypophysis* (*neuro,* meaning "nerve" and *hypophysis,* meaning "lying under"), is very appropriately named, as it is a downgrowth of nervous tissue of the hypothalamus and does lie directly beneath it. Also, two clusters of hypothalamic nerve fibers pass down and end in the neurohypophysis. There is also a set of capillary blood vessels connecting these two areas. The somewhat older term *posterior pituitary* is a misnomer, since this lobe of the hypophysis is a downgrowth of the hypothalamus. The hormones seemingly secreted in this lobe (see Table 3.1) are actually produced in the hypothalamus, move down through the nerve fibers into the neurohypophysis, and then are released into the bloodstream at this point. Only two of these hormones are known to be important in humans: vasopressin (see Table 3.1) and oxytocin, which causes the contractions of the uterus at the time of birth, and the contraction of smooth muscles in the milk ducts of the breasts to release milk.

The *anterior lobe* of the pituitary is an upgrowth from the roof of the embryonic mouth and is true endocrine tissue. This lobe is the *adenohypophysis* (*adenos,* meaning "gland"). It secretes at least seven different hormones (see Table 3.1). Two of these hormones are gonadotropic hormones. One is the follicle-stimulating hormone (FSH), which in females stimulates the growth and maturation of ovarian follicles (containing ova) and secretion of estrogen. In males it stimulates growth and maturation of sperm. Luteinizing hormone (LH in females and ICSH in males) stimulates the production of the male hormone testosterone in males; in females it causes ovulation and stimulates development of the corpus luteum (which produces the female hormone progesterone). Production of progesterone within the corpus luteum is maintained by the *lactogenic hormone* (*LTH*) (Table 3.1). In both males and females, LTH acts like a growth hormone by stimulating a general synthesis of proteins in many areas. This very broad field of action is the major reason it is not classified as a gonadotropic hormone.

As shown in Figure 3.1, these hormones control the relative levels of each other through a negative-feedback mechanism. Another major factor in the release of FSH and LH is the release by the hypothalamus of a group of so-called *hypothalamic releasing factors,* which then flow down from the hypothalamus through a series of capillaries into the anterior pituitary. As shown in Figure 3.6, these factors then cause the synthesis and release of their respective hormones. The negative-feedback mechanism controls the overall levels of FSH and LH, but the hypothalamus, by releasing factors, controls the synthesis of these hormones and

TABLE 3.1 Summary of Hormones from Endocrine Glands Affecting Sexuality

Anterior Pituitary (Adenohypophysis) Hormones	*Secretion Directly Controlled by:*	*Summary of Major Actions*
Growth hormone	Hypothalamic GH-releasing factor	Direct influence on the actions of other hormones involved in metabolic reactions.
ACTH (adrenocorticotropic hormone)	Hypothalamic releasing factor CRF (corticotropin-releasing factor) and cortisol	Stimulates adrenal cortex to produce cortical hormones.
TSH (thyrotropic or thyroid-stimulating hormone)	Hypothalamic TSH-releasing factor and thyroxine	Principal action to stimulate thyroid gland to produce thyroxine.
Lactogenic hormone (LH)	Hypothalamic prolactin-inhibiting factor	Initiation and maintenance of milk production in nursing female. Maintenance of progesterone in corpus luteum. General synthesis of proteins in many areas of both males and females.
FSH (follicle-stimulating hormone)	Hypothalamic FSH-releasing factor; estrogen and progesterone in females, testosterone in males	Stimulates growth of follicle containing ovum and produces estrogen in females. Stimulates production of sperm in males.
LH (lactogenic hormones) Often termed ICSH (interstitial-cell-stimulating hormone) in males.	Hypothalamic LH-releasing factor; estrogen and progesterone in females, testosterone in males	Ovulation, formation of corpus luteum, and production of progesterone in females. Production of testosterone and other androgens in males.
Posterior Pituitary (Neurohypophysis) Hormones		
Oxytocin	Nerve impulses, changes in hypothalamic secretory neurons	Stimulates contraction of uterine muscles during birth. Stimulates contractions of muscles in mammary glands, causing release of milk.
Vasopressin (ADH, antidiuretic hormone)	Neurons of hypothalamus in response to fluid content and blood pressure	Maintains proper water balance and blood pressure in the body.
Gonads: Testes and Ovaries		
Female ovaries: estrogen and progesterone	FSH and LH	Estrogen: secondary sex characteristics, menstrual cycle. Progesterone: maintenance of uterine living, and breast development at puberty.
Male testes: testosterone	LH	Secondary sex characteristics.
Males and females: androgens	FSH and LH	Sex drive.
Adrenal Cortex hormones		
Cortisol	ACTH	Influences glucose-glycogen balances.
Aldosterone	Angiotension and plasma K^+ concentration	Direct control over sodium, indirect control over calcium and potassium (mineralocorticoid).
Adrenal androgens	Not definitely known	Supplement testicular androgens.

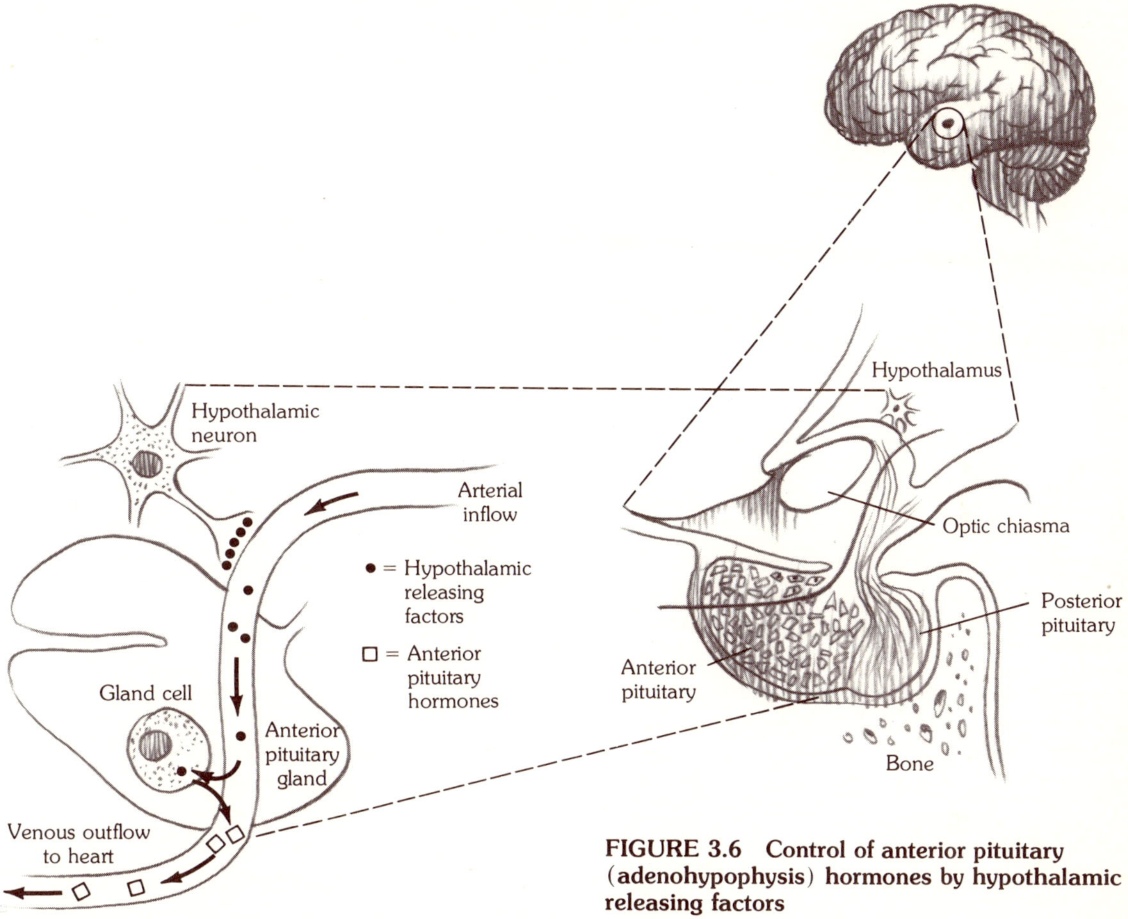

FIGURE 3.6 Control of anterior pituitary (adenohypophysis) hormones by hypothalamic releasing factors

the timing of their release. Consequently, any factor that affects the hypothalamus may also affect these two hormones, and the sexuality of the person.

Biorhythms

Many physical patterns of life are subject to rhythmical variations. The rhythm of light and darkness, the *solar day,* is based upon the revolution of the earth. The *lunar month* (about twenty-nine days) is the time required for the moon to orbit the earth. There are also yearly rhythms, such as the seasons. These rhythms are controlled by variations in the environment. But science has found physiological and behavioral changes within animals (including humans) showing rhythmical patterns controlled directly by internal timing mechanisms or indirectly by external environmental factors. The controls of these rhythms have been called "biological clocks." Actually the sites and mechanisms, whether chemical or physical, are subject to controversy. Most males like to think that they are immune to rhythms while women with their menstrual cycles are not. Scientists now believe that this is not the case.

All humans show biorhythms. Male sexual rhythms in sperm production and hormonal production (adrenal and testicular) have been shown in many animals. These seem ultimately to be controlled by light (either sunlight or artificial light). Androgenic (male) hormones are at their highest in the morning just after sunrise. This may account for the heightened sexual feelings of many men and women early in the morning. Female sex hormones seem to be stimulated by darkness rather than light (Thommen, 1973). Girls usually begin menstruating in the winter. Most women start their monthly menstrual flow early in the morning, after a full night of darkness. Some women with irregular menstrual periods may find that if they keep a light on at night for two or three days, beginning the day before ovulation (usually about the thirteenth day after the beginning of the last menstrual flow), their menstrual cycles will stabilize at a predictable twenty-nine days.

It is thought that there are basic biorhythms that rise and fall at regular intervals in each individual. One such rhythm is the monthly menstrual cycle in women. Often rhythms in both males and females follow the *circadian rhythm* or day-night cycle (*circa,* meaning "about," and *dies,* meaning "day"). Two other basic biorhythms being explored in humans are a twenty-three-day *physical* (or energy) *cycle* and a twenty-eight-day *sensitivity* (or emotional) cycle (Thommen, 1973).

The twenty-three-day cycle is felt to affect physical strength, endurance, energy, and physical confidence. This cycle may help to explain the variation in physical performances of athletes (both male and female). The first eleven and one-half days are believed to be a time when a person feels vigorous and vital, and when endurance is at its highest. The second half of the cycle is a restful period, with a reduction in performance. Individuals tire more easily and do not really enjoy extreme physical activity. During the twenty-eight-day sensitivity cycle the first fourteen days are a period when the person is optimistic, cheerful, and enterprising. The second half (days fifteen through twenty-eight) builds toward irritable and negative feelings.

An attempt to find your sensitivity cycle can be made by making a chart on a piece of paper similar to the chart shown in Figure 3.7. (This is

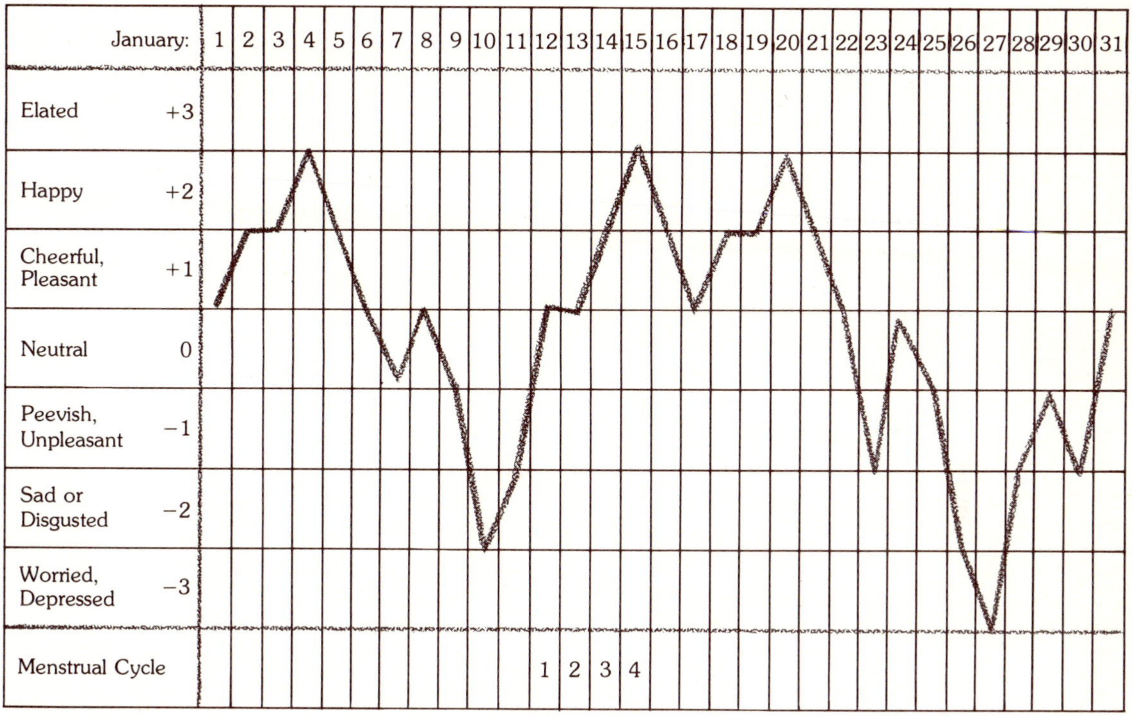

FIGURE 3.7 Chart of a twenty-eight-day sensitivity cycle; hypothetical chart of a woman's feelings throughout a month

a hypothetical chart for a woman, including the beginning of the menstrual cycle.) Various recognizable states of feelings have been arranged on this chart. The feelings are given positive or negative ratings. Neutral has the value of 0, to signify neither positive nor negative feelings.

There are various ways and times to chart your feelings. If you are a person who is grumpy when you awaken, feel better after breakfast or coffee, then cheerful during the morning, and grouchy when you tire in the afternoon, begin by charting yourself three or four times a day. Divide a column into four areas and chart your feelings at 10:00 A.M., 2:00 P.M., 6:00 P.M., and 10:00 P.M. Within a few weeks you should know yourself well enough to use one time as an average of how you feel for the day. The rest of you should relax for a moment in the evening and chart an "honest" estimation of how you felt during the day. After you have charted your feelings over a period of time (a number of months), you can use your chart to help you make decisions on the timing of events in your life.

Women face two problems when charting their emotional cycles. They must also consider their menstrual cycle. Many women experience emotional changes during their menstrual cycles. These feelings may be expressions of the twenty-eight-day sensitivity cycle, hormonal changes of the menstrual cycle, or learned behavior tuned to a society that expects such changes in women. Whatever the reasons for these emotional fluctuations, as shown in Figure 3.7, it may be helpful for a woman to chart her menstrual cycle along the bottom of the chart, counting the first day of her menstrual flow as day 1.

Few people are either continuously happy or continuously depressed. Most of us experience emotional, physical, and social changes. The study of biorhythms is an attempt to explain such observed changes.

Male Sexual Anatomy and Physiology

4

The biological symbol for male is ♂. This symbol is a combination of the O of the shield of Mars and the ↗ of his spear. A factual knowledge of the reproductive anatomy and physiology of both sexes is useful as a basis for understanding the mechanisms of sexual stimulus and response. Many of the problems that arise in sexual relationships result, at least in part, from inadequate knowledge of the biological aspects of sexuality.

Reproductive Structures

Figure 4.1 illustrates the major male sexual organs. The most important include the testes, the epididymis, the vas deferens, the seminal vesicles, the prostate gland, Cowper's glands, and the penis.

FIGURE 4.1 Male reproductive system (front view)

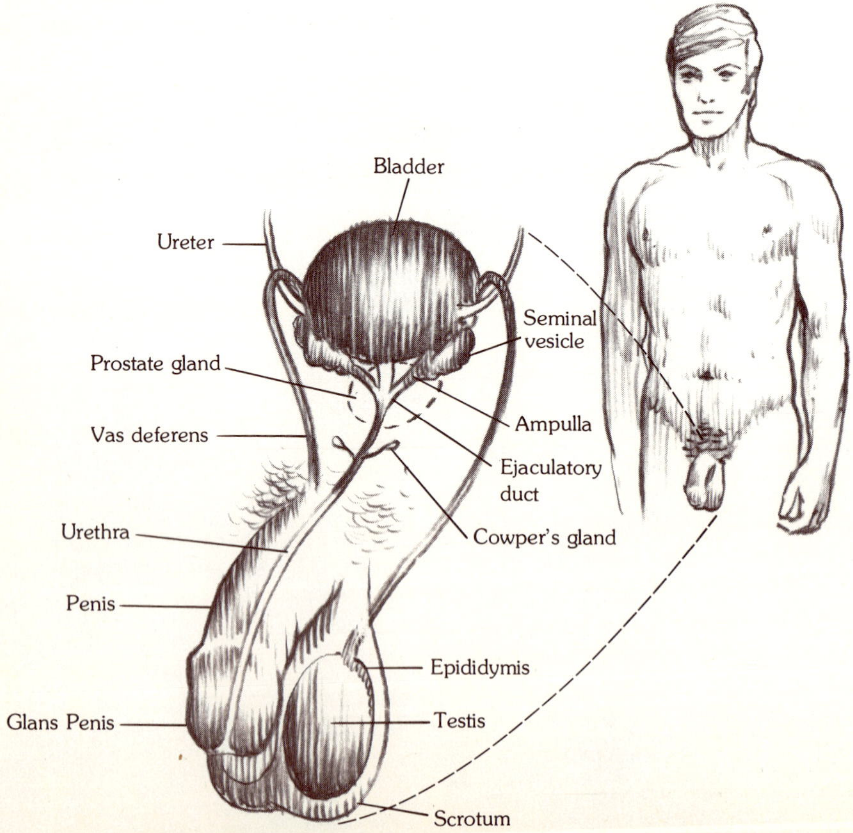

The Scrotum

The scrotum is a muscular sac containing the testes, associated structures, and the spermatic cords. Sperm production cannot occur at normal body temperature (98.6°F. or 37°C). The scrotum allows the testes to be suspended away from the body, serves as a thermostat, and keeps the testes at a temperature two to three degrees (average 2.2 degrees) lower than normal body temperature. This condition appears to be ideal for sperm production. Numerous experiments show that exposure of the testes to heat causes severe damage to developing sperm. Repeated or prolonged exposure to heat may result in permanent damage.

Not only do high temperatures prevent sperm production; they may also destroy sperm cells, causing *infertility* (temporary inability to reproduce) or even *sterility* (permanent inability to reproduce). Extreme low temperatures inhibit sperm production but do not destroy sperm cells.

One mechanism of thermostatic control involves contraction of the scrotal muscles. During cold temperatures, the testes are pulled closer to the body wall and are warmed. In hot temperatures the muscles relax, allowing the testes to be suspended farther away from the body where they will be cooler. The arterial blood of the testes runs countercurrent to the cooler venous blood. By the time this blood reaches the seminiferous tubules its temperature is lower and these tubules are cooled.

The scrotum also responds to sexual stimulation. As sexual response increases, tensing and thickening of the scrotal sac elevates the testes closer to the abdomen.

The Testes

At about the eighth month of embryonic development the previously formed testes migrate from the abdominal cavity, where they were formed, into the scrotum. Failure of the testes to descend leads to sterility. Such a condition is called *cryptorchidism* (*crypt* meaning "hidden" and *orchid* meaning "testis"). The condition may be corrected by surgery.

Within each testis is a great number of very small tubes called *seminiferous tubules* (Figure 4.2). Sperm cells are formed inside these tubules. Beginning during puberty, these sperm cells are produced more or less without letup during the lifetime of the male. Initial production starts slowly, then increases until, in the sexually mature male, 10 to 30 billion sperm are produced each month. The number of sperm produced during a man's lifetime defies imagination.

Each sperm cell is microscopic. The length of each cell is about fifty microns (it would take 480 of them placed end to end to cover an inch). Each cell consists of a head, neck, body, and tail (Figure 4.3). One set of chromosomes (twenty-three in number) is carried in the head. Another

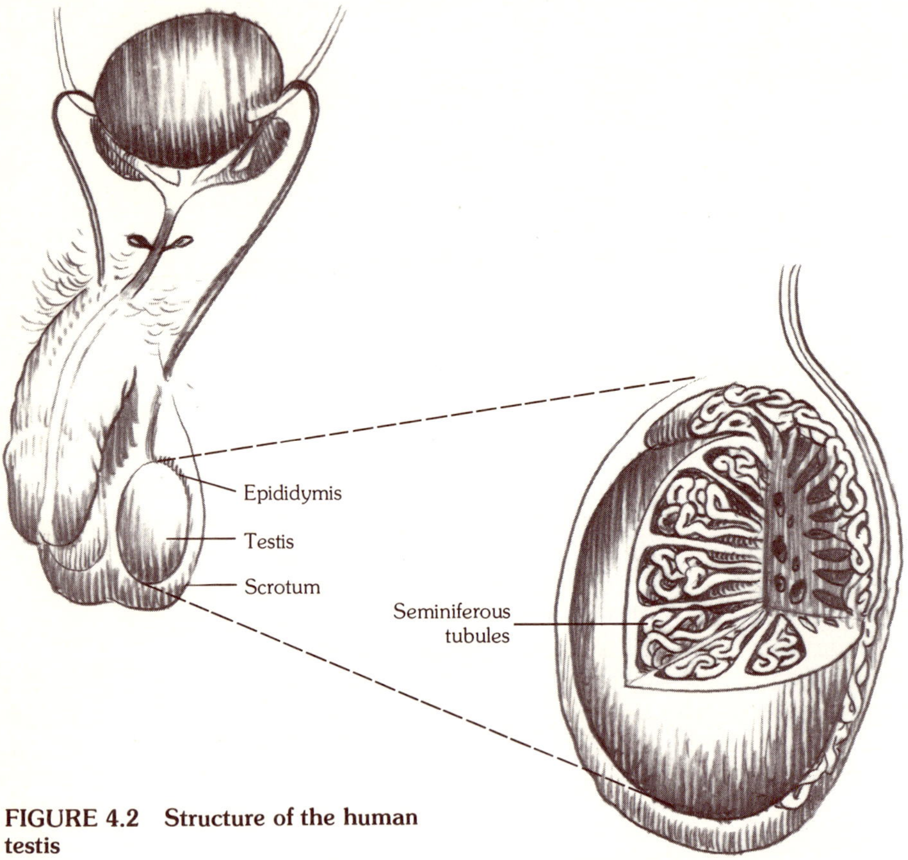

FIGURE 4.2 Structure of the human testis

set of twenty-three chromosomes is carried in the ovum. These chromosomes contain the heredity of a child when the sperm penetrates (fertilizes) a female's ovum. Thus each parent makes an equal contribution to the hereditarial characteristics of the child.

The sex of a child is determined by the sperm. One pair of chromosomes in all human cells is called the sex pair of chromosomes, because they determine whether the person will be male or female. One type of sex chromosome is the Y or *male chromosome.* The other type of sex chromosome is the X or *female chromosome.* Every ovum contains an X chromosome. Some sperm contain X chromosomes and some contain Y chromosomes. If an X-containing sperm fertilizes an ovum, the child will develop into a female (XX chromosomes). A Y sperm penetrating an ovum will produce a male (XY chromosomes).

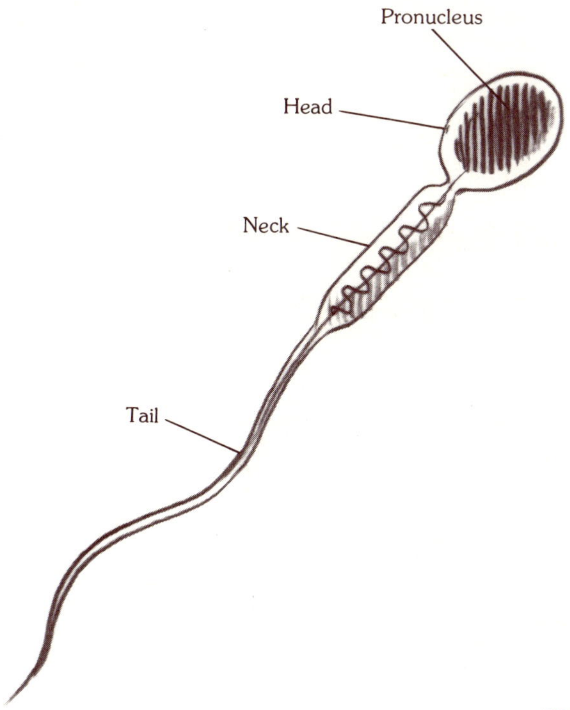

FIGURE 4.3 Human sperm cell

As shown in Table 4.1, abnormal numbers of sex chromosomes lead to specific conditions.

The testes serve as endocrine glands as well. The male sex hormones they produce begin to flow in large amounts at about thirteen years of age. This is the onset of puberty and marks the beginning of the physical changes leading to sexual maturity. Such changes are called *secondary sex characteristics* and include the development of broad shoulders, lowered voice, growth of hair on the face, chest, limbs, and pubis, and development of the male sex drive.

The male sex hormones are collectively called *androgens*. There are several closely related male hormones, all termed androgens. Usually the term *androgen* is used when referring to the general group of hormones, and *testosterone* when referring to the specific hormone of that name. In males FSH and ICSH do not cycle, but testosterone level does show a daily rhythm (highest in the morning). Males often exhibit a heightened sexual drive corresponding to this cycle. Testosterone levels can also be made to vary in response to sexual and social stimuli.

TABLE 4.1 Aberrations of Human Sex Chromosomes

Chromosome Number	*Name of Syndrome*	*Characteristics of Syndrome*
XX	Normal female	
XY	Normal male	
XO	Monosomy X (Turner's syndrome)	Female, stature abnormally short, sexually immature, immature sexual structures, no menstruation, sterile
XXX	Trisomy X (superfemale)	Female; stature ranges from Turner's syndrome to normal, to very tall
XXY	Klinfelter's syndrome	Male; may appear normal, but small testes and often sterile; may be tall and thin; high-pitched voice; occasionally immature sex organs; often mentally retarded
XYY	XYY syndrome	Male; tall, aggressive, and usually normal.
XXXX	Tetra-X syndrome	Female; sterile, often mentally retarded
XXXXX	Penta-X syndrome	Female; sterile, often mentally retarded
XXXXY	Tetra-XY syndrome	Male; sterile, often mentally retarded
XY	XY-female	Female in all respects, but sterile; inability of uptake granules in cytoplasm of embryonic cells to use hormones producing maleness

The absence or removal of the testes will cause hormonal deficiencies in the male. Surgical removal of the testes is called *castration*. The effects of this loss of the hormone testosterone depends upon when the castration was performed. If it occured before puberty, the male fails to develop normal secondary sex characteristics. The penis does not develop and sexual feelings are suppressed. A male who loses his testes prior to puberty is known as a *eunuch*. If the castration occurs after puberty there is often no diminution in his ability to perform sexual intercourse or experience orgasm. Following removal of the gonads, testosterone-like androgens are produced by the adrenal glands and are probably responsible for these sexual reactions.

Spermatogenesis Spermatogenesis is the process of producing sperm in the testes. As shown in Figure 4.2, the actual sites of production are the many long coiled tubes within the testes called the *seminiferous tubules*. Some cells of the walls of the tubules are called the *male germi-*

nal epitheliums. It is from these cells that all sperm are formed. The first cell to develop is the *spermatogonium* (Figure 4.4). Each spermatogonium multiplies and produces a new generation of cells, the *primary spermatocytes.* Each of these cells divides to form two smaller *secondary spermatocytes.* The two secondary spermatocytes then divide into four *spermatids.* The spermatids change directly into sperm. First, they lose some fluid; second, they reorganize the chromosomal material of the nucleus into a compact head; and third, the remainder of the cell collects at one end and lengthens out, forming the tail (Figure 4.3).

FIGURE 4.4 Seminiferous tubule structure and production of human sperm

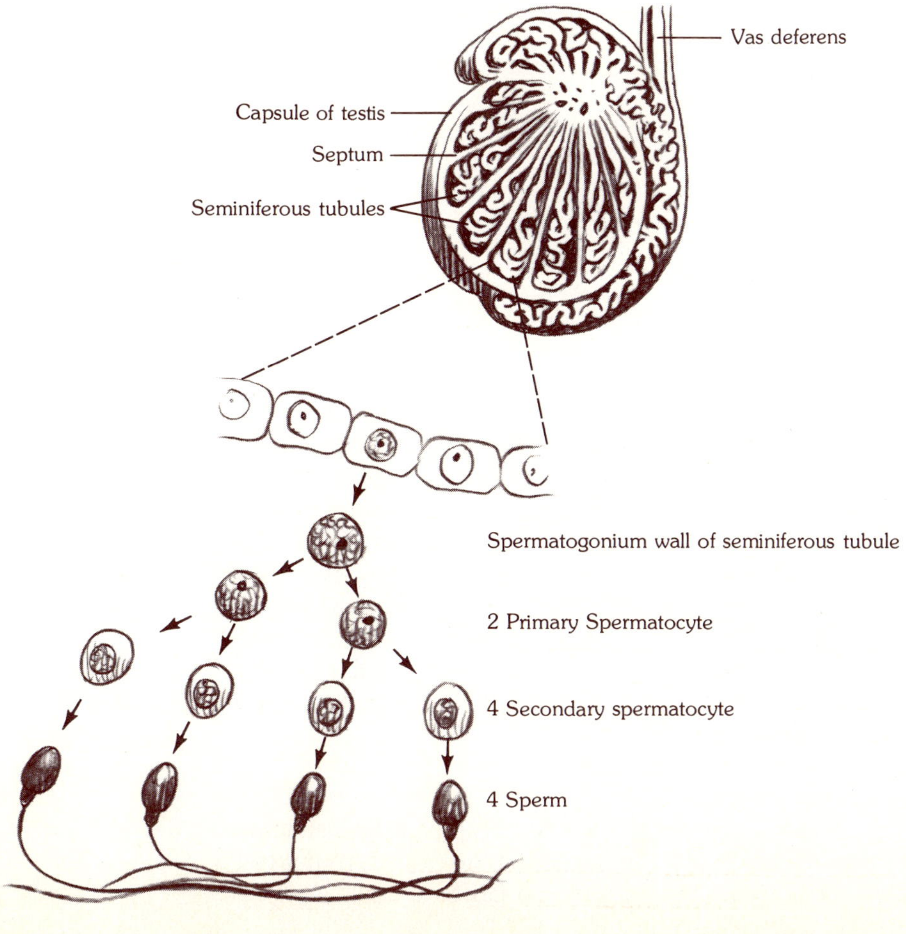

The Epididymis

As the sperm develop they move out of the seminiferous tubules and collect in a coiled tube called the *epididymis* (Figure 4.2). One epididymis lies on the upper side of each testis. Sperm mature and are stored in the epididymis until released from the body by ejaculation or until they disintegrate and are reabsorbed by the seminiferous tubules or by the epididymis itself.

The sperm remain almost totally inactive during the period when they are in the epididymis. During this time changes take place in them that increase their ability to fertilize an ovum. Sperm can stay alive for as long as a month in the seminiferous tubules and epididymis, awaiting ejaculation.

The epididymis of each testis becomes continuous with a duct about eighteen inches long which carries sperm from the epididymis through the abdominal cavity to the *ejaculatory duct* (Figure 4.1). This duct is termed the *vas deferens* or *ductus deferens.* From the epididymis to the body wall the ductus deferens is part of the *spermatic cord.*

The Spermatic Cord On either side of the testes, from the scrotum to the body wall, a firm, rubber-like tube about one-eighth of an inch in diameter may be felt (Figure 4.5). This is the spermatic cord, which consists of the vas deferens, the testicular blood vellels, and nerves bound into this single cord.

After the vas deferens enters the body wall, each duct loops behind the bladder (Figure 4.1) and ends in a spindle-shaped enlargement just before the junction of each vas deferens and the excretory duct of the seminal vesicle. This dilated portion of the vas deferens is the *ampulla,* a storage reservoir for mature sperm.

Adjacent to each ampulla is a saclike gland termed the *seminal vesicle.* The openings of these glands and the two ampullae fuse and form the ejaculatory ducts, which enter the prostate gland.

The seminal vesicles, prostate gland, and Cowper's glands secrete and store a fluid termed the *seminal fluid.* This fluid provides a nutrient medium for conveying sperm into the female. After the sperm have been mixed with the seminal fluid, the mixture is termed *semen* or *ejaculate.* This is the fluid expelled from the penis during the male ejaculation. It is grayish-white and sticky. It contains about 120 million sperm per cubic milliliter.

The Seminal Vesicles

Not all functions of the seminal vesicles are completely understood, but one is the provision of a portion of the seminal fluid. The seminal vesicles secrete a sticky, alkaline fluid that is high in fructose sugar (impor-

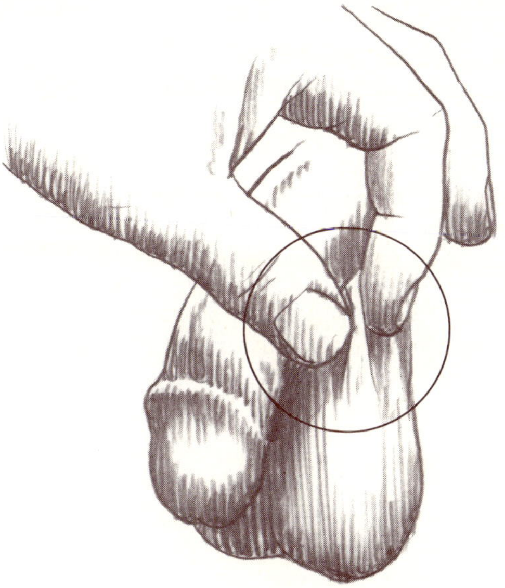

FIGURE 4.5 Spermatic cord; approximate position of one spermatic cord in the testicle

tant in sperm nutrition). The seminal vesicles secrete their fluid directly into the ejaculatory ducts.

As shown in Figure 4.1, the ejaculatory ducts empty their mixture of sperm and seminal fluid into the urethra. At this point these structures are embedded in the *prostate gland,* lying at the base of the urinary bladder. Several ducts from the prostate gland open into the urethra at the same point as the ejaculatory ducts.

The Prostate Gland

The prostate gland secretes much of the seminal fluid. In a sexually mature male the prostate gland continually secretes fluid (the amount depends upon the degree of androgenic hormone stimulation taking place). The normal prostatic fluid is thin and milky; it contains proteins, calcium, cholesterol, electrolytes (in concentrations comparable to those found in blood plasma), and enzymes (including acid phosphatase). Acid phosphatase is important because its presence in prostatic fluid indicates the amount of androgenic hormones being produced.

Several *prostaglandins* (PGs), a group of chemical regulators, have been found in male seminal fluid. These substances have varying affects upon the female genital tract. During the middle phases (ovulatory and secretory) of the female menstrual cycle, prostaglandins enhance the muscular activity of the female reproductive tract. These actions help in the migration of sperm from the vagina into the fallopian tubes, helping fertilization to take place.

Prostatitis Prostatitis, an inflammation of the prostate gland, is a common problem among men. It may be acute (short-term) or chronic (long-term). In the past prostatitis was a common outcome of gonorrhea infections, but with the use of antibiotics in treating gonorrhea, such prostatic inflammations are becoming less frequent. The causes of much of the prostatitis and enlargement of the prostate are unknown, but one of the major causes of temporary enlargement of the prostate gland is infrequent sexual intercourse.

Cowper's Glands (Bulbourethral Glands)

The small *Cowper's glands* (bulbourethral glands) lie on either side of the urethra slightly below the prostate gland (Figure 4.1). These glands produce a secretion that precedes ejaculation and is evident at the tip of the penis as a drop of clear, sticky fluid. This fluid removes any urine that may be in the urethra and also helps to lubricate the vaginal canal during intercourse.

The Urethra

The urethra serves two functions in the male. It conveys both urine and semen through the penis to the exterior of the body. The urethra is approximately eight inches long. It is divided into three divisions: the *prostatic urethra* (the part embedded in the prostate gland), the *membranous urethra* (the following half inch), and the remaining length, the *cavernous* or *penile urethra* (Figure 4.6).

The Penis

The male organ for copulation is the *penis* (Figure 4.6). The penis is used both for urine excretion and, in the erect state, for ejaculation of semen. As with other physical dimensions, the size of the penis varies. The nonerect penis is from three to four and a half inches long. In an erect state it will average about six to seven inches in length and one to one and a half inches in diameter.

Passing through the length of the penis are three columns of erectile tissue, two *corpora cavernosa*, side by side, and a smaller *corpus spongiosum*, beneath. A cross-section of the penis is shown in Figure 4.6. At the tip of the penis, the corpus spongiosum enlarges to form the *glans penis*, or head of the penis. The glans penis is richly supplied with nerve receptors, making it especially sensitive to external stimulation. A free

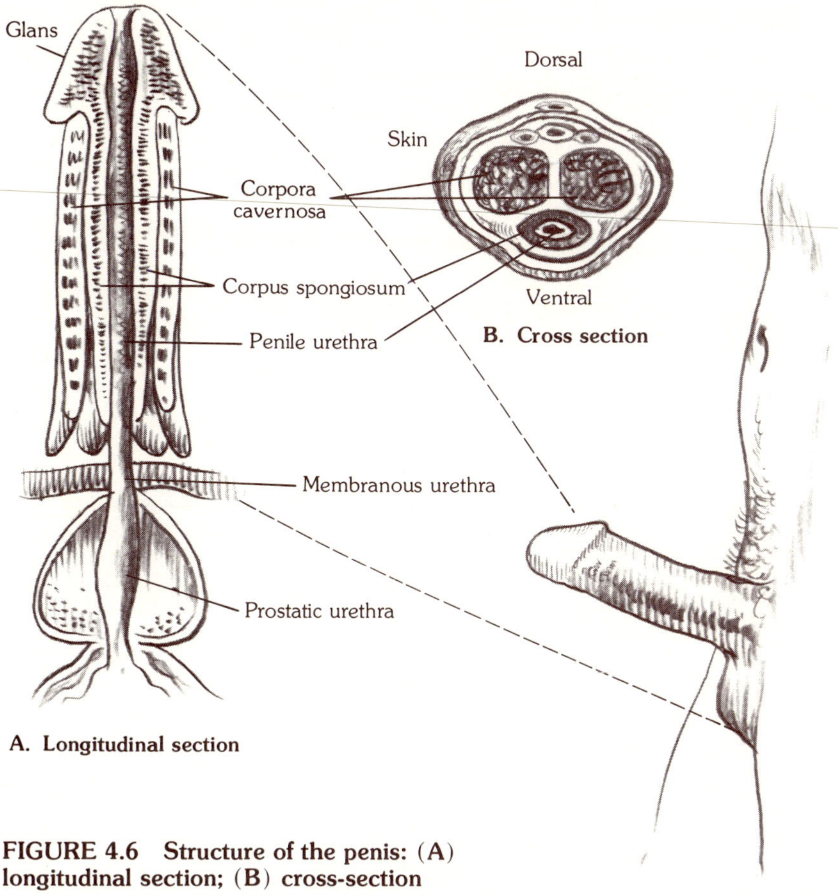

FIGURE 4.6 Structure of the penis: (A) longitudinal section; (B) cross-section

fold of skin, the *foreskin* or *prepuce,* overhangs the glans when it is relaxed (Figure 4.7). Sweat glands under the foreskin *(preputial glands)* discharge a white, cheesy substance called *smegma.*

Smegma should be removed because there is strong evidence that penile smegma harbors organisms that may cause a variety of infections in the female genital tract after sexual intercourse. One group of viruses that may be passed to women during sexual intercourse are the *herpes simplex* (type II) viruses, which may play a role in cervical cancer. Surgical reduction of the foreskin is known as *circumcision.* One of the major reasons for circumcision is to keep smegma from collecting under the foreskin. In a noncircumcised male smegma may be removed by pulling back the foreskin and washing the glans penis.

Erection The corpora of the penis are richly supplied with blood vessels. Erection of the penis is produced when the corpora (Figure 4.7) become engorged with blood. The inability to attain erection is called *impotence.* This should not be confused with *sterility,* which is either an insufficient number or total lack of sperm cells in the semen. A man may be sterile yet fully potent.

After erection, the return of the penis to the soft (flaccid) state is called *detumescence.* This occurs when the blood flow through the corpora of the penis returns to normal.

Mechanisms of Erection The mechanisms of erection seem to be more complicated than previously supposed. Nerves from the spinal column, in the small of the back, supply the penis and its arteries and veins. Stimulation of these nerves increases blood flow into the arteries supply-

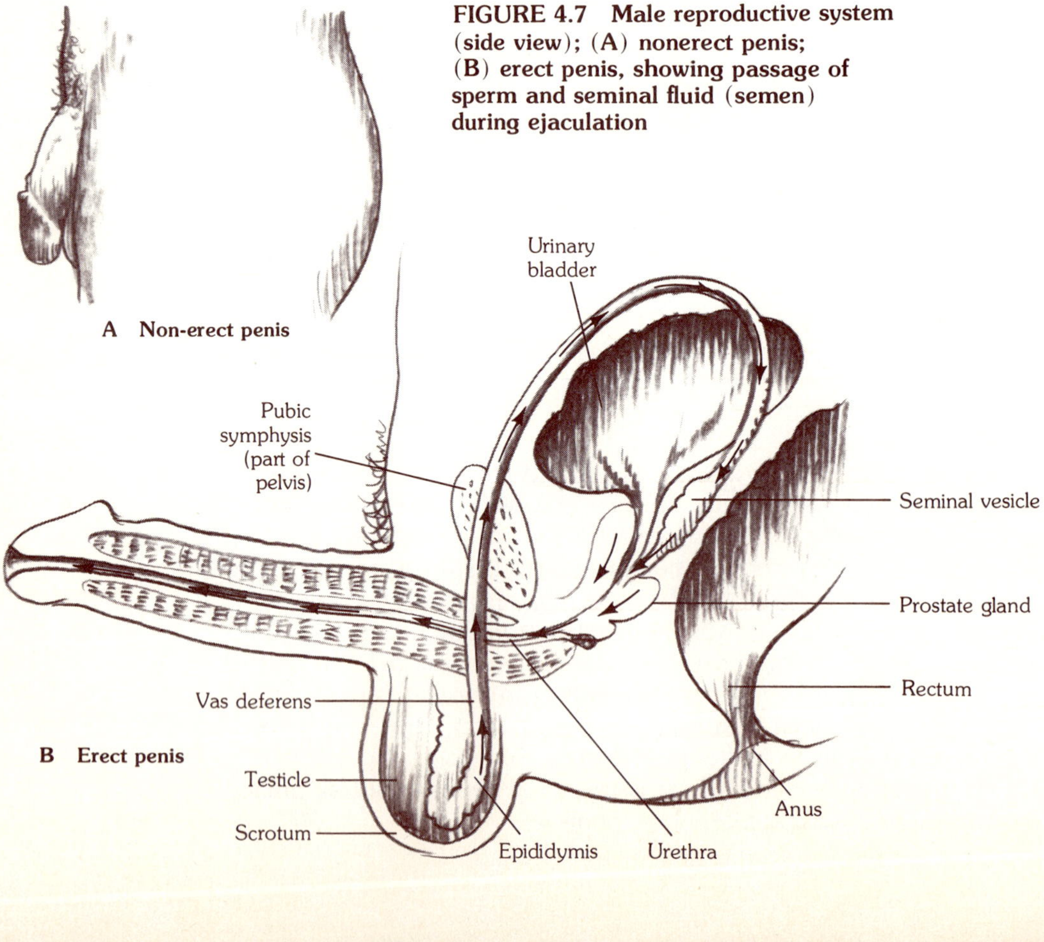

FIGURE 4.7 Male reproductive system (side view); (A) nonerect penis; (B) erect penis, showing passage of sperm and seminal fluid (semen) during ejaculation

ing the corpora. In the past it was felt that this stimulation completely blocked the flow of blood from veins draining the erectile tissue of the corpora, maintaining the erection. It has since been shown that during an erection there is flow of blood both into and out of the erectile tissue. During erotic stimulation, blood flows into the erectile tissue (Figure 4.6) from coiled arteries at the base of the penis. The increasing blood pressure and flow uncoils and straightens these arteries. Spaces in the erectile tissue fill with blood, causing the penis to become enlarged, turgid (stiff), and erect. The erection is maintained by this increased flow of blood through the erectile tissue.

Stimulation of the nerves causing erection can occur in three or four basic ways. First, direct physical stimulation of the penis produces a nerve-reflex arc with the spinal cord, causing stimulation of the coiled arteries, increasing blood flow and producing an erection. Tactile stimulation of other body parts, such as the male's breasts, will also stimulate the nerves controlling the blood vessels and produce erection. Higher centers of the brain may stimulate erection in response to the sight, smell, or touch of another person. Any stimulus that is erotic to an individual (including fantasizing) may produce erection.

Maintenance of erection is more complicated. Nervous stimulation must be maintained between the spinal column and the blood vessels of the erectile tissue to continue an erection. Often, if this nervous stimulation is disturbed or destroyed, no amount of stimulation, physical or emotional, will reinstate the erection. Loss of erection, in normal males, is completely under involuntary nervous control.

Ejaculation Physical stimulation of the penis not only causes it to become erect, but finally results in the forcible expulsion of semen, called *ejaculation*. Ejaculation usually results in the discharge of about three milliliters of semen. In sexual intercourse ejaculation occurs at the climax and sperm cells are placed in the vaginal canal. Ejaculation is usually accompanied by a feeling of intense sexual excitement and emotional release, called *orgasm*. Shortly after ejaculation the orgasm subsides, the penis usually becomes limp, and the male feels sexually satisfied.

Self-stimulation of one's reproductive organs to the point of orgasm (ejaculation in the male) is called *masturbation*. Involuntary ejaculation occurring during sleep is called a *nocturnal emission* ("wet dream"). This is accompanied by an orgasm.

Upon ejaculation the sphincter muscles (internal and external) of the urinary bladder close, preventing urine from entering the bladder or the penile urethra.

Ejaculation occurs in two stages. First there is contraction of the accessory organs (seminal vesicles, prostate gland, and Cowper's glands). Then there is contraction of the entire genital tract.

In the first stage, seminal fluid begins to accumulate in the ejaculatory duct by expulsion of prostatic fluid from the prostate gland. Then the contents of the ampulla are discharged into the ejaculatory duct accompanied by simultaneous expulsion of the contents of the seminal vesicles. During ejaculation prostatic fluid is added to the seminal fluid by regularly recurring contractions of the prostate gland.

The second stage of the ejaculatory process begins with the relaxation of the external sphincter of the bladder, which allows the semen to flow into the penile urethra. The ejaculate is then propelled from the prostatic urethra along the penile urethra to the outside of the penis by the muscles of the groin and penis. The prostatic urethra and ejaculatory duct contract regularly, aiding ejaculation of the semen. Seventy-five percent of all sperm are found in the first third of the semen. Following ejaculation, semen coagulates and then in several minutes liquefies. Sperm are relatively inactive until liquefaction occurs; then the sperm assume maximal motility. By the time of liquefaction the sperm are well established within the vagina of the female.

Ordinarily males become sexually mature sometime between eleven and fourteen and a half years. At this time a male first experiences nocturnal emissions, though masturbation almost universally begins in infancy. The male's sexual ability can often continue throughout life. Sperm production and ability to maintain erection decreases somewhat in older men, but in most males it never completely ceases.

The Male Climacteric

Is there a male menopause: No. Menopause is the cessation of menstruation, which occurs only in women. Between the ages of 48 and 68, however, many males (up to 35 percent) will experience a significantly diminishing gonadal function. This can be defined as *male climacteric* (Kupperman, 1974). Beginning signs are decreasing ability to achieve erection or experience ejaculation, inability to maintain erection for an adequate length of time, and infrequent erection. Older men may complain of inability to perform sexually or to achieve erection while fantasizing. During the male climacteric, pituitary gonadotropic hormone levels increase, while testosterone levels decrease.

This stage in some men's lives is not so specific and definite as the female menopause, but it can be much more disrupting and disturbing. Men may experience the same "hot flashes" that some women do. Sleep is often disturbed, and the man may be less positive, less forceful, more irritable, and generally difficult to live with. The sexual implications of the male climacteric will be discussed in Chapter 11, after we have considered female anatomy and physiology and other aspects of our sexuality.

Female Sexual Anatomy and Physiology

5

The biological symbol for female is ♀. One explanation for this symbol is that it represents the "mirror of Venus," the Greek goddess of love. Unlike the explanation of the male symbol, this gives a sexual connotation to the symbol for femaleness. In this explanation love is equated with reproduction. Biologically, the reproductive function of the female is to receive sperm from the male and form offspring from the union of sperm and ovum.

Reproductive Structures

The female *genital* or *reproductive organs* are both internal and external. The inner organs of the female reproductive systems are the ovaries, fallopian tubes, uterus, and vagina.

FIGURE 5.1 Uterus and related organs (front view)

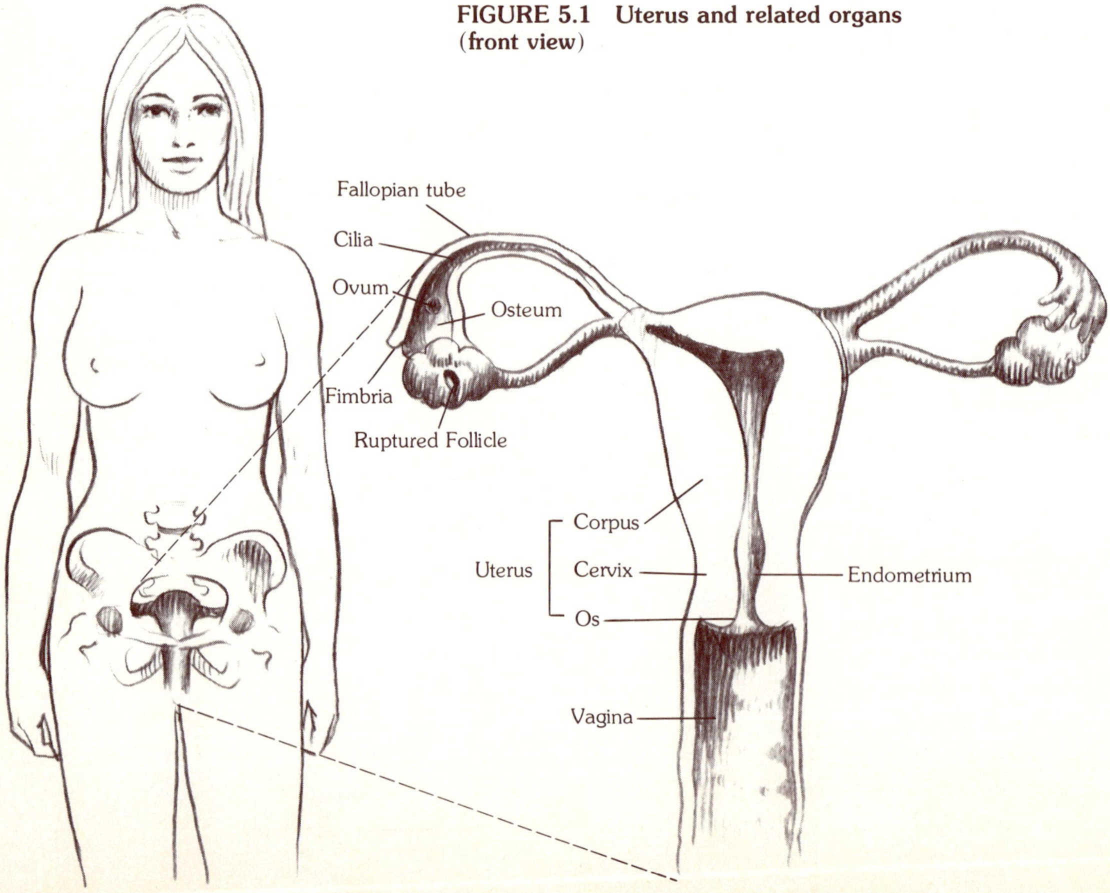

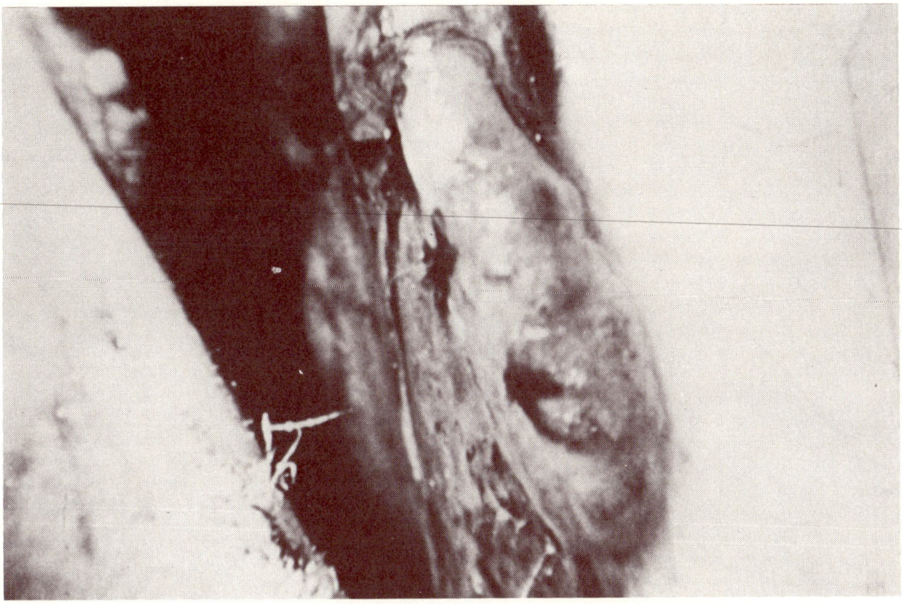

FIGURE 5.2 Single frame of time-lapse motion picture recording ovulation (in a rabbit)

Ovaries

The ovaries (female gonads) are situated deep in the pelvic cavity, one on either side of the uterus (Figure 5.1). Each is attached to the uterus by a ligament.

The ovaries serve a dual function, producing both eggs (ova) and hormones. Within the ovary are many vesicles called *ovarian follicles.* Beginning at puberty, these immature follicles ripen or mature at the rate of one about every twenty-eight days (menstrual month) and develop into *graafian follicles.* Each month, approximately midway between menstrual discharges, a graafian follicle ruptures and releases a mature egg. Since the reproductive life of the female extends about thirty-five years (from about ages twelve to forty-seven) and about one ovum is produced every twenty-eight days (or thirteen per year), usually only about four hundred to five hundred eggs ever mature.

Each graafian follicle begins development near the center of the ovary. As it enlarges, it moves outward until it finally appears like a little blister on the surface of the ovary (Figure 5.2). Near the midpoint between menstrual discharges the graafian follicle ruptures and releases the egg (ovum) enclosed within it, a process called *ovulation.* Ovulation

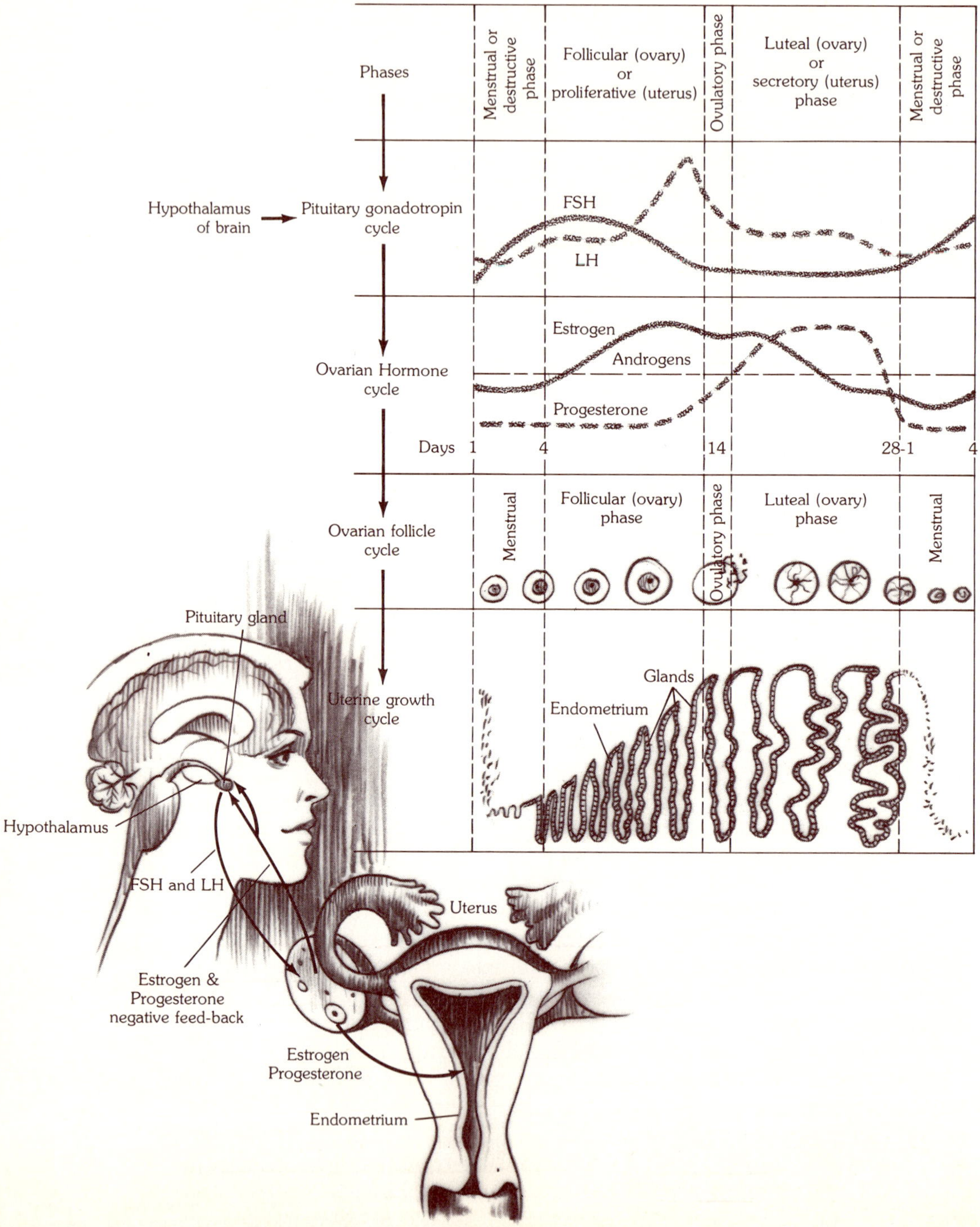

FIGURE 5.3 Diagram of events of menstrual cycle

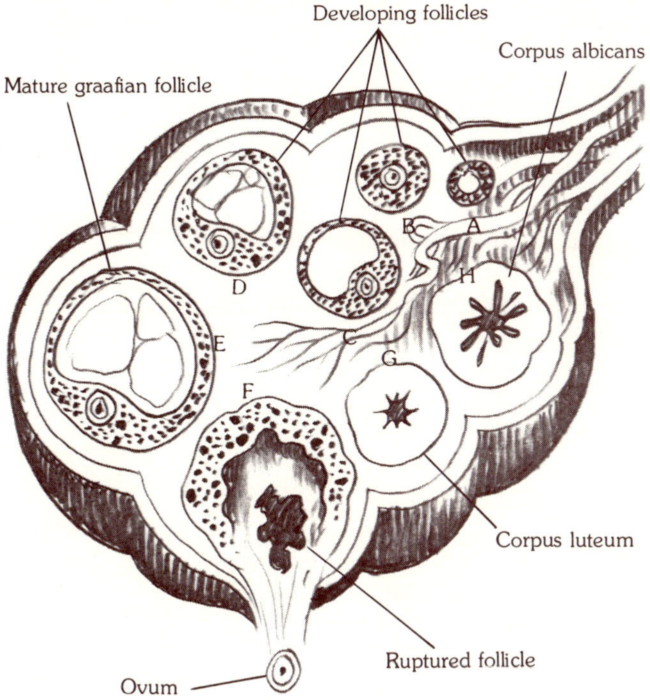

FIGURE 5.4 Cross-section of ovary showing complete events of a menstrual cycle: A through E, follicular phase; F, ovulatory phase; G, corpus luteum; H, corpus albicans

may occur as early as the eighth day of the cycle and as late as the twentieth day (Figure 5.3). A small blood clot forms at the point of ovulation on the surface of the ovary (Figure 5.2). After ovulation, this tiny blood clot is soon replaced by yellow-colored cells and is called the *corpus luteum* (Figure 5.4 G). This body of tissue remains about twelve days, after which it degenerates.

Fallopian Tubes (Oviducts)

The fallopian tubes are two funnel-shaped tubes, about four inches long, extending between the uterus and the ovaries. The outer end of each tube is fringed. The finger-like fringes, called *fimbria,* are adjacent to each ovary (Figure 5.1). The waving of the fimbria is believed to play a role in helping the ovum enter the funnel opening (*osteum*) of the fallopian tube. When the ovum ruptures through the wall of the ovary it can float freely in the peritoneal cavity for a short time, but quite soon the current produced by the fimbria catches the ovum and passes it into the fallopian tube. The inner lining of the fallopian tube is covered with minute, hairlike structures called *cilia.* Once inside the fallopian tube, the ovum is propelled toward the uterus by movements of the cilia and by contractions of the walls of the tube. An ovum has no movement of its own. If the ovum is fertilized by a sperm, it will normally travel down the fallopian tube and become embedded in the lining of the uterus.

Normally the ovum is picked up by the fallopian tube on the same side as that on which the ovulation occurred (Figure 5.4). It has been clearly shown that on occasion ova have been pulled across the pelvis to be picked up by the fimbria of the opposite tube. On rare occasions, an ovum may fail to be drawn into the fallopian tubes. Sperm from recent sexual intercourse may be present at the time of ovulation and may fertilize this ovum outside of the fallopian tube, in the pelvis itself. If this fertilized ovum is not picked up by a fallopian tube, it may become embedded in the pelvic cavity. A fertilized ovum may also become embedded in the wall of a fallopian tube itself and develop there. The development of a fertilized ovum anywhere outside of the uterus is called an *ectopic pregnancy.*

Uterus

The uterus, a thick-walled muscular organ, is about three inches long and two inches wide in the *nulliparous* woman (one who has never borne a child). It is a hollow, pear-shaped organ located slightly above and behind the bladder, but in front of the rectum (Figure 5.5).

The upper half of the uterus is the *corpus* (body), the lower half is the *cervix,* and the opening of the cervix is the *os.* A portion of the tissue lining the body of the uterus (*endometrium*) breaks down approximately once a month, causing the *menses* (*menstrual flow* or bleeding).

The endometrium is richly supplied with blood vessels and glands. After fertilization the developing embryo becomes embedded in the endometrium within four or five days after entering the uterus (or seven to eight days after fertilization). During pregnancy the uterus, often called the *womb,* stretches to over twelve inches in length to accommodate the growing baby.

The uterus normally tilts forward, opening into the upper surface of the vagina (Figure 5.5). It is loosely suspended in this position by several ligaments. Loosening of these ligaments due to childbearing may cause it to tilt backward. Other causes for tilting or displacement may be congenital deformity or pelvic disease (such as cancer).

Vagina

The vagina is a muscular tube from four to six inches long extending from the vaginal opening inward, at a 45-degree angle, toward the small of the back. As shown in Figure 5.5, it lies between the urinary bladder and the rectum, slightly below and in front of the uterus. It connects the uterus with the exterior of the body.

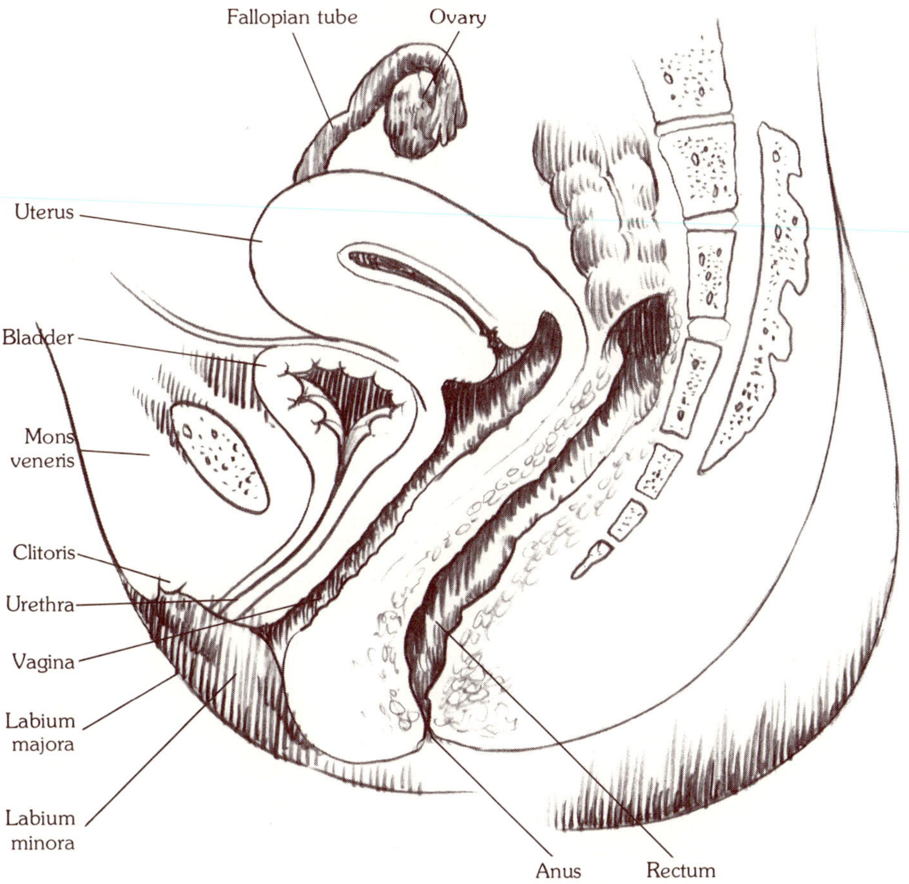

FIGURE 5.5 Female reproductive organs (side view)

The vagina is the excretory duct for the menses (menstrual flow), the female organ for sexual intercourse, and the birth canal in childbirth. The fluids present in the vagina come from several sources: the wall of the vagina, glands in the uterus and cervix, and Bartholin's glands. There are no moisture-producing glands in the wall of the vagina; the mucus-like material produced there arises from the network of veins in the vaginal walls. This fluid is secreted through a process similar to sweating during sexual arousal. The Bartholin's glands in the labia minora, near the entrance to the vagina (see Figure 5.6), produce only a drop or two of fluid late in sexual arousal. This fluid has a minimal effect on vaginal lubrication.

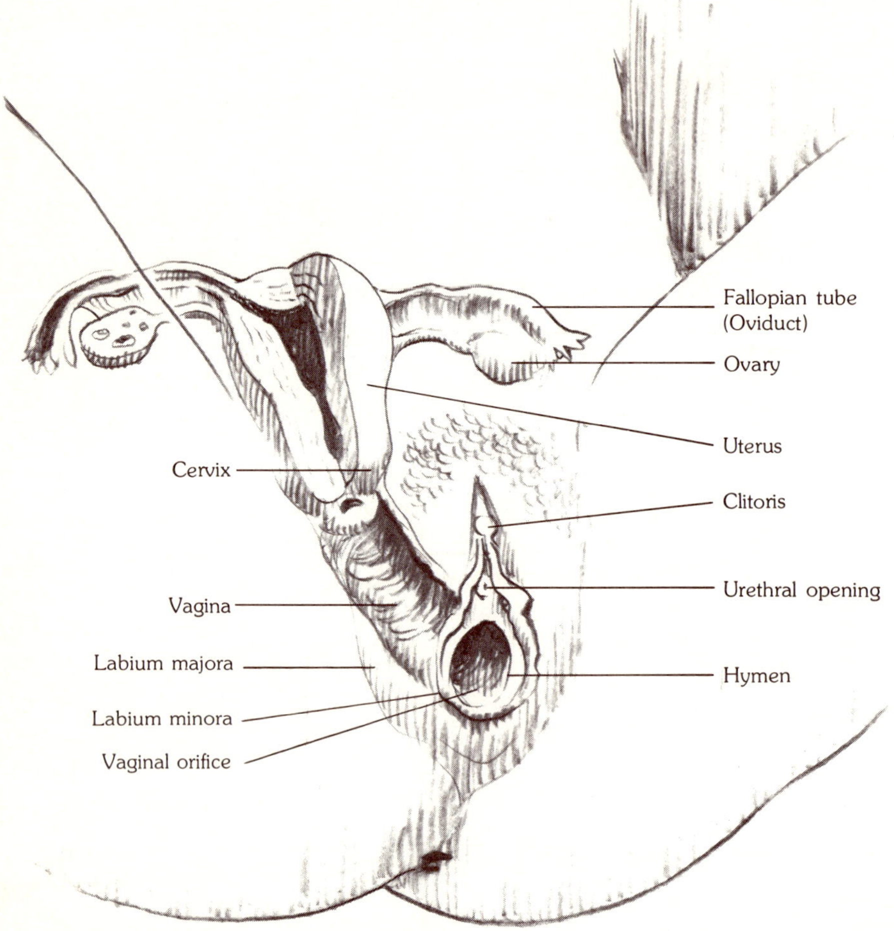

FIGURE 5.6 Female external genital organs

During the climax of intercourse, rhythmic contractions of muscles begin in the vaginal area and spread throughout the pelvic area. These contractions, along with relief from the vasocongestion of erectal tissues, physiologically contribute to an intensly pleasurable sensation called *orgasm.* Orgasm is a complex physiological-psychological reaction of the total body. The physiological reaction of the muscles and blood supply are the only constant factors.

The external genitals of females are given the general name *vulva* (meaning covering). The vulva include the pubis, labia, and clitoris.

Pubis

At the junction of the thighs and torso is the *mons pubis.* This rounded pad of fatty tissue lies over the pubic bone and cushions it during sexual intercourse (Figure 5.6).

The mons pubis becomes covered with hair at puberty. As shown in Figure 5.6, the female pattern for such genital hair is a triangle with the apex pointing down.

Labia

Below the mons pubis are two pairs of liplike structures that surround the external openings of the urethra and vagina. The outer pair are the *labia majora* (major lips). As shown in Figure 5.6, the labia majora are thick folds of skin and fatty tissue covered with pubic hair. The *labia minora* are smaller folds of skin and fatty tissue, free of hair, lying inside the labia majora, and usually concealed by them.

The space between the labia minora, into which the vaginal passageway and the urethra open, is the *vestibule.* The area behind the vaginal opening and before the anus is the *perineum.* This is the area that is usually cut surgically during childbirth to prevent its being torn during delivery, since a surgical slit heals much more easily than a jagged tear. This surgical incision is called an *episiotomy.* Above the urethral opening, the labia minora meet and form the *prepuce* (or hood), a covering over part of the *clitoris.*

Clitoris

The clitoris lies at the top of the labia minora just under the prepuce. Like the penis of the male, the clitoris has a shaft and a glans. The shaft of the clitoris is hidden under the prepuce. The glans protrudes from the prepuce and looks like a small bump (Figure 5.6).

The clitoris contains erectile tissue (corpora cavernosa) that fills with blood and makes the clitoris stiff and erect during sexual arousal. The erect clitoris measures one to one and one-half inches in length, though most of it is buried under other tissue and not visible. It contains many sensory nerve endings and is sensitive to touch, especially during sexual arousal. If a woman is not sure where her clitoris is (see Figure 5.6), she should feel her genitals until she finds a very sensitive spot at the front terminus of the labia minora. This is the clitoris.

Hymen

Stretched partially across the vaginal opening is a fold of tissue called the *hymen* (Greek for "thick skin"). Hymen is also the Greek god of marriage, who is usually pictured as a young man carrying a bridal torch.

The hymen varies in thickness and extent. It may be totally absent or so thick that it must be broken surgically before sexual intercourse. This is a painless procedure, when done with a local anesthetic.

Contrary to common belief, rupture of the hymen does not always produce bleeding. The use of tampons (vaginal insertions used during menstrual discharge), vaginal medical examinations, finger manipulation and participation by women in active sports often destroy the hymen prior to sexual intercourse. Hence absence of a hymen should not be taken as a sign of lack of virginity. Also, sperm deposited between the labia can pass the hymen, enter the vagina, and propel themselves through the uterus and into the fallopian tubes, making it possible for a woman who is technically a virgin to become pregnant.

Breasts (Mammary Glands)

The breasts, or mammary glands, are present in both sexes. They are modified sweat glands and are exocrine (ducted) glands. Similar breast development is found in both males and females up to the time of puberty. In the male the breasts then atrophy and are nonfunctional. In the female they continue to develop, reaching their functional maturity after pregnancy. Breast development in a girl during puberty is closely related to her reproductive maturity and dependent upon female hormonal ac-

FIGURE 5.7 Human female breast; lower half dissected to show internal structures

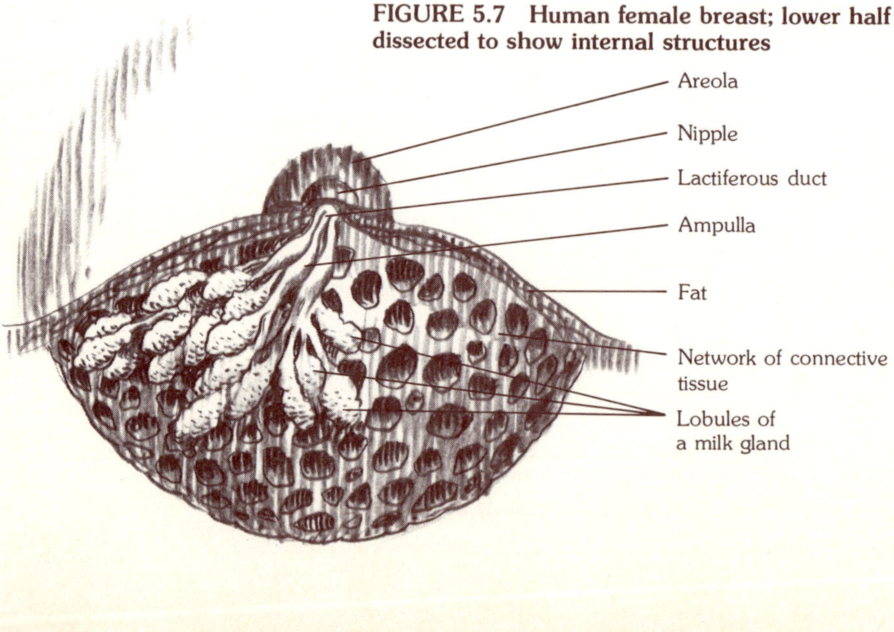

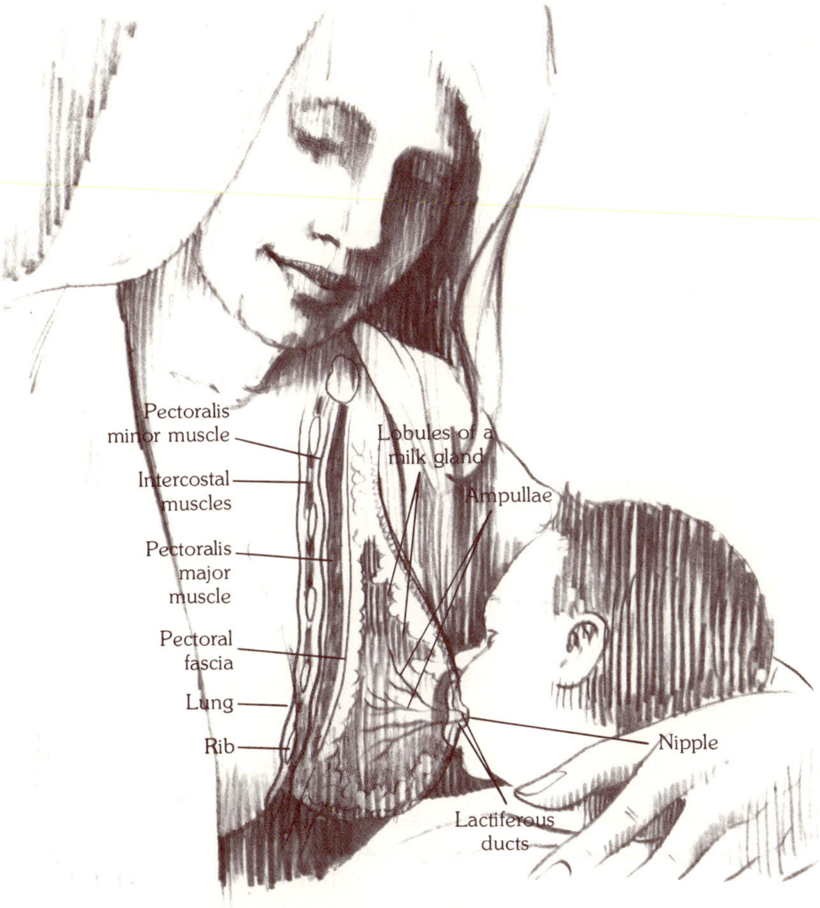

FIGURE 5.8 Cross-section of a human female breast

tivity. Although breasts are not directly related to reproduction, they are considered secondary sex characteristics and are closely related to human sexual responses.

The breast of an adult woman (Figures 5.7 and 5.8) may assume any of a number of shapes, from conical to hemispherical. The left breast is generally larger than the right one. Some women have hair in the cleavage between the breasts or surrounding each nipple. Such hair is normal and does not indicate any hormonal imbalance. The *nipple* at the center of the breast contains fifteen to twenty openings from which milk exudes in drops at the time of lactation. The nipple also contains erectile tissue. Stimulation causes it to become engorged with blood, firm, and extended (Figure 5.8), assuming the shape of the artificial nipple used on baby bottles.

Surrounding the nipple is a circular area of markedly darker color and different texture than the rest of the breast. This is the *areola.* The roughness and wrinkledness of the areola is caused by the openings of various glands. These glands produce a fluid that protects the areola and nipple from the irritating effects of an infant's saliva during suckling.

Internally the female breast consists of fifteen to twenty multilobed milk glands arranged radially around the nipple opening. Connective tissue hold the glands in place. Fatty tissue is also distributed among the lobes. The size and shape of the breast is largely dependent upon the amount and distribution of fatty tissue present. As shown in Figure 5.7, each milk gland is a number of lobules drained by small ducts that come together and form a major *lactiferous* duct. The lactiferous duct ends in the ampule (a reservoir for milk) just before opening on the surface of the nipple. The milk produced by these glands is a combination of water, minerals, fat, sugar (lactose), and protein (casein).

During puberty the hormones estrogen and progesterone from the ovary induce the development of the milk-producing tissue and breasts. During pregnancy the amounts of the ovarian hormones increase. They cause greater development of the milk-producing structures and are responsible for the increased size of the breasts at this time. But the ovarian hormones apparently inhibit the actual production and flow of milk.

After childbirth and removal of the placenta, estrogen and progesterone are reduced to extremely low levels for a time, permitting the release of LTH or *prolactin* by the pituitary gland. LTH acts upon the secretory cells of the milk glands to stimulate milk production. At other times the *hypothalamic prolactin-inhibiting factor* keeps this hormone from being produced.

The production of milk and the release of milk are two separate processes. Prolactin causes the production of milk, but the hormone *oxytocin,* from the pituitary gland, activates the flow of milk. Suckling after birth causes the secretion of oxytocin. Oxytocin contracts the muscle cells surrounding the smaller milk ducts. This contraction injects the milk into the larger milk ducts and the ampullae, where the milk can be removed by the suckling baby. The process is known as milk "letdown." When a baby first sucks a nipple, no milk is present in the breast. It takes forty-five to sixty seconds for the production of new milk and the letdown of milk already produced. Suckling causes sensory impulses to pass up through the nervous system to the hypothalamus of the brain. Hypothalamic prolactin-inhibiting factor is reduced, permitting the release into the bloodstream of prolactin by the anterior pituitary. Oxytocin is produced in the pituitary gland and is released into the bloodstream. The hormones flow back to the breasts, causing the production and letdown of milk. As long as the breast is emptied of milk, this circuit continues to operate. There is a gradual increase in prolactin (LTH) secretion, which increases the production of milk as the child grows. Lack of suckling stops the activity of the hypothalamus and milk production stops. If a baby is breast-fed, return to regular menstrual cycles may not occur for several months. If suckling does not occur, menses begin immediately or within twelve weeks after delivery.

There is no correlation between breast size and the ability to breast-feed an infant. Psychological reactions are known to affect a woman's ability to produce and let down milk. A woman undergoing emotional trauma may be unable to breast-feed. Her reactions to the idea of breast-feeding can also influence her ability to breast-feed. Some women let down milk as soon as they hear their children's cry.

The Menstrual Cycle

Human females do not have breeding seasons. They are sexually receptive throughout the year. Their sexual desires depend largely upon psychic stimuli, but one group of hormones seems to exercise a great amount of influence on a female's sexual receptiveness or sexual drive. Testosterone or testosterone-like substances (*androgens*) are not found exclusively in males. Some of these are found in normal females. These androgens are produced primarily in the adrenal glands and they play several roles in females, mainly stimulation of body growth and maintenance of sexual receptiveness. During several diseased states the female adrenal gland may secrete abnormally large quantities of androgens, producing a *virilism* that may result in facial hair, male body-hair distribution, a lower pitch to the voice, a loss of female fat distribution, an enlarged clitoris, or reduced breast size. In extreme conditions sterility may result.

Although there is no breeding season, women do have a physiological cycle that plays a vital role in their reproductive physiology and sexual receptiveness. This biocycle is the *menstrual cycle,* the advent of which is the sign of sexual maturity.

Two female hormones, estrogen and progesterone, are secreted from the ovaries in cycles. *Estrogen* actually is a general term used to include several closely related female sex hormones: estrone, estriol, and estradiol. *Progesterone* is a specific substance. The cyclic secretions of estrogen and progesterone are controlled by two pituitary hormones (Figure 5.9), *follicle-stimulating hormones* (FSH) and *luteinizing hor-*

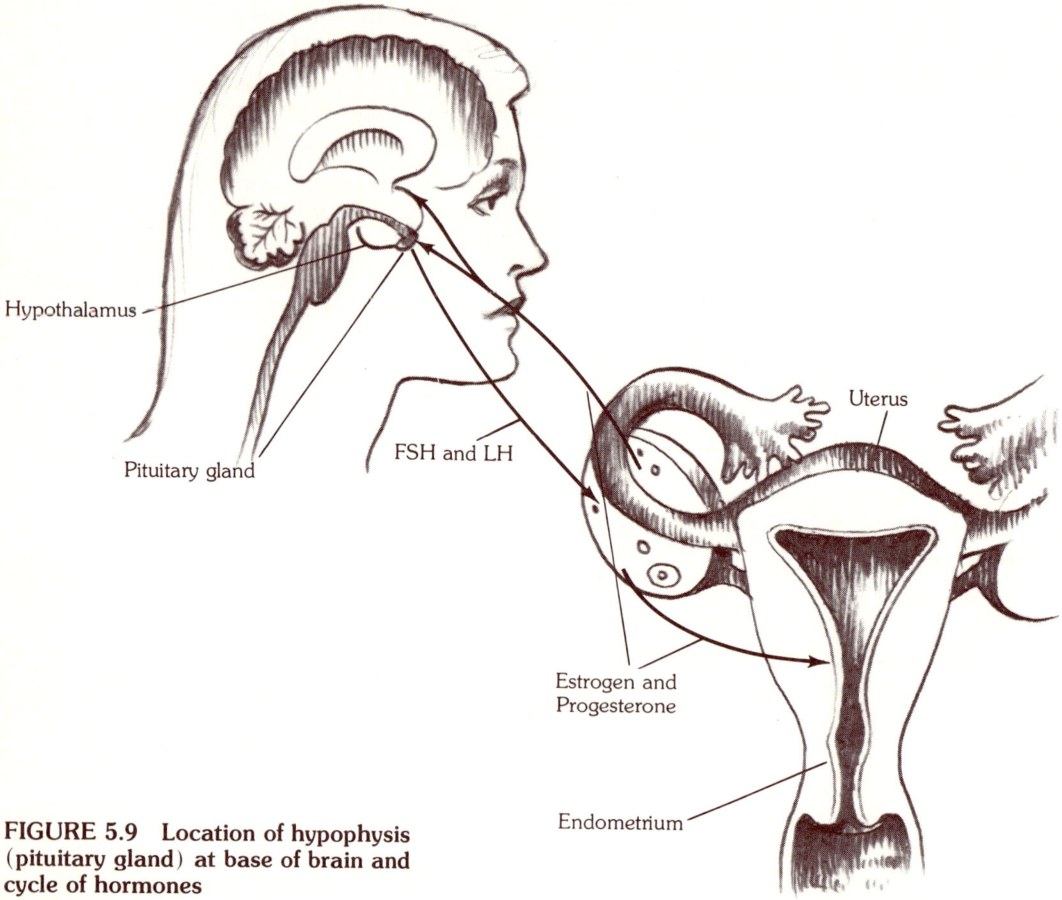

FIGURE 5.9 Location of hypophysis (pituitary gland) at base of brain and cycle of hormones

mone (LH). The interaction of these four hormones produces the menstrual cycle. As explained in Chapter 3, there are four organs that are important in the menstrual cycle: the brain, the pituitary gland, the uterus, and the ovaries.

The major visible evidence of the menstrual cycle is *menstruation*. Menstruation is the periodic discharge through the vagina of blood, mucus, and cellular fragments from the uterine endometrium (see Figure 5.5), occurring at more or less regular intervals (except during pregnancy and lactation) from menarche to menopause.

The first menstruation is referred to as *menarche*. This usually occurs between the twelfth and thirteenth years, but it may occur as early as the tenth year or as late as the sixteenth year. Since puberty involves a broad range of physical changes occurring between childhood and maturity, menarche represents just one sign of puberty. The cessation of menstruation is termed *menopause.* Menopause occurs in the late forties or early fifties (the mean age in the United States is forty-seven years). About half of all women cease menstruating between forty-five and fifty years of age, about a quarter before forty-five, and about a quarter after fifty. Just as menarche represents only one sign of puberty, menopause is just one sign of the *female climacteric,* sometimes referred to as the "change of life."

As shown in Figure 5.9, the hypothalamic portion of the brain triggers the pituitary to secrete FSH and LH in a cyclic manner. This cycling of the pituitary begins during puberty and continues until menopause unless it is upset, delayed, or stopped by physical or emotional stress or pregnancy.

The two control systems of the body, the endocrine system and the nervous system, interact through the pituitary and affect the menstrual cycle. The hypothalamus of the brain secretes specific chemicals called *hormone-releasing factors.* One of these releasing factors causes the pituitary to produce FSH to initiate the monthly menstrual cycle.

As shown in Figure 3.6, the hormone-releasing factor is secreted by nervous tissue in the hypothalamus and flows down the blood vessels between the hypothalamus and the pituitary gland, causing the release of hormones (such as FSH and LH) into the bloodstream. Because the hypothalamus is part of the brain, any nervous stimulus that affects the hypothalamus may affect the menstrual cycle. Emotional upsets can precipitate or delay the menstrual cycle.

Menstrual Phases

The cycle of events from the beginning of one menstrual discharge until the next is called the *menstrual cycle.* Although the menstrual discharge most commonly occurs every twenty-eight days, women vary considerably in the length of their menstrual cycles. Some women are known to have cycles as short as twenty-one days and others as long as thirty-eight days. Many women have menstrual cycles of varying lengths. As shown in Figure 5.3, four phases can be observed in the uterus during the typical twenty-eight-day cycle: (1) the menstrual or destructive phase, (2) the proliferative or follicular phase, (3) the ovulatory phase, and (4) the secretory or luteal phase.

Menstrual or Destructive Phase The first day of the menstrual flow is counted as day 1 of the menstrual cycle. When the menstrual flow begins, the lining of the uterus (the endometrium; see Figure 5.5) has grown nearly twice as thick as it will be at the end of the menstrual flow.

The menstrual flow is the shedding of a portion of this thickened lining. This layer has a very rich blood supply, and with the death of endometrial cells both blood and cell fragments are discarded as the menstrual flow. The average amount of blood lost ranges from thirty to sixty milliliters during each menstruation. The total blood and tissue loss in each menstruation ranges from 60 to 180 milliliters (about four to twelve tablespoonsful). The duration of the menstrual flow is usually four to six days, but periods ranging from two to eight days may be considered normal.

The shedding of the thickened endometrium is caused by the sudden drop in the level of progesterone in the bloodstream (see Figure 5.3). At the beginning of this phase the supply of progesterone drops drastically, and within two or three days the network of tiny blood vessels in the endometrium begins to shrink, depriving it of support and nourishment. The upper two-thirds of the layer gradually becomes detached and small pieces of the lining start to shed. Within the next few days each tiny vessel empties droplets of blood, the layer detaches, and the combined material flows out of the body.

As the old lining is shed and washed away, the blood vessels seal and return to their original size. The former thick, spongy, deep-red lining is now a thin, smooth, pink surface ready for new growth. As the phase ends, the FSH begins to be secreted from the pituitary in increasing amounts (Figure 5.3), causing new growth in the uterus and in the ovary, and starting the new month's menstrual cycle.

In the past there was a strong taboo against sexual intercourse during menstruation. It was based upon the misconception of the "uncleanliness" of menstrual blood. Most women, however, feel a heightened sexual arousal during the menstrual flow, and intercourse during this time can be very pleasurable. These feelings may be in response to androgen levels, which are more effective at this time because of the low levels of progesterone and estrogen (see Figure 5.3).

Proliferative or Follicular Phase As shown in Figure 5.3, during the menstrual phase the pituitary hormones FSH and LH and the ovarian hormones estrogen and progesterone drop to their lowest levels. After menstruation has stopped, the endometrial lining (and the vaginal lining) is thin and dry. The glands contained within the endometrium are straight, short, and narrow.

As the follicular phase begins, one of the follicles (containing an ovum) grows faster than the others in the ovary. At first the estrogen levels in the bloodstream are low, causing the increasing FSH levels shown in Figure 5.3. The increased FSH levels in turn stimulate the follicle to grow and secrete increasing amounts of estrogen (Figure 5.3). The estrogen causes active growth (or proliferation) of the endometrium, producing a dense, thick lining in the uterus.

This phase lasts about nine or ten days, and by the midpoint the increasing amounts of estrogen reverse the pituitary action and diminish FSH secretion. The amount of FSH in the blood decreases so that by day 12 or 13 the blood FSH levels are low and the estrogen levels are high. This combination of hormone levels causes the fast-growing follicle to move to the surface of the ovary, forming a blister-like bump on the surface of the ovary (see Figure 5.2).

Ovulatory Phase During the follicular phase the egg follicle has grown from a mere pinpoint to nearly a third of an inch in diameter. The endometrium of the uterus has thickened in preparation for implantation of a fertilized egg.

As shown in Figure 5.9, the estrogen also feeds back to the pituitary gland and, while inhibiting the production of FSH, *stimulates* the production of LH. There is a surge of LH, and when the LH level in the blood reaches a certain critical level, the now mature follicle bursts through the blister on the ovary. This is *ovulation*—the expulsion of the ovum into the abdominal cavity, where it is picked up by the fimbria of the fallopian tube (see Figure 5.1).

Ovulation occurs an average of fourteen days after the beginning of menstruation, although it commonly takes place anywhere from the eighth to the twentieth day. In rare cases, ovulation has been known to take place outside of these limits—even during menstruation. As shown in Figure 5.3, the ovulatory phase is very short and covers only the period of ovulation, whenever it happens.

Secretory or Luteal Phase As shown in Figure 5.4, as soon as ovulation takes place (F), the empty follicle, under the influence of the high level of LH, recloses, heals, and becomes a structure known as the corpus luteum (G), which means "yellow body". Under the direction of the LH the corpus luteum produces increasing amounts of the hormone progesterone. The progesterone serves to prepare the endometrium of the uterus for implantation and to prevent its sloughing off (menstruation).

Progesterone began to increase slowly at day 10 of the cycle, but until now estrogen has been the dominant hormone. Under the influence of this estrogen, the uterine wall (endometrium) has become richly supplied with blood vessels, thick, and filled with fluid. This tissue is ready for a fertilized egg to implant and grow into an embryo. If the egg is fertilized, it usually implants on day 21 or 22.

This phase begins with the formation of the corpus luteum and the secretion of increasing amounts of progesterone into the bloodstream. The corpus luteum also produces small amounts of estrogen, although progesterone is the dominant hormone during the secretory phase.

At the beginning of the secretory phase, immediately after ovulation, there is a slight drop in body temperature, which is caused by the increase in estrogen (shown as the first increase in Figure 5.3, around day 14 or 15). This drop in body temperature is followed by an increase in body temperature, often to slightly above normal, lasting throughout the remaining days of the menstrual month. This increase in body temperature is due to the progesterone.

After ovulation, the corpus luteum secretes increasing amounts of progesterone until day 21 or 22. After day 22 the progesterone level in the blood declines slowly until day 25 or 26. Then, in preparation for the following month's menstrual phase, or menstruation, the progesterone declines very rapidly (days 26 through 28).

This phase of the menstrual cycle lasts thirteen to fourteen days (from day 16 to day 28). If the ovum is not fertilized, the corpus luteum folds in (Figure 5.4 H) and becomes inactive. This reduction in the activity of the corpus luteum reduces the progesterone in the bloodstream, causing the death of the cells and glands of the endometrium and producing the menstrual flow of the next month's menstrual phase.

If the egg is fertilized, it continues down the fallopian tube, dividing and redividing into two cells, then four, eight, sixteen, and so on. By the time it reaches the uterus it consists of a hollow ball of cells resembling a tiny mulberry. Within ten days after fertilization the now developing embryo implants itself in the uterus by digesting the upper cell layers of the endometrium.

Soon after implantation the embryo begins to produce a *gonadotropic* hormone that functions much like LH in stimulating the corpus luteum to continue to grow and produce progesterone and estrogen for about the first twelve weeks of pregnancy. This high, sustained level of estrogen causes the endometrium to continue growing, instead of degenerating and sloughing off. It also prevents further egg-follicle development in the ovary and resulting ovulation.

Biorhythm Moods of the Menstrual Cycle

There are a number of mood and emotional changes that seem to be closely related to the different phases of the menstrual cycle. Some have been linked to physiological factors. Others have been linked to speculation or theories that have grown out of animal studies but which have not always been verified in human studies. Many may be linked to the twenty-eight-day sensitivity cycle explained in Chapter 3. The great majority of these mood and emotional changes, when they occur, probably result from a combination of the physical makeup of the woman involved, hormonal and other cyclic chemical changes, social attitudes and training, and emotional stability.

Most physical menstrual changes are linked to the relative levels of estrogen and progesterone in a woman's bloodstream. Any accompanying emotional changes may be traced to the same source. Women who are large-breasted usually have less body hair, and it usually is fine in texture. These women are considered to have higher levels of estrogen than small-breasted women with more and courser body hair, who are believed to have higher levels of progesterone. Consequently, many of the physical and emotional effects of estrogen and progesterone may be due not to the absolute levels of either hormone but to the balance between the two. Also, some women are more sensitive to estrogen while others are more sensitive to progesterone.

A class of chemical regulators called *prostaglandins* regulate relative levels of hormones. These substances often influence the balance of hormones in the body. Prostaglandins work in pairs. A specific pair seems to work on the uterus. One member of the pair relaxes the muscular layer while the other allows this layer to constrict (inducing labor or producing abortion). These actions seem to work during differing phases of the menstrual cycle. Early in the cycle one of the pair relaxes the muscular layers while later in the cycle the opposing prostaglandin allows muscular contractions to occur, causing cramping.

During the proliferative phase (days 5 through 13) the endometrium of the uterus is growing from a thin, smooth layer into a thick, dense layer. This growth may take much of a woman's energy. Often a woman will not feel like overexerting herself physically at this time.

Estrogen rises and peaks in the bloodstream the last day or two (day 12 or 13) of the proliferative phase. This high level dips slightly at ovulation (usually day 14) and then returns until about day 16. Estrogen is the "feminine" hormone, and some women may exhibit what are thought of as "feminine" characteristics to a high degree during peak estrogen days (days 12 through 16). You may have to revise some of your ideas about "femininity," though. Don't expect a woman to choose a dress of tender pink on these days; she's much more likely to prefer a bold red. Color sense has been found to be strong during this time. Her energy levels are heightened now, too.

At the time of ovulation (ovulatory phase, Figure 5.3) estrogen drops drastically. During this drop in estrogen some women feel a strong sexual drive. Since this is the time of ovulation, these feelings may increase her chance of conceiving. Sexual feelings seem to be caused by a rise in the androgen (malelike hormones) level in the blood, either from the ovary or from the adrenal gland.

During the early and middle part of the secretory phase (days 15 through 22) the heightened energy levels persist. This may be a time for physical recreation and projects. If there are no other outlets for these energy levels by the end of the secretory phase, it is not unusual for a woman to devise some sort of project in which she can become absorbed, such as refinishing a piece of furniture or cleaning the complete house in one or two days.

The feelings of self-esteem, well-being, happiness, and heightened energy levels during the middle part of the cycle occur when estrogens, progesterone, and androgens are high. At about day 22 the estrogen and progesterone begin to drop to their lowest levels. The rapidly declining estrogen and progesterone are believed to cause the emotional depression, anxiety, irritability, weepiness, and fatigue that sometimes occur after the twenty-second day of the cycle, and have been termed "premenstrual tensions."

Premenstrual tensions, when they occur, reach their height about two days before the menstrual flow (days 26 through 28). The depression, irritability, and weepiness that may occur at this time can affect male-female relationships to such an extent that the last two days before the menstrual flow (days 26–28) may be known as "fight time." At the same time, because of high androgen levels during this period, many women experience heightened sexual feelings, which make it "make-up time," along with "fight time." These tensions are not inevitably and universally strong or even noticeable.

There are three times in the life of a woman when there are sharp declines in estrogen and progesterone: during the secretory phase of the menstrual cycle (especially days 22 through 28), just after childbirth (which may help to produce what is called postpartum psychosis and the well-known "baby blues") and during menopause. The latter two are also periods in which women experience strong social pressures. As the mind, emotions, and body are interrelated, social training, traditions, and sexual attitudes and expectations, as well as changing hormonal levels, have significant influences upon the personality fluctuations in women.

Physical Menstrual Problems

The physically painful menstrual flows that some women experience are known as dysmenorrhea. These painful periods are classified as either *spasmodic dysmenorrhea* or *congestive dysmenorrhea*.

Spasmodic dysmenorrhea occurs most often in younger women and often after a pregnancy. Symptoms include mild to severe low back pain, uterine cramps, tenderness of the breasts, and/or skin eruptions such as pimples or blotches. This type of dysmenorrhea is due to a high ratio of progesterone to estrogen. Spasmodic dysmenorrhea may be treated by using birth-control pills (preventing ovulation also prevents the high amounts of natural progesterone), pain-killing drugs, or muscle relaxants, or by increased exercise and physical activity.

Congestive dysmenorrhea occurs at all ages. Its symptoms include noticeable bloating and weight gain before menstrual flows (caused by sodium retention and excess body fluids), headache, and breast tenderness. All of these symptoms seem to be in response to high levels of estrogen. Congestive symptoms may be treated separately, such as with a diuretic (which removes sodium and excess water from the body) for weight gain and aspirin for headache, or with birth-control pills, which may either decrease or increase the symptoms, depending upon the woman's individual sensitivity to the estrogen in the pills.

Menopause

The functioning of the ovaries reaches its peak before the age of thirty. After thirty a woman's ovarian functions gradually decline. As shown by Figure 5.10, there is a decreasing ability of aging ovaries to respond to

FIGURE 5.10 Excretion of estrogen in the urine of women as indicator of blood concentration of estrogen

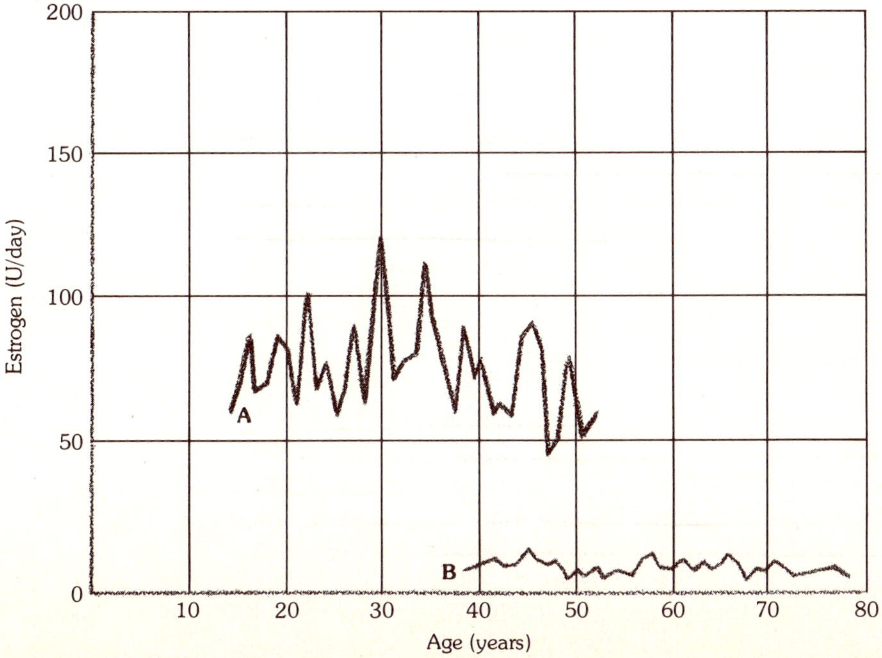

the pituitary hormones FSH and LH. When the average woman reaches the age of forty-five or fifty her ovaries cease to produce ova, and the monthly shedding of the endometrium of the uterus (producing menstruation) stops, usually gradually but sometimes suddenly. This cessation of the menstrual cycle is termed the *menopause*.

At the time of birth the ovaries of the average woman contain about 400,000 immature egg follicles (see Figure 5.4). During her reproductive years one egg follicle matures per menstrual cycle for a total lifetime production of from 400 to 500 eggs (ova). The remainder of the immature follicles gradually degenerate, until by the time a woman is forty-five to fifty no ova remain to respond to the FSH and LH of the hypophysis. Since the high production of estrogens by the ovaries depends upon maturing follicles, estrogen drops to a very low level.

As menopause develops, ovulation and menstrual periods become irregular. But as long as any menstrual periods are occurring, however erratically, there still remains some chance that a woman can become pregnant. If a woman has not had a menstrual period for a year she can be reasonably sure that ovulation has ceased and conception is impossible.

The hormonal imbalances that occur during this time are usually associated with a number of instabilities in women. One of these is in the circulatory system, which causes irregularity in the diameter of blood vessels. This permits periodic erratic flowing of blood, which may cause feelings of heat or marked sweating, alternating with periods of coldness. The warm periods are termed "hot flashes," and may last anywhere from a second or two to several minutes. They are common among menopausal women but by no means universal. Other instabilities such as fatigue, dizziness, headaches, insomnia, sleepiness, and emotional depression are also common during menopause, but their causes are generally unknown. Generally, the better the emotional, social, and personal attitudes of the woman before menopause, the fewer unpleasant symptoms occur. But severe emotional disturbances can occur during menopause. The physical fluctuations of the period of change, awareness that reproductive potential has ceased, hot flashes, and emotional upsets can be extremely disturbing to any woman.

As shown by line A of Figure 5.10 some estrogen generally continues to be produced beyond menopause. This estrogen seems to come from the tissues of the body and not from the ovary. Such tissue estrogen, shown by line B, is inadequate to maintain the estrogen-dependent organs and tissues of the body. The breasts and genital organs shrink in size (atrophy) and a thinning of the skin and bones occurs. These changes can be reduced by use of supplemental estrogen beyond menopause but this greatly increases the chances of the woman developing cancer of the body of the uterus. Ovarion estrogens protect women, during their reproductive years, from uterine cancer and cardiovascular diseases. The tissue-estrogens seem to reverse this protection. The heavier a woman at menopause the more of these estrogens she produces; consequently, she shows fewer menopausal difficulties but increases her chances of developing uterine cancer or some cardiovascular conditions.

Another important aspect of menopause is the relationship between estrogen and *plasma cholesterol.* Lipids, such as plasma cholesterol, have been linked with atherosclerosis and heart attacks. Ovarion estrogen significally lowers plasma cholesterol. This, or some related effect, may explain why women have much less atherosclerosis than men before menopause, but have the same incidence as men after menopause.

It has been frequently said that the sex drive of a woman increases with age, and that the postmenopausal woman is likely to enjoy sexual intercourse more, and more frequently, than in the past. Some scientists feel this is because androgens are relatively more prominent in her blood (see Figure 5.3) and levels of estrogens and progesterone are reduced. Others link this increased sex drive with the removal of the fear of pregnancy. Still others deny that the sex drive does necessarily increase after menopause. Many women have no need to wait for the menopause to enjoy sex fully and frequently. Those who do find greater enjoyment after menopause may be influenced by the many articles that have been published about this "phenomenon"—articles that originally served the good purpose of exploding the myth that a woman's sex life was over with the menopause, but which now may be perpetuating a myth of their own.

Sexual Development

6

Until recently the fields of sexual physiology and sexual behavior were among the least advanced of all sciences affecting humans. One of the primary reasons is that most mammals exhibit similar physiological reactions, except when it comes to reproductive physiology and behavior. In these respects humans are often unique. This fact greatly reduces the usefulness of other animals for research into physiological and behavioral comparisons between males and females. Besides, until comparatively recently there was little research into sexual response, particularly in females. These questions are now being studied and knowledge is advancing very rapidly.

Anatomical Relationships

The sex of an individual is determined at fertilization. The XX chromosomal combination results in a female and the XY chromosomal combination will become a male. But these chromosomes directly determine only whether the individual will have testes or ovaries. All of the remaining sexual development depends upon the correct functioning of these testes or ovaries. Early in embryonic development embryos are bisexual and have the potential of becoming either male or female. The testes and ovaries are produced from the same tissues. Until the sixth week of development there is no gonad at all. There is no indication of sex until the seventh week, when the gonads begin to acquire sexual identity. During this seventh week, in the genetic male, the testes begin to develop. In the genetic female, the ovaries do not begin to develop until several weeks later. After development begins, the embryonic gonad (either testis or ovary) regulates the remainder of the individual's sexual development.

Female and male organs are often *homologous* (both develop from the same embryonic tissue) and sometimes *analogous* (perform similar functions). Table 6.1 lists some of these relationships of the reproductive systems.

The undifferentiated gonad becomes the ovary in the female and the testis in the male. In the ovaries masses of cells form primary follicles surrounding one to several cells, which swell and become *oogonia* (see Figure 5.4). These oogonia undergo rapid cell division by twenty weeks of development of the embryo. By this time some 7 million oogonia are present in the developing ovaries. At this time cell division ceases and no further ova are ever produced. These 7 million start to degenerate to about one million at birth, and less than 400,000 by puberty (beginning of ovulation, menstruation, and active sexual maturity). Only about 450 of these ova are ovulated during a woman's reproductive lifetime. All the rest degenerate. In the male testis, sperm development does not begin until puberty.

TABLE 6.1 Relationships of Reproductive Systems

Male Derivative	*Female Derivative*	*Homologous*	*Analogous*
Testis	Ovary	+	+
Epididymis	Fallopian tubes, uterus, vagina	+	
Scrotum	Labia majora	+	
Corpus spongiousum	Labia minora	+	
Bulbourethral glands	Bartholin's glands	+	+
Penis	Clitoris	+	+
Corpora cavernosa of penis	Corpora cavernosa of clitoris	+	+
Glans penis	Glans clitoris	+	+
Prepuce of penis (foreskin)	Prepuce of clitoris (hood)	+	+

In the male embryo a system of thin tubules develops from the gonad to become the vas deferens and the epididymis. In females, the tubules that would become the vas deferens in the male degenerate and disappear. The tubules that develop into the epididymis in the male fuse in the female into the fallopian tubes, uterus, and part of the vagina. The remainder of the vagina forms from a part of the tissue that becomes the urinary bladder and urethra in both male and female.

As shown in Figure 6.1, the labia majora of the female develop from the same embryonic tissue as the male scrotum. The labia minora of the female are derived from the tissue that forms the corpus spongiosum in the male. Both of these structures contain erectile tissue and become swollen during sexual arousal. Where the labia minora meet in front they fuse to form the hood (or prepuce) that covers the clitoris. This hood is the same tissue that forms the foreskin (or prepuce) of the male's penis (Figure 6.1).

The clitoris of the female is homologous to the penis of the male. Both the penis and the clitoris consist of a shaft and a glans. The shaft of the clitoris is hidden under the hood, but the glans protrudes from the hood and appears as a small bump on the female (see Figure 5.5). Both structures contain hollow areas (corpora cavernosa) that fill with blood and are the means of erection during sexual arousal. The clitoris and the penis also contain many nerve endings and are very sensitive, especially during sexual excitement.

Hormonal Control of Development

It is possible to remove or destroy the area from which the gonads will develop in the embryos of some animals (such as rabbits, monkeys,

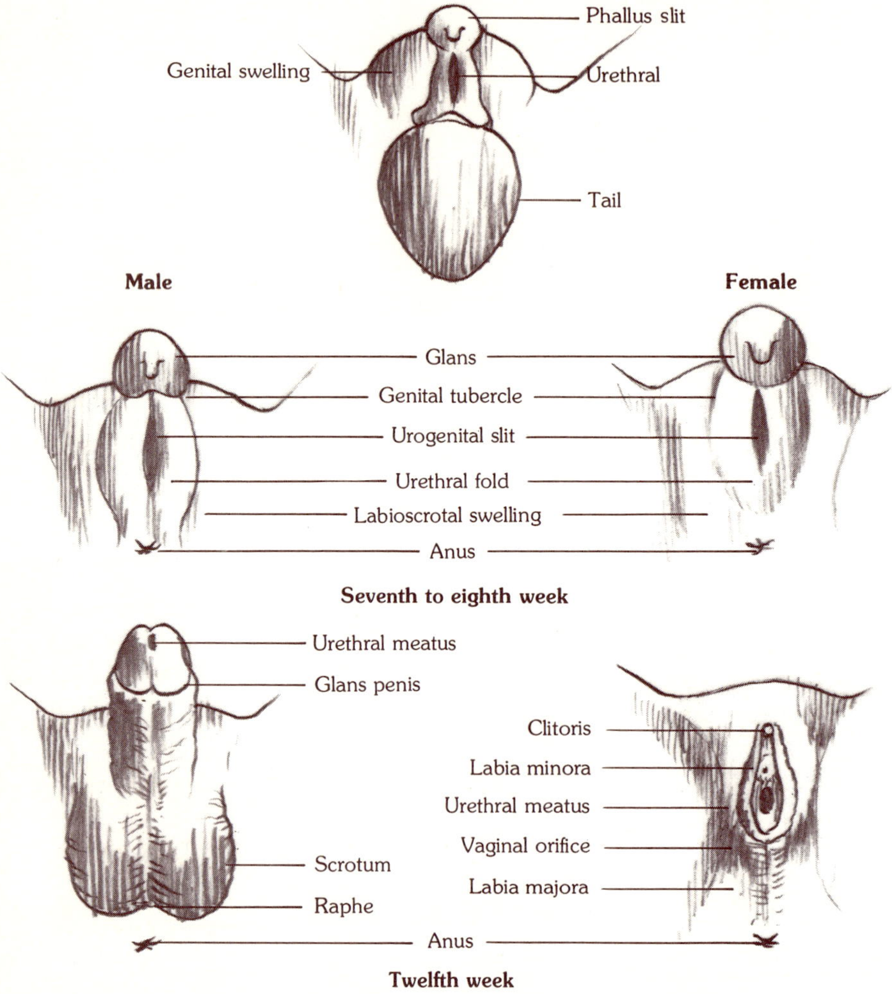

FIGURE 6.1 Homologous development of the labia and the scrotum. The male and female external genitalia form from similar structures in the embryo. (In the absence of androgenic hormonal stimulation, female development will always occur.)

and sheep) without killing the embryo. When this is done, regardless of the genetic sex of the developing individual (whether XX or XY), the now gonadless embryo develops into a female. Consequently, the presence of a normally functioning testis is essential in inducing development of the male sex organs. But a female gonad (ovary) need not be present for the female organs to develop. The testes produce an androgenic hormone that induces development of the male sex organs and also stops the cyclic production of female sex hormones (estrogen and progesterone) in the male. The pituitary gland secretes FSH and LH in a cyclic manner (Figure 5.9), unless these androgenic hormones act upon it during embryonic development. In infant boys, testosterone, or a testosterone-like androgen, acts upon the anterior pituitary and keeps it from cycling later in life. In girls, the fetal lack of androgens permits the pituitary to cycle later in life. Also, during the critical period of gonadal development and testicular control, a normally functioning testis is needed for normal male sexual development. In some genetic males (XY) a failure of gonadal function during critical periods of organ development can cause the development of female external and internal genitalia. Such people can vary in appearance from male pseudohermaphrodites (Figure 6.2) to sexually complete but sterile females (Figure 6.3).

FIGURE 6.2 Male pseudohermaphrodite, showing male and female external sexual characteristics

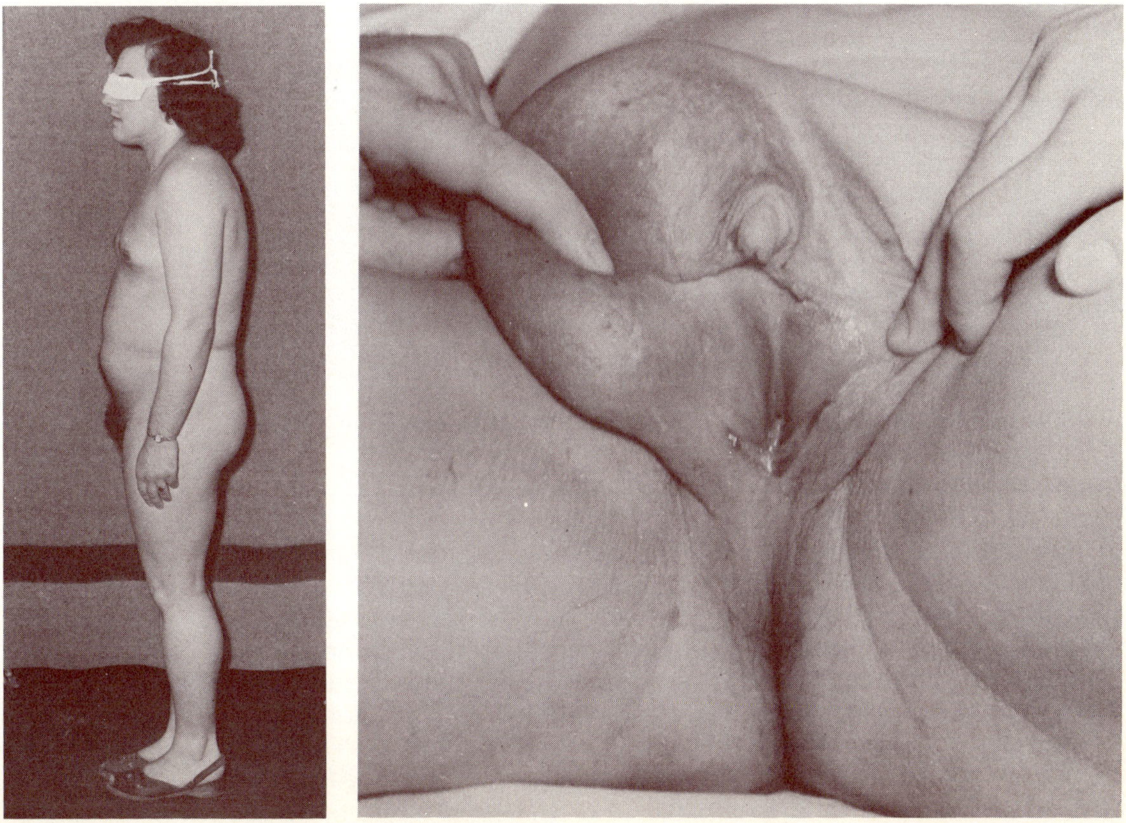

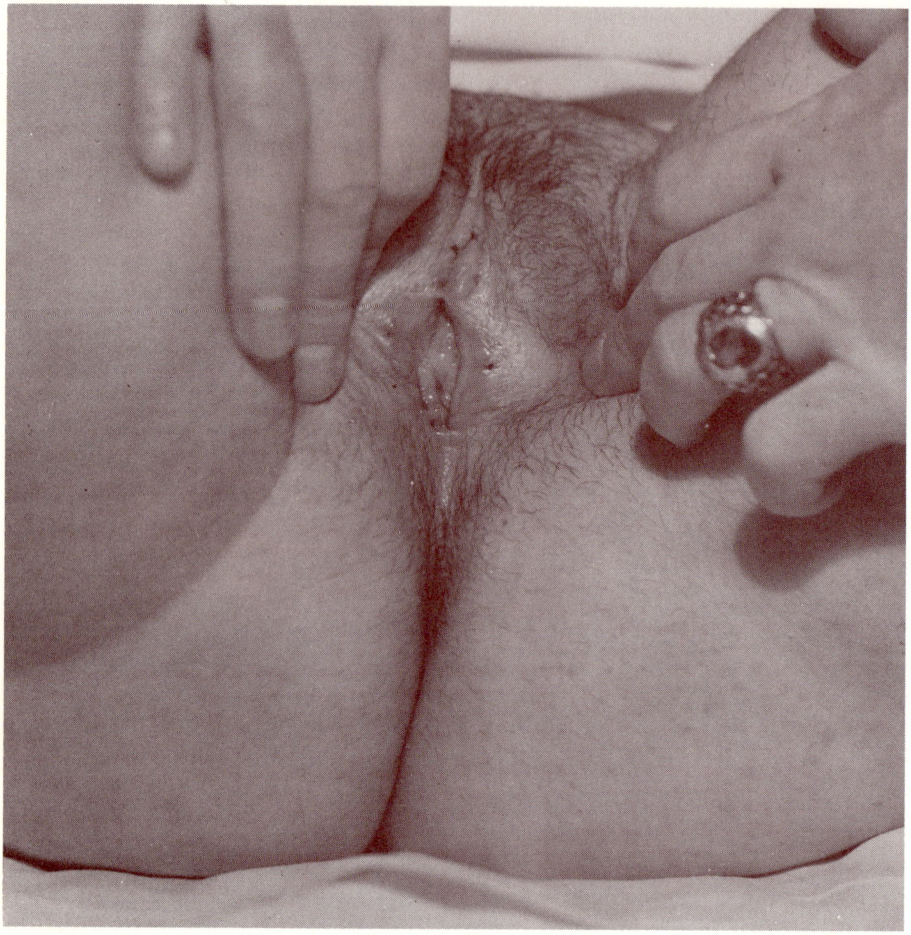

FIGURE 6.3 Female development of a genetically XY male. This female shows normal secondary sexual characteristics but is sterile.

A gonadless embryo will develop female sex organs, but normal anatomical and functional sexual development will not occur. An individual who receives only one X chromosome from her parents never develops gonads and consequently never menstruates and cannot bear children. The condition is known as Turner's syndrome (Figure 6.4). Apparently both X chromosomes are required for normal ovarian growth during embryological development and overall female development throughout life. At least one X chromosome and one Y chromosome are needed for normal male development.

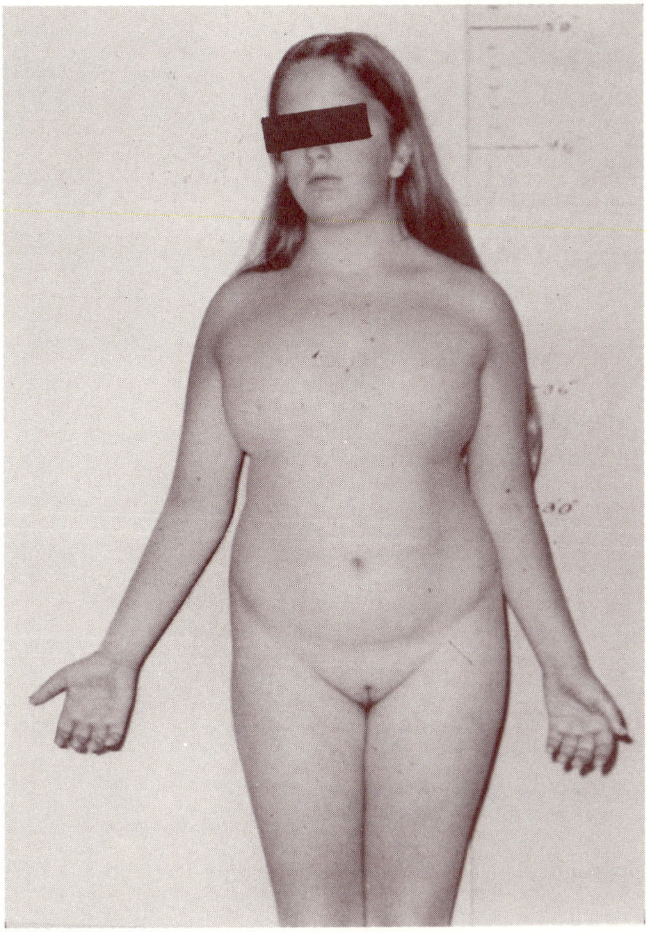

FIGURE 6.4 Turner's syndrome. Genetically the individual has only one X chromosome. Sexual characteristics are abnormal.

Postnatal Development

Anatomical development does not cease at birth. The genital organs are only partly formed. As shown by Figure 6.5, the body proportions of an infant are quite different from those of an adult. Each organ of the body has its characteristic rate of growth, but the growth rates of various organs follow definite patterns (Figure 6.6). The growth patterns follow three broad postnatal growth curves. Figure 6.7 shows the *neural curve,* representing the growth of the head, brain, spinal cord, and sensory organs. Neural growth is rapid during infancy and slow in adolescence. As shown in Figure 6.7, these areas are nearly adult size by nine years of

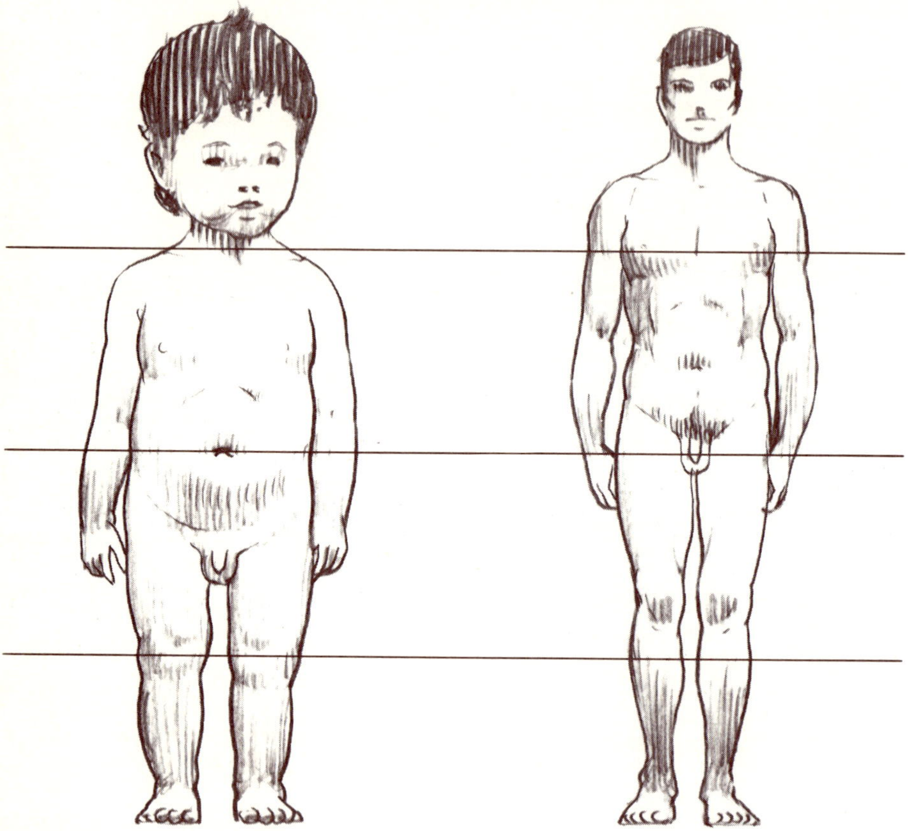

FIGURE 6.5 Relative differences in body proportions between a young child and an adult

age. The *sexual* or *reproductive* pattern follows a different growth curve. Figure 6.8 illustrates the growth of the primary sex characteristics (genital organs, ovaries, and testes). The secondary sex characteristics (breasts, body and facial hair) show a similar growth pattern. These organs grow very slowly until about age eleven in females and thirteen in males, when they undergo rapid growth. This period of rapid growth is termed *puberty*. Following puberty, growth tapers off throughout adolescence (period between puberty and complete sexual maturity), although the testes continue to grow until the twenties.

The third growth pattern represents the overall body growth. It is usually called the *somatic* (body) growth curve, representing the growth of arms and legs, chest and abdomen, shoulders and hips, some internal organs, and height and weight. As shown by Figure 6.9, growth is rapid

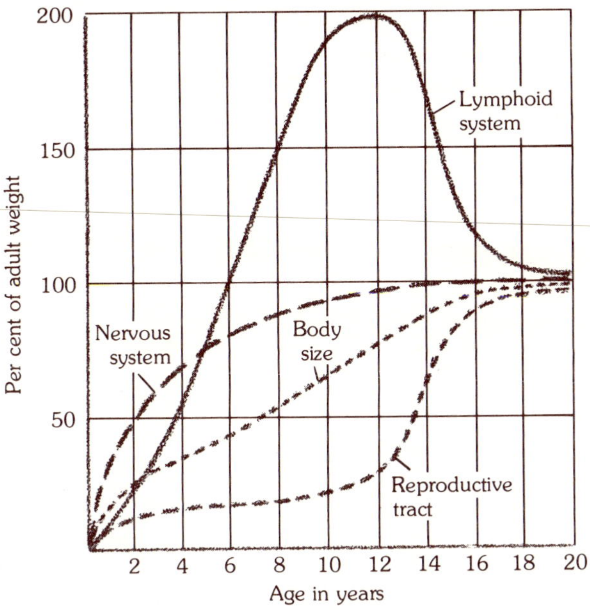

FIGURE 6.6 Diagram of relative growth rates of several different body systems during human development

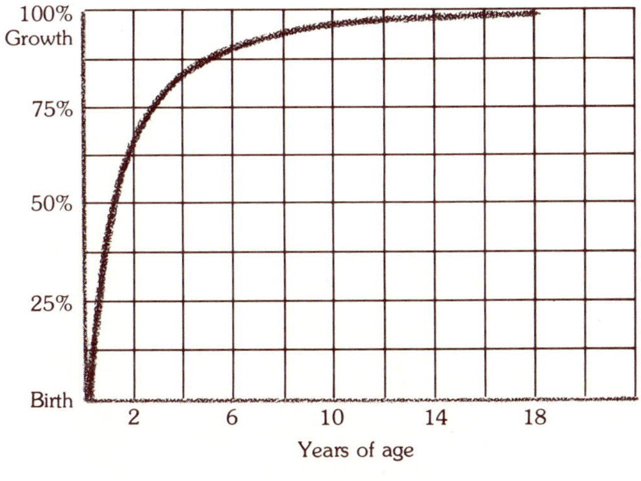

FIGURE 6.7 Curve of development and growth of the organs of the nervous system

during infancy, slowing slightly to puberty. At pubescence there is a spurt of growth in girls (shown by the solid line in Figure 6.9). The spurt of growth is usually seen in boys about a year later and is less pronounced (shown by the broken line in Figure 6.9). Both males and females then show a moderate gain followed by a slow year-by-year increase through late adolescence.

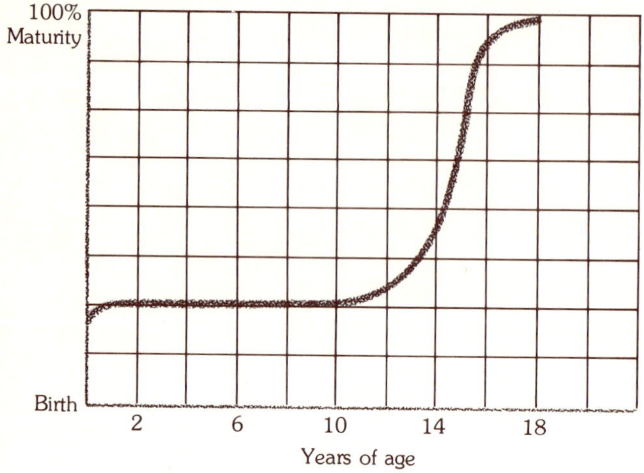

FIGURE 6.8 Growth curve of the development of primary sex characteristics

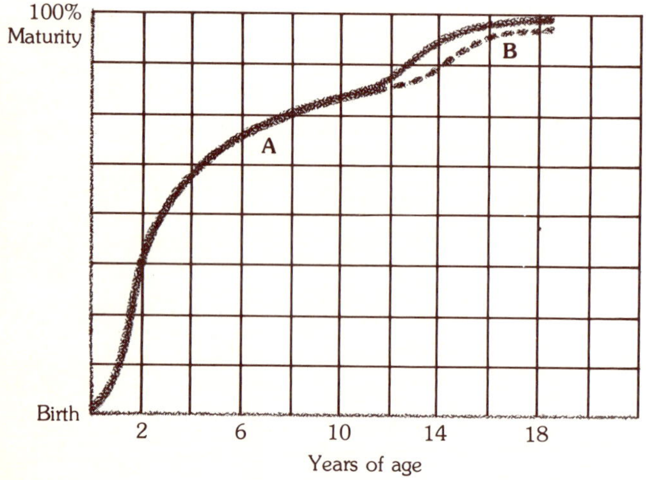

FIGURE 6.9 Somatic or body growth curve: (A) female growth curve, (B) male growth curve

Puberty

Puberty is the period during which the reproductive organs mature and reproduction becomes possible. As shown by the three growth curves, puberty is the beginning of maturity. The period of time needed for complete physical maturity to take place is termed adolescence. Preadolescent boys and girls have both estrogen and androgens. These hormones probably come from the adrenals instead of the testes and ovaries. Small but equal amounts of estrogen are found in the urine of both sexes until about the age of ten. At this time estrogen increases rapidly in girls, but remains constant in boys. The androgen levels remain the same in boys and girls until the middle teens, when they increase rapidly in the males. The relative changes in both of these hormones seem to produce the widening differences noted between boys and girls during adolescence.

The actual cause of prepubertal sexual dormancy is the lack of *hypothalamic releasing factors* in the brain. The onset of puberty, shown by these changes in estrogen and androgens, is produced by an unknown alteration in brain function that causes the secretion of releasing factors producing FSH and LH. The hormones then induce estrogen and testosterone production in the ovaries and testes. The increased levels of sexual hormones induce the changes associated with puberty: menstrual cycle, growth of secondary sex characteristics, penis enlargement, and initiation of sexual drive. In males, the seminiferous tubules of the testes begin to produce sperm, the penis enlarges and becomes sexually functional, and sexual drive is initiated. All of these changes are the direct results of testosterone levels. In both males and females the hypothalamus is the critical site of control.

The events of puberty and adolescence proceed in an orderly sequence, but the ages at which they occur vary according to sex and from individual to individual. Puberty occurs in females about two years earlier than in males, and the changes in body form are more noticeable in females (see Figure 6.10). Appearance of breast buds is usually the first indication that puberty is beginning. Pubic hair may appear slightly before, at the same time as, or slightly after the appearance of breast buds. Next comes a noticeable spurt of total body growth (Figure 6.9), which peaks and passes by age thirteen. Menarche, the first menstrual period, usually occurs after this total body growth spurt has passed (the average age of menarche is thirteen). The early menstrual cycles are commonly not accompanied by ovulation, so conception is often not possible until twelve to eighteen months after menarche. Secondary sex characteristics and the female body form begin with the breast buds and continue to respond to estrogen and progesterone levels throughout the lifetime of the individual.

In males, the signs of puberty are acceleration of growth of testes, scrotum, and penis. Pubic hair appears first; axillary and facial hair appears later. Growth of the penis begins at about thirteen years (eleven to fourteen and a half) and is complete by fifteen (thirteen and a half to seventeen). Because of the overlap in ranges of development, it is not unusual for some males to be completely sexually mature while others of the same age are still prepubescent. This difference can produce a wide range of social and psychological pressures in peer groups.

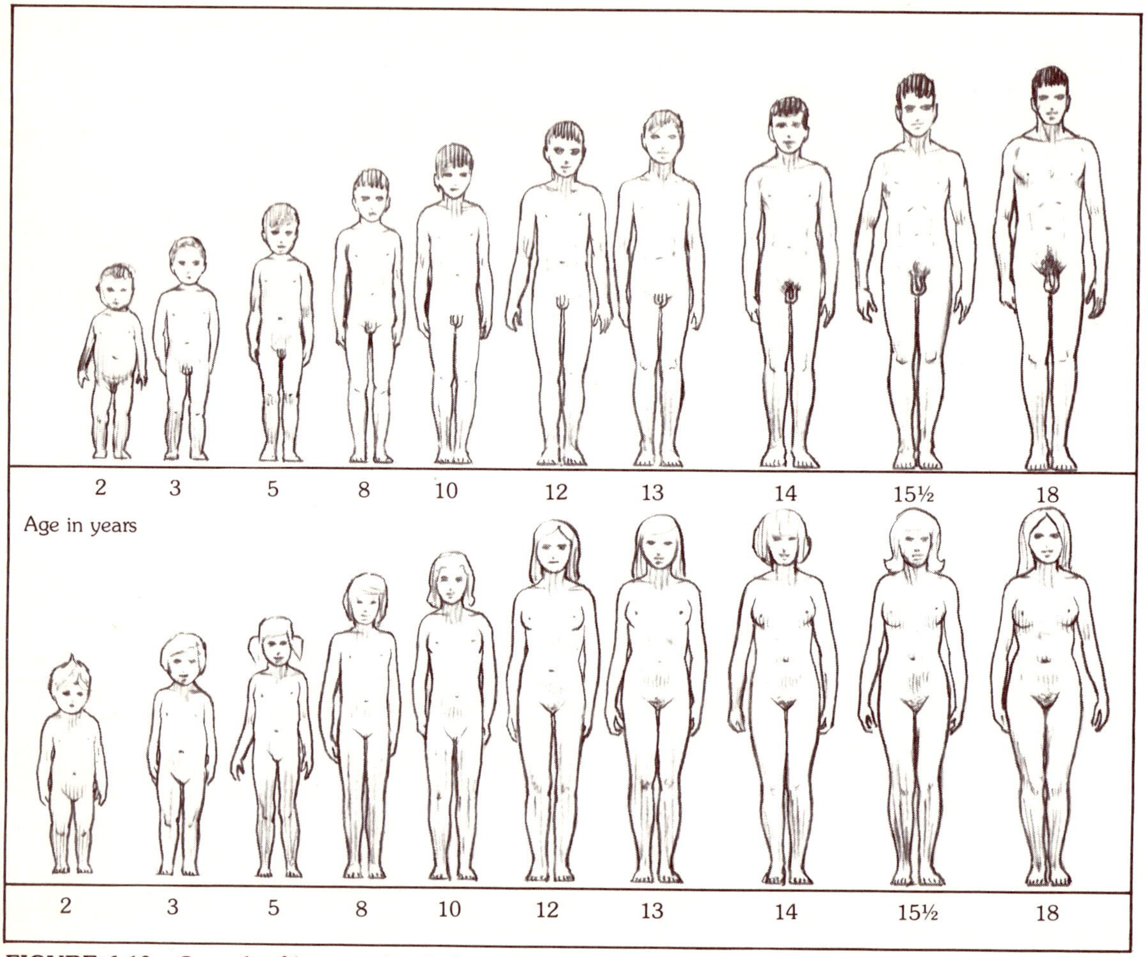

FIGURE 6.10 Growth of boys and girls from 2 to 18 years of age

Identity

Usually the first thing parents want to know when a child is born is its sex — "What is it?" "A girl!" "A boy!" The child has begun to assume an *identity*.

The obvious structural differences between males and females can only have biological origins; they cannot be culturally induced. Most of a man's height is usually in his legs and chest. His lungs usually have a greater capacity than a woman's, his heart is larger, and his chest and shoulders are broader. Much of a woman's height is in her abdomen, to accommodate her uterus and her larger abdominal organs. She has broader hips, and the muscles supporting the hips are the only ones that are larger than the corresponding muscles in a man. A woman has a subcutaneous layer of fat and a metabolism more sensitive to temperature changes. Her metabolic rate decreases more rapidly than a man's in response to a rise in environmental temperature, causing her to perspire less than a man.

There are also less obvious differences that are biologically induced. Diseases afflict and kill more men than women in any age group, and the life expectancy for men is six years below that for women (seventy-two years for women, sixty-six years for men in the United States).

As growth takes place and social influences are brought to bear, one is deemed a male or female by the way he or she behaves as well as looks. Are sex differences in behavior determined biologically or culturally? Men have successfully masqueraded as women and women as men for years. Often these masquerades have been carried out by individuals who were biologically male but felt that they were female, or who were biologically female but felt that they were male. The individualized sex image that one has of oneself as either male or female is termed *gender identity*.

Interactions between society's attitudes and an individual's own emotional reactions and physiological controls (hormones) determine one's sexual identity. Achievement of gender identity and the learning of the appropriate or socially acceptable ways of expressing that identity are purely socialization processes.

Sexual Identity

The presence of normally functioning testes in an embryo represses the development of the female genitalia and induces development of the male sex organs. The testes exert these effects by secreting androgens (the major inducer androgen is testosterone), which act upon the developing embryo. Evidence on the role of male and female hormones in behavior of humans and other animals is now accumulating.

A genetically female monkey (XX) whose mother had been given large doses of testosterone during the critical period of external genitalia development was born with a scrotum and a markedly enlarged clitoris, resembling a penis. This monkey, along with others treated in the same manner, also exhibited a high degree of masculine play behavior during growth and pronounced masculine sexual behavior as an adult.

As shown in Figure 6.11, the androgen hormones or the lack of them play a crucial role in determining one's sexual identity before and shortly after birth. After this initial surge, testosterone drops to a very low

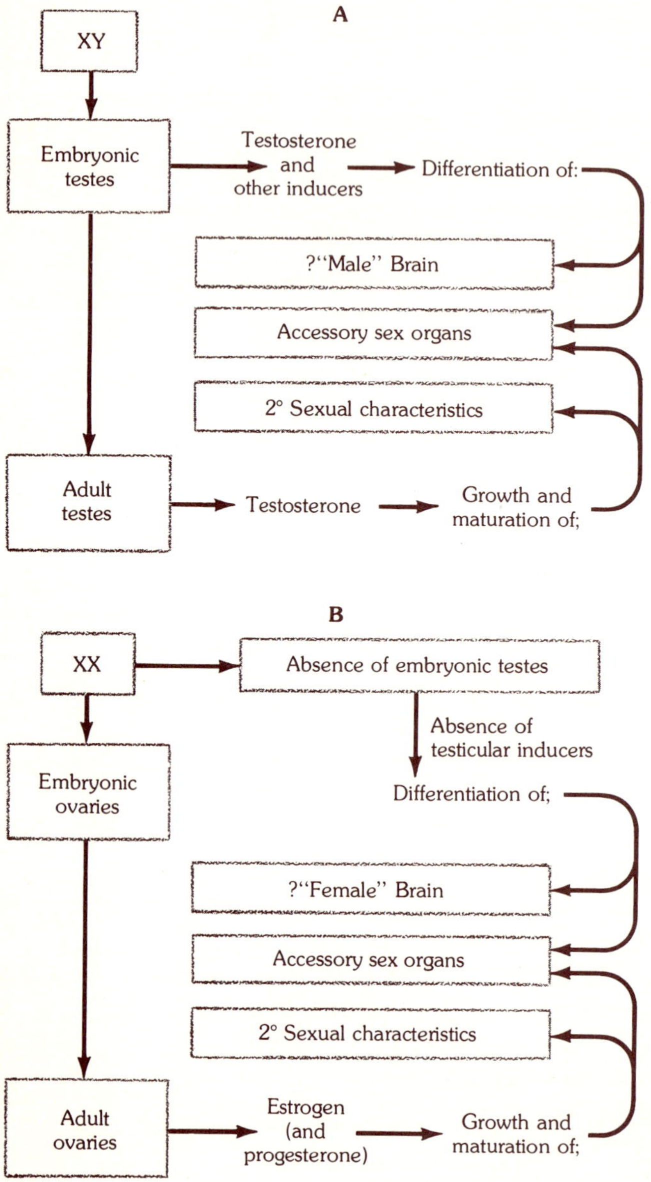

FIGURE 6.11 Hormonal influences on sex differentiation in humans: (A) male, (B) female

level until once again it increases in the male to stimulate the organs it previously helped to develop. In females estrogen takes little if any active part in the early development of female reproductive organs, which require only the absence of testosterone and other androgens. But at puberty, and through adolescence into adult life, estrogen is the major stimulating agent in female sexual growth.

Gender Identity

The most powerful factors determining gender identity (sexual differences in social, psychological, and behavioral identity) are social behavior and social experiences. These influences, however, play upon a range of sexual potentials previously established within an individual. The physical differences between males and females are obvious, but gender identity is less so. Learned behavior accounts for the great diversity of gender identities found among humans. Yet people hold strong beliefs about gender roles, even when their beliefs fail to have any scientific support.

As boys and girls grow and develop, there are some observed similarities and differences in social, psychological, and cultural responses. The vast majority of these are learned through the expected reactions of other children and adults. The similarities and differences between male and female roles begin at a very early age. By the time a child starts to verbalize (usually between eighteen and thirty-six months), gender identity has begun. Subtle attitudes expressed in the color and texture of clothing, the way an infant is handled by parents, and sexual references made to a child, such as "That's my big boy," or "What a cute little girl!" are the beginning of gender identity.

The first ten years of a child's life are usually dominated by the mother, and her attitude tends to be a strong factor in the distinct role differences between boys and girls. Children of both sexes are equally interested in social contact, and both learn by imitating people they observe around them.

Group pressures are very important in establishing gender differences later in life. Both sexes are susceptible to group pressures, but there are some differences in reactions. Girls are more likely to adapt their judgments and feelings to those of a group than boys. Boys are less bothered than girls when group values conflict with their personal judgments and feelings. They do not feel it necessary to change their values in order to enjoy membership in a group.

Both girls and boys have similar feelings of self-confidence and self-satisfaction in their early school years. But by the high school years, males in our culture tend to feel more confident of their ability to influence their own fate, as opposed to being the victims of chance. In the classic feminine role, girls and women are expected to be submissive, and submissiveness is not compatible with self-confidence. One of the positive aspects of the women's liberation movement is its effect in helping women to understand that they can and should have confidence in their ability to direct their own lives.

When youngsters begin to reach the age of social play, boys are more physically competitive than girls. Dominance appears to be more of an issue in boys' groups than in girls'. This need for dominance seems to be the basis of the aggressive behavior classically associated with masculinity. In all cultures in which aggressive behavior has been observed, males are more aggressive physically and verbally. Both sexes lose aggressiveness with age, but men in our culture generally remain more aggressive than women throughout life.

All human societies govern the sexual behavior of their members. The most common method of control is monogamous marriage. Every society defines husband-wife duties and responsibilities for child care. But sexual morality and behavior are so variable that it is impossible to consider any specific behavior as normal for all societies at all times. Behavior that is considered masculine in one society is considered feminine in another, and work that is considered appropriate for men in one society is performed only by women in another. The only constant is a division of labor according to sex.

Cultural patterns of masculinity and femininity and gender identity are based upon sexual identity. It is quite evident that childhood interactions are vital in developing the characteristics that tradition attributes to masculinity and femininity.

Current trends in our society are easing traditional conformity to male and female roles. Men are beginning to feel freer to be tender, and women are finding it easier to be more assertive. Barriers against demonstrations of warmth and affection between friends of the same sex are being removed. Rules of sexual conformity are easing, and problems of gender identity may be fewer in the future. We can look forward to better sexual adjustment and mutual concern and satisfaction when men can be manly and tender and women can be womanly and self-confident. We will all be happier when men and women can acknowledge need for each other without shame and without insisting that one partner must always be dominant while the other must always be submissive.

Sexual Intercourse

7

One of the constructive effects of the relaxing attitudes on sexual expression in this country has been that many people are increasingly unashamed to acknowledge that lovemaking is beautiful and highly pleasurable. They are discovering that this more open approach is making them more receptive to each other as individuals. There is a new openness in expressing sexual needs, and in communicating feelings about sex and love without embarrassment.

To understand sexuality we must learn to respond to the hopes, fears, hesitations, and joys of others. We must feel free to express our sexual needs and to communicate without apology our feelings about sex and love. We must learn to admit our need for help in developing sexual sensitivity. We must rise above the current obsession with sex as *performance.* So long as sex is used only to demonstrate one's prowess and so long as one is afraid of being found lacking in sexual achievment, there can be no genuine opening of the self to another, no truly mutual relationship.

Such an understanding of sexuality puts intercourse in a new context. The whole body is appreciated for its own worth, in contrast to the goal-oriented attitude that misleads so many in Western society. Some describe it as a "recovery of the natural sexuality of childhood," the pursuit of pleasure through the activity of any and all organs of the body.

Most important is the sensitivity of each partner to the needs of the other. Sexual relations can be viewed as a sharing of one's body with another in a mutual journey of discovery, including an exploration of the pleasures of sex.

Intercourse is thus viewed as one of a series of mutually enjoyable experiences rather than a target or a concession. Mature sexuality does not exclude the unique and supreme satisfaction of mutual orgasmic pleasure, yet it is not viewed as an isolated goal. "Sexuality should be a matter of joyous exploration. Kissing, fondling, caressing, and petting should be enjoyed for their own value as means of interpersonal union, rather than checked off on a list of foothills to be scaled as quickly as possible before conquering Mount Climax" (Hettlinger, 1975).

A lack of awareness of or a refusal to admit to both your own needs and those of your partner readily leads to the misuse of sexual intercourse. In fact, it may also lead to a detour around many of the mutually enjoyable nonorgasmic experiences.

Sexual enticement for nonsexual reasons may reflect questionable motives. If the misuse is flagrant, it may bring social disapproval and even legal intervention. More commonly it violates no laws and is not easy to detect. Unfortunately, sexual intercourse for the wrong reasons often leads to sexual difficulties of all kinds as well as maladjustments in human relationships.

A person may passionlessly engage in intercourse as a duty or obligation, perhaps out of a sense of promise or indebtedness. Sexual intercourse may be used in an attempt to capture and retain another's interest, thus revealing one's low self-esteem. A person may feel coerced into intercourse to repay or secure a favor, or to guarantee the continuity of favors, thus risking developing feelings of resentment.

Sexual intercourse may be demanded as proof of loyalty. While intercourse may express love, it is impossible for it to prove love. A man may use sexual intercourse to prove masculinity and power, making it a conquest of the victor over the vanquished. Or a person may use intercourse to attempt to prove maturity and sophistication. Neither the participation in nor the abstinence from sexual intercourse proves one's success in assuming adult responsibilities.

"The new sexuality seeks to transcend the traditionally antagonistic and defensive stances that reduce sex to role-playing or to goal-oriented maneuvering. Many of today's college men and women desire open, honest relationships in which each is treated as a person, not as a thing; as a Thou, not as an It" (Hettlinger, 1975).

Sexual Seduction

An intriguing part of the ritual of lovemaking is the art of seducing or allowing oneself to be seduced. There is the need to signal to the other person one's feelings of sexual urgency. Sexual seduction has both psychological and physical components.

Psychological Stimuli

Sexual seduction must begin by the setting of a mood. This may develop spontaneously; at other times it must be encouraged through intentional interaction between the partners. Mere closeness can be helpful in creating sexual responsiveness in one's partner—spending time together, touching each other. The response may arise from kind words, gestures, or expressions of love. It may come from the relaxation of having dinner together, observing each other's bodily movements, looking into the eyes, undressing your partner, watching him or her in the nude.

Physical Stimuli

Sexual arousal can result from any of a multitude of physical stimuli.

Earlobes Particularly for women, the skin areas of the earlobes, behind the ear, and on the back of the neck are often erogenous areas. In fact, for a few women, caressing of the earlobes can induce full climax.

Kissing Lip and tongue kissing is highly tantalizing and stimulates widespread arousal. Kisses belong anywhere on the body—mouth, neck, eyes, legs, breasts, genitals. They can be given with the lips, tongue, eyelashes, penis, or labia. Kissing may be transient or it may continue throughout intercourse. This is one reason some couples prefer face-to-face positions.

The mouth kiss may be intense and meaningful, but it does not need to be crushing. It helps if your teeth are brushed and your breath is pleasant. The problem of persistent mouth odors after eating certain foods can be avoided if both partners eat the same thing. Many prefer tongue kissing, imitating the entry and thrusting of the penis or imitating penile rhythm. Some explore the mouth parts, probing all corners of the mouth.

The breasts and nipples of many people of both sexes are quite sensitive to oral stimulation. Encircling the areola and particularly the nipple with the tip of the tongue, a gentle nibbling with the lips and tongue, or gentle sucking are pleasurable to many people.

Using the mouth to stimulate the genitals may produce the highest kind of arousal, often including orgasm. Cunnilingus (stimulation of a woman's labia and clitoris by a man's tongue) and fellatio (sucking and licking of a man's penis by a woman) can produce some of the most intensely pleasurable moments of all love play.

Breasts While breasts aren't the primary target in lovemaking, they may receive some of the first caresses. Although they vary considerably in both size and responsiveness, there is no relationship between size and sensitivity.

The tip of the tongue, the glans of the penis, and the balls of the fingertips are ideal tools to caress the nipples gently. Massaging or soft kneading with the hands, soft biting or sucking are good starters. A woman can use some of these same techniques with a man's breasts. Breast play at the same time as clitoral or vaginal stimulation causes intense arousal in many women. Some women experience orgasm from receiving breast stimulation alone, particularly with penis-breast massage. This can all be prelude to intercourse or may result in mutual orgasms without intercourse.

Buttocks Although the buttocks are not the erogenous zone the breasts are, lovers find satisfaction in having their buttocks held, caressed, or tickled. Some men are able to have intensified ejaculation if their partners hold their buttocks firmly while they thrust vigorously. Holding the woman's buttocks firmly not only holds her pelvis closer for firmer penetration, but may tend to intensity the man's own arousal. The buttocks can also be a visual stimulus for both partners. Viewing a partner's buttocks through a mirror during intercourse can be highly pleasurable. An attraction of the rear-entry position for some men is being able to view the woman's buttocks and feel them warmly nestled in his lap.

Genitals Many women find real enjoyment in stimulating the penis—holding it, varying the amount of pressure and movement, letting the tempo of their caresses coincide with the man's feelings. They may stimulate it in various ways. Most effective is holding it just below the groove behind the glans with the skin pulled far back. It may work well to use both hands—one to fondle the scrotum and hold the base of the penis, the other to make a ring to stroke the penis. By varying the caressing a woman can hasten or retard the arousal, and when desired can stimulate ejaculation.

The man receives the greatest tactile sensation in the outermost inch of the penis. The attention given a man's penis is most important in determining the type of response he makes, for men tend to be penis-centered. Their view of themselves often depends upon their penile performance in sexual activity. (Since their own feelings are concentrated in their genitals, men instinctively tend to start their sex play with fondling of the woman's genitals, even though she may prefer to begin with nongenital play.)

Women should learn to play with the penis—exposing it, caressing it to erection, handling it, making it pulsate and ejaculate. This boosts the man's ego and helps him to feel that he is a good sex partner.

For the man's caressing of the vulva, an effective method is to place the flat of the hand on the vulva with the middle finger between the lips, with its tip moving in and out of the vagina, while the ball of the hand presses hard just above the pubis. Steady, rhythmic movement is important. Stretching the lips, then working the clitoris and its hood with the forefinger or little finger, with the thumb thrust into the vagina, works wells. Some women respond to caresses with both hands one holding the lips open while the other works gently with all fingers. As the clitoris becomes aroused and retacts under the hood, it becomes highly sensitive and is best massaged indirectly from the side rather than from directly atop it. Skillful stimulation can often arouse a woman to such an extent that she demands intromission.

Genital Sizes Like all other physical dimensions, vaginal and penile sizes vary. Yet rarely is a woman's vagina too small or too large for exciting sex. In Masters and Johnson's clinical experience, women who have exceptionally small vaginas are able to accommodate a large penis when they are sufficiently stimulated by their partners (Figure 7.1). The only times they reported experiencing difficulty was when intromission occurred before high levels of excitement had been reached. Thus small women making love to large men should have no fears of pain or discomfort because of dissimilarities in the sizes of their genital organs, nor should men fear that the penis will be hurt by a narrow passage. If ever the woman were to experience temporary vaginal discomfort from the penis, the man has only to be careful not to thrust too deeply until he knows the thrusting does not hurt her.

On the other hand, some women naturally have large vaginas; and vaginal dimensions tend to enlarge as the result of childbirth. If there seems to be a loose fit between the penis and the vagina, the couple can compensate for this. One method is for the woman to learn control of the pelvic muscles, as described later in this chapter. Another is for the couple to choose a coital position that seems to give each of them the greatest intensity of feelings. It's a rare couple indeed for whom pleasurable adjustments are not possible.

While women may be concerned over the sizes of their vaginas and breasts, men are often concerned over the size of the penis. The average

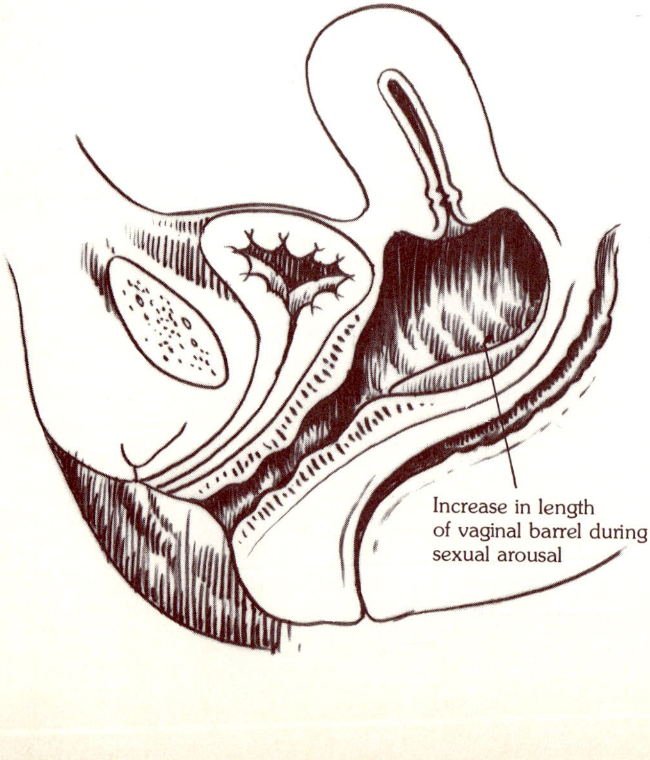

FIGURE 7.1 **During sexual arousal increase in length of the vaginal barrel is sufficient to accommodate an erect penis of any length.**

erect penis is about six inches long and about three and one-half inches around, but don't be dismayed if your penis is smaller or larger. Various sizes work equally well. Masters and Johnson have found that the smaller relaxed penis increases more in erection than the larger relaxed penis. So ignore the myth that the larger the relaxed penis, the larger it will be when erect.

Since the penis is not a muscular organ, there is no way to increase its length through exercise. Anxiety over its length and shape is totally unwarranted. A man should prize it and view it as a pleasurable organ. A woman should speak only favorably of a man's penis, particularly since erection is so largely a psychological matter.

Oral-Genital Arousal A man may approach a woman from any of various positions—a reverse position atop her, a reverse position on their sides, between her open legs, and so on. As the man's tongue is applied to the labia and clitoris in cunnilingus, he may detect the slightly salty taste of the woman's genitalia and a distinctive odor that often reinforces his arousal. He may use his tongue in a flipping action on the clitoris and labial walls. By using a combination of tongue-lip-tooth massage of the clitoral area he may produce a response many women may find particularly arousing. It's possible to bring a woman to orgasm repeatedly this way.

A woman may take the man's penis into her mouth in the act of fellatio. As she takes the glans of the penis and as much of the shaft of the penis as she prefers, her lips can feel the throbbing of the penis, and she can enjoy its distinctive smell and taste. She may or may not prefer to bring him to ejaculation orally. As with other forms of sexual arousal, response to oral-genital arousal is an individual matter. A couple may wish to share cunnilingus and fellatio simultaneously.

A couple should have no fears of experimenting with oral-genital stimulation. It is neither dirty, abnormal, nor perverted, and the great majority of couples engage in it.

Pubic Hair While some people prefer the hardness of the bare pubis, many find pubic hair decorative. It does have some useful purposes. Brushing or caressing a woman's pubic hair, twirling or kissing it, pulling it and playing with it so that it moves the whole pubis can bring her to orgasm. Couples should decide together whether they prefer to shave it off, trim it, or leave it alone. Like all other human hair, it will grow back after being shaved.

If a man uses a condom, hairs on the shaft or around the base of the penis may tend to get caught up and rolled into the condom. He may need to shave off those hairs in the affected area. It is best to shave the hairs rather than pulling them out, unless the man receives pleasure from pain.

Personal Cleanliness Few things enhance the mood for lovemaking more than a soap-and-water bath or shower beforehand. It far exceeds the commercial perfumes, deodorants, and after-shave lotions, which smell a bit too unreal and taste worse. The replacement of odors from smoking, underarm perspiration, oily hair, and cloistered genitals with the aroma of skin freshly bathed is a stimulus. Some people are more sensitive to skin contaminants than others.

The aroma of cleanly bathed skin is soon replaced in lovemaking by the odor of fresh genital secretions as the woman becomes aroused. Later, different scents become apparent when intercourse has begun, and still others after intercourse is complete. While women may have the sharper sense of smell, men are more aroused by the sequence of new odors in lovemaking.

Tenderness

It is most important that each partner have a deep awareness of how the other person feels. Each must want to know ways to heighten sexual response in the partner and then patiently practice. Sex partners are not mind readers. Partners should let each other know, both verbally and nonverbally, when they are being satisfied and when they are not.

Tenderness starts with an inner desire on the part of each to please the other. Masculinity should not be equated with brutishness. Not all individuals are naturally adept at tenderness. Many men, and some women, need to learn how to stimulate their partners progressively. Many women respond to very light brushing of the skin and hair. Although a man may feel like grabbing his partner's breasts or genitals with his whole hand, such an approach may bring less arousal than a light touch. The greater the arousal, the greater stimulation the body can tolerate until strong, forceful actions are desired. What may be painful to a woman early in arousal may be highly pleasurable once she is aroused or has had orgasm. Although a man's strength may itself stimulate a woman, what she will prize in him is an ability to be tender.

Momentary dissatisfaction is sure to occur. Longer periods of dissatisfaction should be reconciled. But first, know your partner's emotional state before expressing dissatisfaction. Everyone has periods of special stress, or moments when self-confidence is lowered. Complaints are not well received at such times. Do not mix nonsexual conflicts with sexual interaction. Clear up nonsexual conflicts, and temporarily forget them in order to concentrate on the passion of sex.

Coital Positions

The positions that can be used for sexual intercourse are many and varied. No one position is more normal or acceptable than any other. Any positions that give pleasure and satisfaction to both partners should be used. Since the only way of finding preferred positions is through experimentation, it is in the interest of a couple to try many different positions.

Experimentation provides many rewards to a couple. Variety in coital positions makes intercourse special and unpredictable. Certain positions are more relaxing, or provide more freedom of movement, or more opportunity for caressing the partner's breasts, face, buttocks, or genitals. One's likes and dislikes will change from time to time, depending upon a variety of factors, such as weight, pregnancy, health, fatigue, and age. The chosen position may also depend upon where lovemaking is taking place, how much time is available for lovemaking, the time of day, and the amount of privacy available. The stature of both partners, their weight, and the size of their genitals will also enter into the choice of position.

Some married couples may do more experimenting during their first years of marriage than later. Others find great excitement in increased experimenting later in life, after the children are older, living conditions are more comfortable, and each is more relaxed with the other and with their goals in life. If lovemaking is unhurried, the couple may enjoy various positions at different times during a given coital session. The man may make initial penetration atop the woman, they may then roll over on their sides or intertwine their legs in various ways, and they may then resume the original position with the man above for the intensity of orgasm. Or they may fall asleep on their sides, face to face or in a rear-entry position. Variation is the spice and freshness of open lovemaking.

The only "should nots" are those positions that violate the coital enjoyment of either partner. Any play or position that violates the comfort or pleasure of either partner should be discontinued. Since the sex play and positions a couple chooses to follow are the concern of no one but themselves, there is not the slightest reason for either to feel guilty, ashamed, or hesitant about any type of play or intercourse that provides pleasure to both of them. There are too many methods of lovemaking that can easily be used for any person to become insistent on a given technique. The positions that provide the greatest satisfaction should be readily communicated to one's partner. Each partner should be guided by the comfort and sexual satisfaction of the other.

Of all the many variations in positions, the four most common positions are the frontal position, man above; the frontal position, woman above; the side position, face to face; and the side position, rear-entry.

Frontal Position, Man Above

The traditional position in America and Europe, and the one apparently most preferred, is the man atop with the woman on her back (Figure 7.2). Because it is so widely accepted in this country, some even consider it to be the "normal" position. Many couples report they never have intercourse in any other position.

This position has various advantages. Entry of the penis into the vagina is easily achieved with the woman on her back, legs spread apart. If guidance of the penis into the vagina is necessary, either the man or the woman can give this assistance. It is easy for the man to apply pressure on the front part of the vagina, and thus add pleasure by squeezing the clitoris against the pubic bone. The woman can be relaxed, while the man takes the initiative. If the weight of the man is too much for the woman, he can support himself on his elbows and knees. The woman is free to change her position, spreading her legs out flat, bending her knees, wrapping her legs around his buttocks or back, spreading her legs and throwing them in the air, putting her legs over his shoulders, or wrapping their legs around each other's. The man-above position facilitates caressing and kissing of the breasts and face of each partner and, if there are lights, watching each other's facial expressions. Masters and Johnson point out that this position is particularly good for impregnation. With the entrance of the vagina tilted upward, there is improved containment of the sperm high in the vagina following ejaculation. After orgasm it is easier for the man to maintain prolonged intromission if he is in this position.

On the other hand, there are several disadvantages to the man-above position. The woman may find penile penetration too deep for comfort, or the man's weight too much for her if he is heavy or does not support himself, or she may find her movements too restricted. Some men find this position too stimulating if they are troubled with premature ejaculation. It may also not be the best position for intercourse during later stages of pregnancy.

FIGURE 7.2 Frontal position, man above

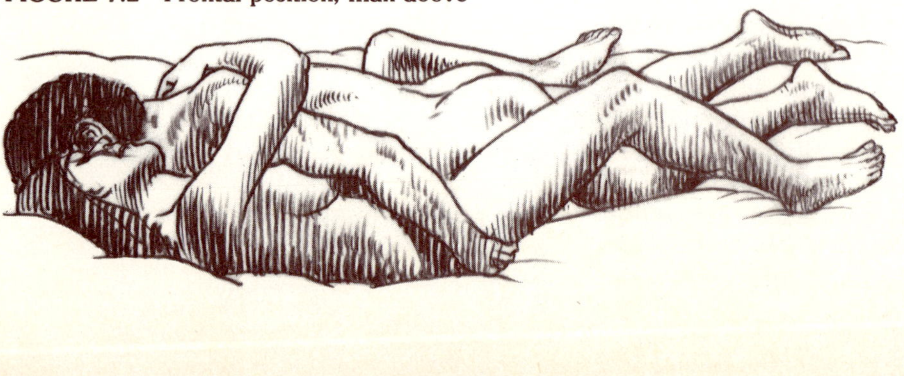

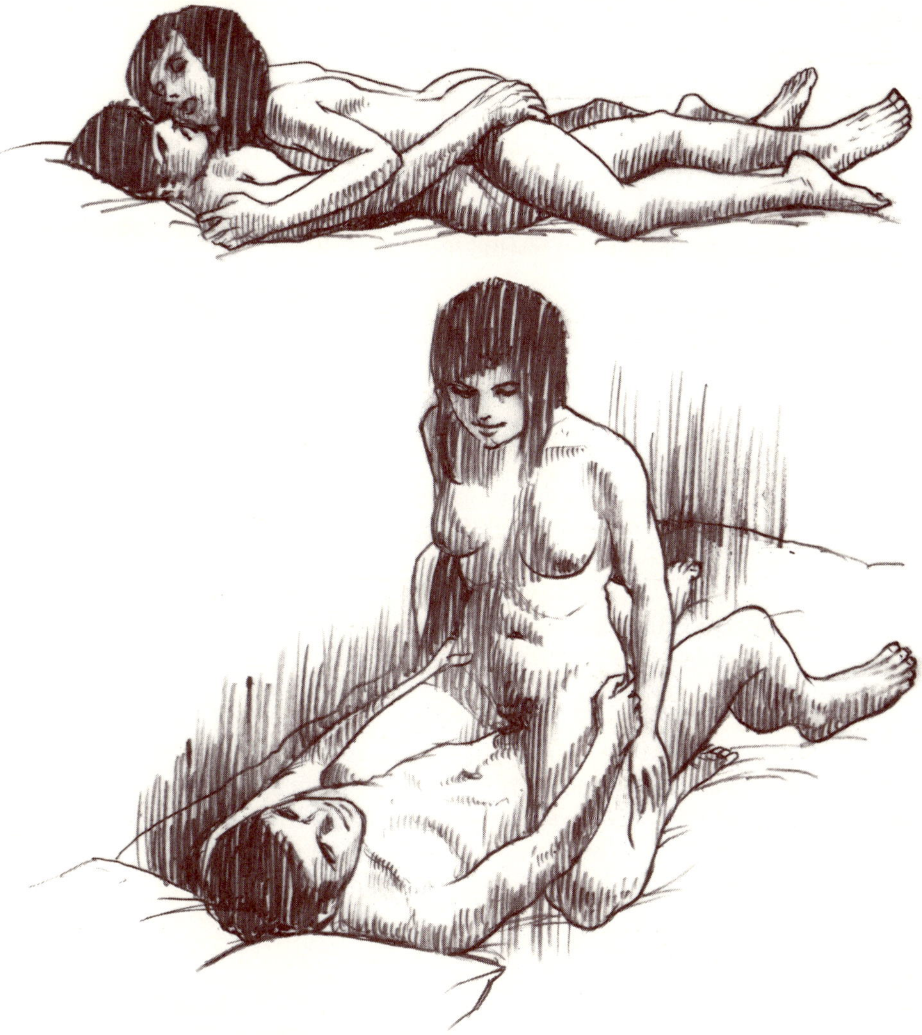

FIGURE 7.3 Frontal positions, woman above

Frontal Positions, Woman Above

A pleasing reversal of the first position is the woman atop with the man on his back (Figure 7.3). The main advantage of this position is that the woman is not nearly so passive, but can more aggressively regulate activities. She can control the tempo of the thrustings, the depth of penetration, and the degree of pressure against the clitoris.

While the man lies flat on his back, the woman can straddle him in a sitting position with her knees bent. If necessary, she can lower her body over the penis for intromission. His hands are free to play with her breasts and face, and to embrace her. She can lean forward for breast and mouth kisses. As she bends forward or backward she can adjust for clitoral pressure as she pleases. She can move her hips in various directions. He may raise his knees for her to lean back on, or he may rest on his elbows. She may wish to lie flat on him with her legs outstretched, thus giving more body contact.

In this position, the woman does not need to contend with the man's weight; it may be a good position if she is decidedly smaller than he. Since the man is in a passive position, it may be less stimulating for him, allowing more delayed ejaculation; thus it may be useful for men bothered with premature ejaculation. It is an ideal position for talking with each other and watching each other's face while orgasm is delayed. Since the man is in a more passive position, the woman may achieve orgasm once or repeatedly before he ejaculates. Since this position works best with a stiff erection, some couples prefer it in the morning when the man may have harder erections.

A disadvantage of this position is that it is easier for the penis to slip from the vagina. Another is that following ejaculation, the semen more easily seeps out of the vagina, thus reducing its value as a position for impregnation.

Some women do not feel comfortable in the "aggressor" role, and some men feel threatened when they assume a more passive position. There is no good reason for either of them to feel this way. There are few things more erotically stimulating to a man or more satisfying to an aroused woman than the free movement that this position makes possible to her.

As with other positions, the couple can easily roll over into another position without withdrawing the penis. Or they may easily move into this position from a man-atop or a side-by-side position.

Face to Face, Side Positions

When the partners are lying on their sides facing each other, intercourse can be very restful and undemanding for both. The beauty of this position is that neither partner needs to be either passive or aggressive—both share the control of movements. They may be fully stretched out, or one partner may be largely on his or her back with the other partner resting partly on the other, or the woman may have her upper leg flexed over the hip or leg of the man (Figure 7.4). The couple may gain intromission and perhaps even experience orgasm in another position and then fall asleep in this position. Or they may achieve intromission in this

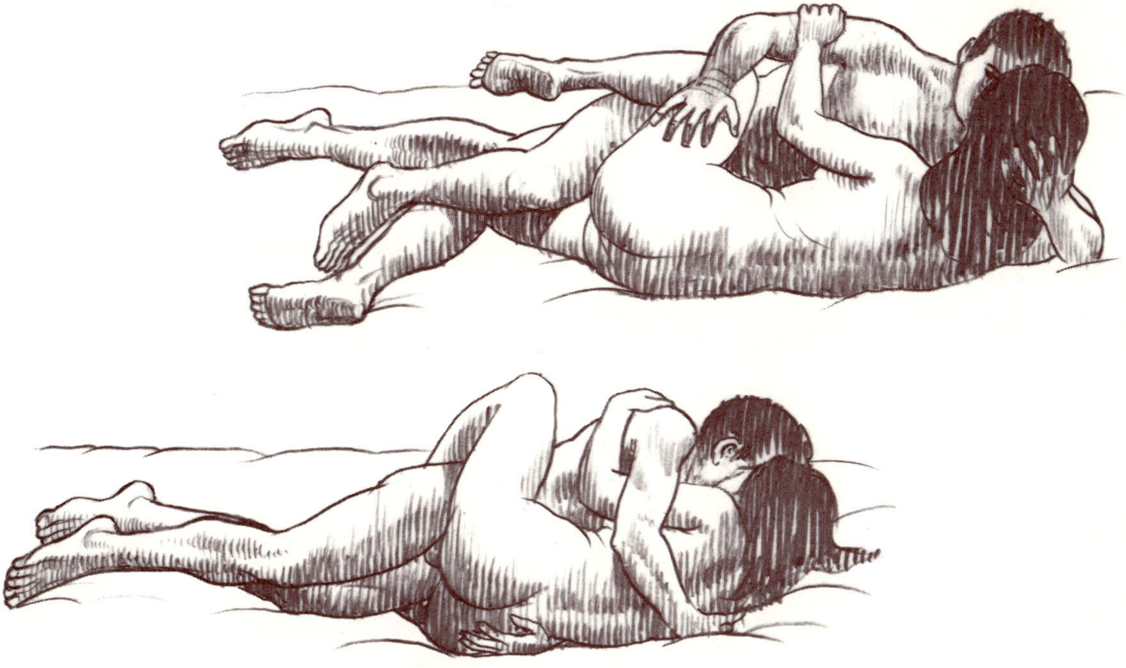

FIGURE 7.4 Face to face, side positions

position and, as they become deeply aroused, roll into another position in which violent thrusting is more easily accomplished, with one or the other above. An advantage of this position is the great amount of maneuverability of the arms, hands, and legs, giving many variations to the basic position.

Other advantages to this position are that it allows for prolonged coital embracing until well after ejaculation, without one partner needing to bear the weight of the other or one having to support his own weight. With the deep relaxation that follows orgasm, it is common for a couple to maintain coital embrace interlocked in each other's arms, and shortly to fall asleep. It is a good position for a couple that wants to extend coital rhythm for an extended time without the man's ejaculating. The man can more easily regulate his pelvic thrusts and delay ejaculation by lying still. There are times when a couple wants a long savoring of the delight of coital contact or wishes prolonged conversation at the same time. This position is ideal for later pregnancy, since there is no weight on the woman's abdomen. At the same time, couples may find the pelvic movements are not so vigorous in this position, penile penetration is not so deep, and there is less stimulation in the vulval areas.

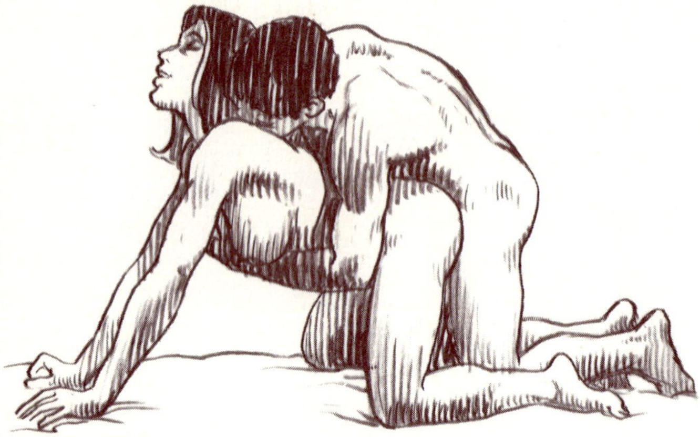

FIGURE 7.5 Rear-entry position

Rear-Entry Position

Another side position is the rear-entry. It works well with the couple standing, lying, kneeling, or sitting, or with the woman astride the man (Figure 7.5). While they are less able to see each other's face, the penetration is extra-deep and the physical intensity may be more intense than usual. The man may be excited by the sight or feel of the woman's buttocks, and at least one of his hands is free to cup a breast or massage the clitoris. If they are standing, the woman may need something to lean on—a bed, chair, desk, or table. Or they may be kneeling at the side of the bed or beside a chair. The reason penetration feels deeper in this position is that as the woman brings her legs forward, the vagina is shortened, carrying the penis into the deeper recesses. If penetration is too deep and the woman tells him it is painful, the man can easily withdraw to some degree. In some rear-entry positions, such as standing or kneeling, the movements can become quite vigorous. When they lie on their sides in bed, this position is very restful for both, particularly if they are tired, yet desire coital embrace. After orgasm it is considered by some to be the best position in which to fall asleep. Because it in no way interfers with the abdominal enlargement of late pregnancy, it is ideal at this time.

The main disadvantage to this position is that it may appear less personal. Some women feel it is "animal-like" or object to being unable to see the man's face. Some dislike it because it appears to resemble anal intercourse, which of course is something else altogether. For a woman whose vagina is unusually short, the deep penile entry may be too uncomfortable.

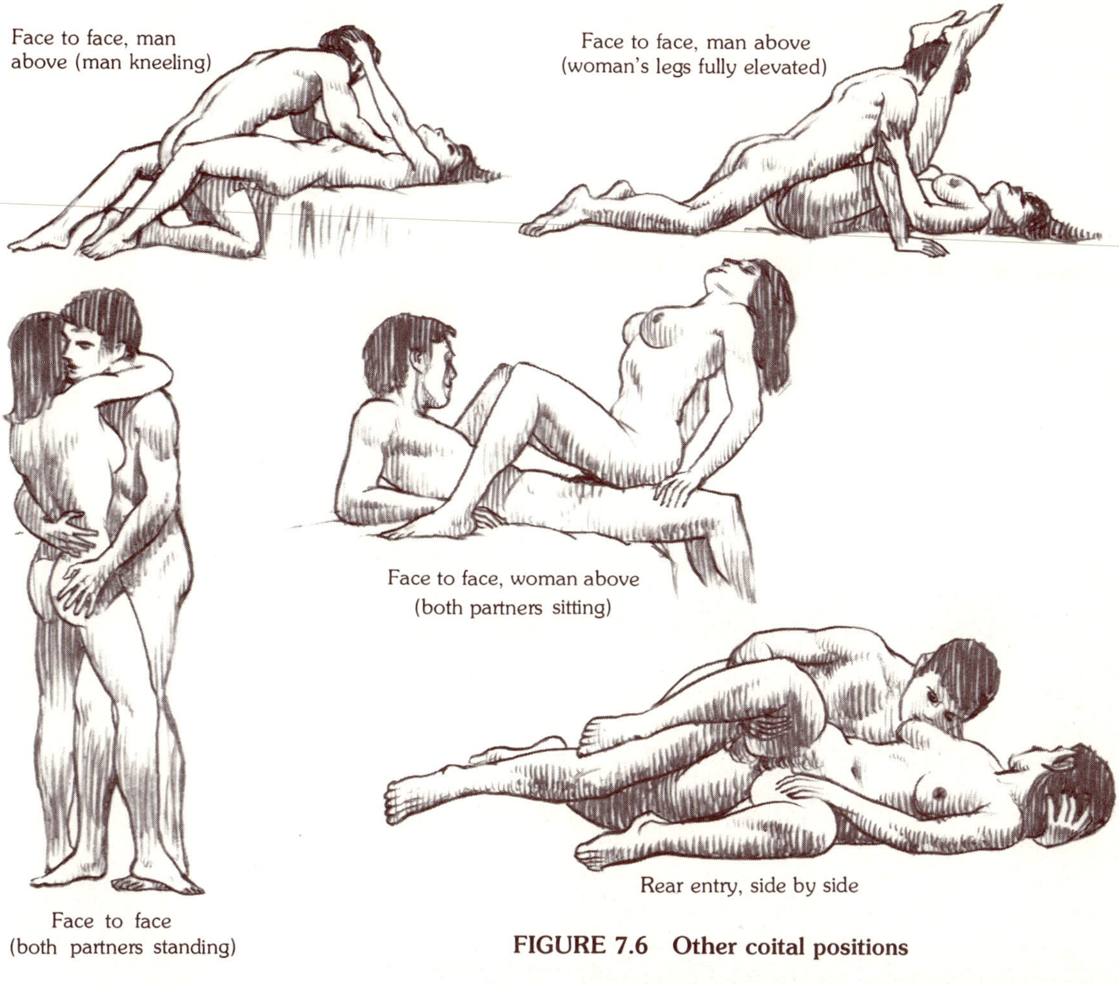

FIGURE 7.6 Other coital positions

Other Positions

If the height of the partners is similar, or if there is something a shorter partner can stand on, intercourse while the partners are standing facing each other can be highly sensual. It may be undertaken with the woman against a solid object such as a wall, or it can be done free-standing with legs apart and arms clasped around each other's buttocks (Figure 7.6). In this position it is exciting for both to watch the penis thrusting into the vagina. While standing, the woman may be lifted up so she can clasp her legs around the man's hips and her arms around his neck, letting her slide into intromission.

For prolonged intercourse some couples prize the X or scissors position. Starting with the woman sitting facing astride the man, the woman lies right back until each partner's head and trunk are between the other's wide-open legs, and they clasp hands. Slow, rhythmic wriggling movements can keep the man erect and the woman close to orgasm for prolonged periods. By either one sitting up, they can switch to other positions without withdrawing the penis.

Positions: Summary

There are other basic positions and more variations on each of these. All are acceptable. The emotionally secure person is capable of experimentation in coital positions. A couple should not worry about the "how" of intercourse while engaging in it. It must be free and spontaneous. Yet is does not need to be a gymnastic feat or an endurance contest. Nor is a person in any way committed to what other couples enjoy or what any book recommends. There is no single ideal position. Those techniques that bring the greatest enjoyment should be freely practiced and enjoyed. Any technique in love play, intercourse, or postcoital caressing that makes either partner feel tense or anxious should be stopped at that point. To maximize the enjoyment of intercourse both partners must recognize their right to sexual pleasure.

Anal Intercourse

A type of intercourse about which quite a bit is said but which may not be so rewarding as has been implied is anal intercourse. It is also known as *sodomy,* and may be referred to as *pederasty* when it is engaged in with boys. If a couple is to attempt it, the glans of the penis must be carefully lubricated with an oil or petroleum jelly, since the anus lacks the natural lubrication of the aroused vagina. Entry must be made slowly, preferably with the woman in a kneeling position. It is best never to enter more than the tip of the penis. The problem is that prolonged practice may produce a dilated, weakened anal sphincter, as well as fissures inside the anus that may easily become infected. In some cases such continued anal trauma has apparently resulted in the formation of neoplasms. The penis should be washed before vaginal intercourse, because of the chance of spreading infective bacteria from the anus into the vagina.

Frequency of Intercourse

The only rule on frequency of intercourse is to have sex as often as both of you enjoy it. Forget all of the written guides that recommend once every other night, or three times a week, or whatever. Although two or three times a week is common, the frequency you choose for intercourse is as personal as the frequency with which you have your hair cut. It's impossible to have too much sex. Some couples may prefer it daily, or several times daily, which is thoroughly normal and healthy as long as both agree and the frequency creates no anxiety. Some prefer a definite schedule, like every other night. Other couples are quite irregular in their lovemaking—perhaps once or twice a day for several days, then not at all for several days. Some couples tend to have more sex when they are in their forties than they did when they were in their twenties. Generally, however, frequency will taper off with age, although you do not need to make this a self-fulfilling prophecy. So your frequency *is* different from that of your best friend. This says *nothing* about your happiness or fulfillment. People have different needs here, just as they do in their eating and sleeping habits. One is no better than another. Fatigue or preoccupation with personal concerns may reduce your interest in sex for a while. The beauty of really caring is that at such times the partners can refrain from enforcing a time schedule on each other.

Sexual activity costs a person relatively little in energy. One study determined that the total energy expenditure for preorgasmic, orgasmic, and postorgasmic periods was around fifty to seventy-five calories, similar to the energy demands of a brisk walk on a level street, or climbing one or two flights of stairs. A dieting book suggests that one way to become and stay slim is to have vigorous sexual intercourse. The author, Abraham Friedman, says that if a person were to have intercourse once each day for a year, he or she would lose about twenty-one pounds (if everything else, of course, remains constant). To stay slim, he suggests, "reach for a mate instead of a plate."

Variety in Lovemaking

As with the new and unexpected dish at mealtime, variety adds excitement to lovemaking. There can be variety in the time and place of lovemaking as well as in the kind of sex plan and coital positions.

Much of the time a couple will make love at times when they would be in bed in any case—in the evening or in the morning. But frequently longer sessions are enjoyable. Weekends and holidays may give you more time and allow you to be more relaxed. At other times you may feel more urgency—in the middle of the night, when your mate comes home after several hours away, before the dishes are done, on the living-room floor, in the woods on a moonlit night, in the middle of the morning, after lunch, or while showering together. If there are no other immediate demands on your time—no appointment to keep, no one waiting for you—

you should feel free to respond when you feel yourself becoming aroused and when privacy is assured.

There are many sex manuals, some of which give a variety of possibilities as to position, time, place, and nature of sex play. Some suggest sterile routines or rigid patterns. Look upon all of them only as possibilities to consider. Some kinds of love play won't interest you, some locations may not put you at ease, some positions will seem too acrobatic. You choose. There is no right and no wrong way to make love. It is wrong *only* if it is not satisfying to both partners. Nothing is normal or abnormal if both of you enjoy it. And nothing is right if one of you dislikes it. Don't hesitate to experiment with new situations. Occasionally try something new. Some of your experiments you may wish never to repeat. But some, you will find, add spice and freshness to those methods you already both enjoy.

First Intercourse

Eventually nearly all of us find ourselves irreversibly propelled toward sexual intercourse. First intercourse usually involves a mixture of exciting expectations and fearful apprehensions. While there may be some difference of opinion over the timing of first intercourse, there can be no question that it should be as positive and apprehension-free as possible. Some basic information on what to expect and ways to plan for it should help make it a positive experience.

An area of some concern to first intercourse has been the presence of the hymen. This functionless rim of membrane extends around the vagina near its entrance, very much like the webbing between the thumb and the index finger, except that the hymen is more or less circular. Its development varies widely. In adult virgins its thickness may vary from fragile to relatively firm, and the size of its opening ranges from very small to large enough to admit one or two fingertips. Occasionally it may be cribriform (Figure 7.7) or imperforate (closed entirely). An imperforate hymen may not be noticed until menstruation seems late in beginning. A physician can nick the hymen, opening it for both menstruation and intercourse.

Contrary to male myths, many girls do not bleed to any extent on first intercourse. The hymens of many girls are stretched beforehand by the use of tampons, exertion during physical exercise, accident, or insertion of fingers or objects into the vagina during masturbation or sex play. Usually first intercourse pushes it aside, tearing it in several places. Some hymens are flexible and are pushed aside during intercourse without tearing. If the hymen is imperforate, cribriform, or quite firm, it is best to

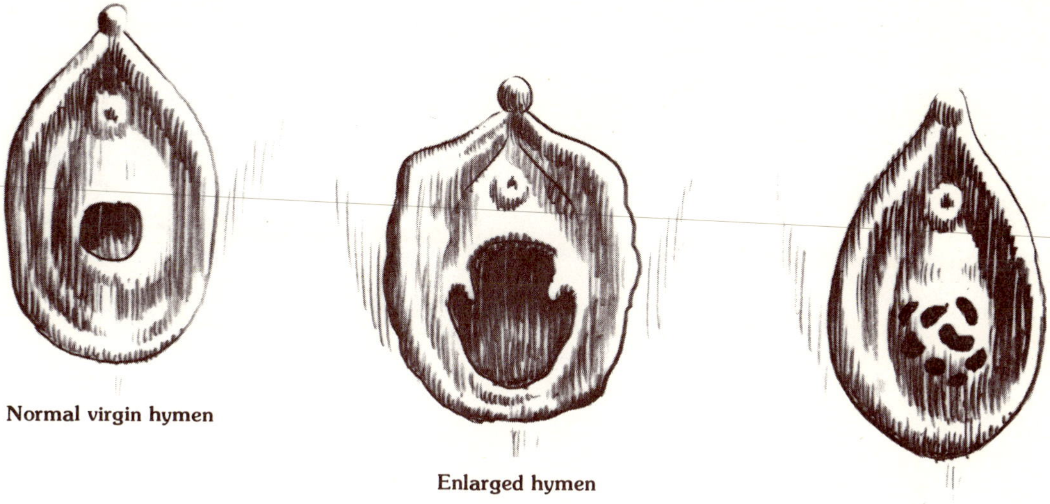

FIGURE 7.7 The hymen

have it cut surgically, to eliminate pain on first intercourse. A young woman would be wise to check the condition of her own hymen beforehand. If her vaginal opening cannot accommodate two fingers, it would be a good idea to have it cut by a physician.

Another possible difficulty in first intercourse is *vaginismus*, a spastic contraction of the vaginal outlet (Figure 7.8), which usually stems from fear—of pain, of pregnancy, of intercourse itself. As long as fear remains, the spasms will occur when intercourse is attempted, in spite of the woman's best intentions. Forcing intercourse in such a case can cause great pain to both partners. This difficulty, however, is much less common than the male problem of premature ejaculation. The first time a man attempts intercourse he may well reach orgasm before he intends to, perhaps as soon as his penis touches the woman's genitals. He will then lose his erection, but it can usually be regained in a few minutes with stimulation of the penis.

Attempts at entry should be delayed until the vagina is well lubricated, which it will be as soon as the woman is sufficiently aroused. When she is highly aroused she is anxious for entry and may communicate this to her partner verbally or by directing the penis toward the vagina. As the man makes initial attempts at entry, he must proceed slowly. If the hymen is resistant, he may apply gentle pressure as long as she does not indicate pain. If he encounters dryness in the vagina, he should make

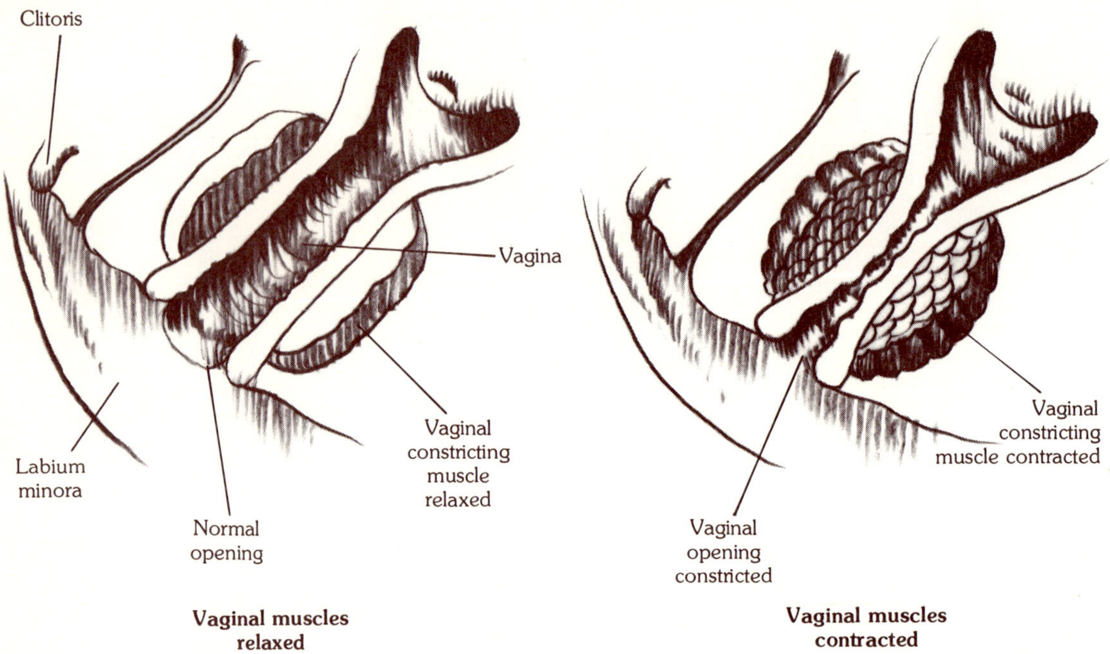

FIGURE 7.8 Vaginismus

short thrusts until it is sufficiently lubricated. The penis slides very easily into a well-prepared vagina. If undue resistance is encountered, he should penetrate no farther than his partner finds comfortable. It is not necessary to achieve full penetration at first intercourse. He may make deeper penetration another time, and after several attempts he should be able to make full entry. His patience will be grandly rewarded. A woman is slow to forget gentleness at first intercourse, especially if she has any expectations of pain or discomfort.

The woman may not attain orgasm the first time. The man may have orgasm and not be able to achieve erection again after a first or second ejaculation. The first experience is seldom totally satisfactory, particularly if it is the first intercourse for both partners. With mutual loving consideration and patience, minor irregularities in their techniques should soon be corrected.

Be prepared for unexpected reactions on the part of either partner. Some women and men groan, gasp, or cry, particularly during orgasm. Don't be disconcerted. Your partner isn't crying with disappointment or gasping in pain or groaning out of agony. Strange as it may seem, the expressions of ecstasy are commonly the same as the expressions of torment.

The beauty of first intercourse is not destroyed by planning for it and making proper arrangements. If you and your partner are unmarried and undecided about intercourse, openly talk it over. Look at the implications and responsibilities of yourselves and each other. Do it only if both partners feel comfortable about it. Refuse it if you feel your partner is engaging in threat, bribe, or coercion. The agreement must be mutual and voluntary. If the decision is to go ahead, be sure that at least one of you visits a physician or clinic such as those run by Planned Parenthood for a supply of contraceptives and reliable instruction in their use. Better yet, go together. Do this before first intercourse. Pregnancy can *definitely* occur at first intercourse. Most women feel safer—and *are* safer—if they assume responsibility for contraception themselves. When a woman visits a doctor or clinic for advice on contraception, she can have a physical examination at the same time to make sure the hymen and other genital structures are ready for intercourse.

Find a suitable location where there is privacy and where both of you can be completely disrobed. First intercourse involves enough apprehensions and misgivings without adding fear of staining clothing or upholstery with semen, fear of severely wrinkled clothing that has not been taken off, or fear of interruption. It should be a place where both persons feel comfortable, such as a home, a dormitory room, or a motel room. Take a shower beforehand, both of you, with particular attention to the genitals. The room temperature and lighting (or darkness) should be comfortable. Give yourselves time, several hours at least, all night if you can arrange it. Do not be overawed or in despair at your performance. Don't be embarrassed if your partner appears to have had more experience than you. On the contrary, consider yourself fortunate; experience is a great teacher.

If great feelings of guilt or discomfort develop, there is no need to go on before these feelings are resolved. Guilt is too uncomfortable. Outside of marriage no one owes coitus to another. If you are married, try to talk over the problem and resolve it. If there is a question you cannot seem to settle, consult a physician, a friend who wishes both of you well, or a counselor.

Both partners deserve full gratification in sexual intercourse. Starting with first intercourse the relationship should be free from fear and guilt, with adequate protection against pregnancy, in a proper setting, with sufficient time, and with mutual concern for the maximum enjoyment by both partners. These make sexual intercourse one of the most beautiful of human experiences.

Strengthening the Sexual Muscles

Some women rarely or never achieve satisfaction from sexual intercourse. In their wish to increase their enjoyment of sex and improve the sensations of intercourse, couples sometimes want to know what they can do to gain control over the sexual muscles. Certain exercises that are recommended to help women who have the inconvenient tendency to release small amounts of urine at inappropriate times when they laugh, cough, or move suddenly may also be helpful in strengthening the sexual muscles.

Vaginal Muscles

There is a floor of strong muscles between a woman's legs that holds the vagina in place. These muscles form a kind of sling from front to back, supporting the urinary bladder, part of the rectum, the vagina, and the uterus (Figure 7.9). Three passages—the rectum, vagina, and urethra—penetrate this floor. These muscles are designed to help control the voiding of urine, help hold the vagina and related structures in place during the stress of intercourse and childbirth, and help control the process of defecation.

These muscles fall into two groups. The first are superficial, the second deeper. A muscle of the superficial group is the vaginal sphincter muscle (*bulbocavernosus*), which is split into two halves, one on each side of the vaginal opening. When the muscle is relaxed, so is the opening. The other muscle in the outer area is the urethral sphincter muscle (*external urethral*), which closes the urethra and thus shuts off the flow of urine when urination is completed. It is possible for a woman to learn to improve her control over these muscles by concentrating on the kind of effort she makes when she holds back her urine. This conscious drawing inward of the pelvic muscles strengthens them and improves control over them. She should firmly pull inward and then hold for several seconds, repeating the exercise twenty to thirty times a day for several weeks. This exercise strengthens both sphincter muscles and improves tension on the vaginal opening, as well as improving bladder control.

The second and deeper group of muscles relating to improved sexual enjoyment is known as the *levator ani,* and includes the pubococcygeus, puborectalis, and iliococcygeus muscles. Extending from the rectal-anal area to the pubic bone, they surround the deeper parts of the vagina. As these strong muscles are constricted, the walls of the vagina are brought together. To develop these deep muscles further, the woman should make the same muscular effort she makes to hold back a bowel movement. This causes the constriction of this group of deep muscles. She should firmly pull in on these muscles and then hold for several sec-

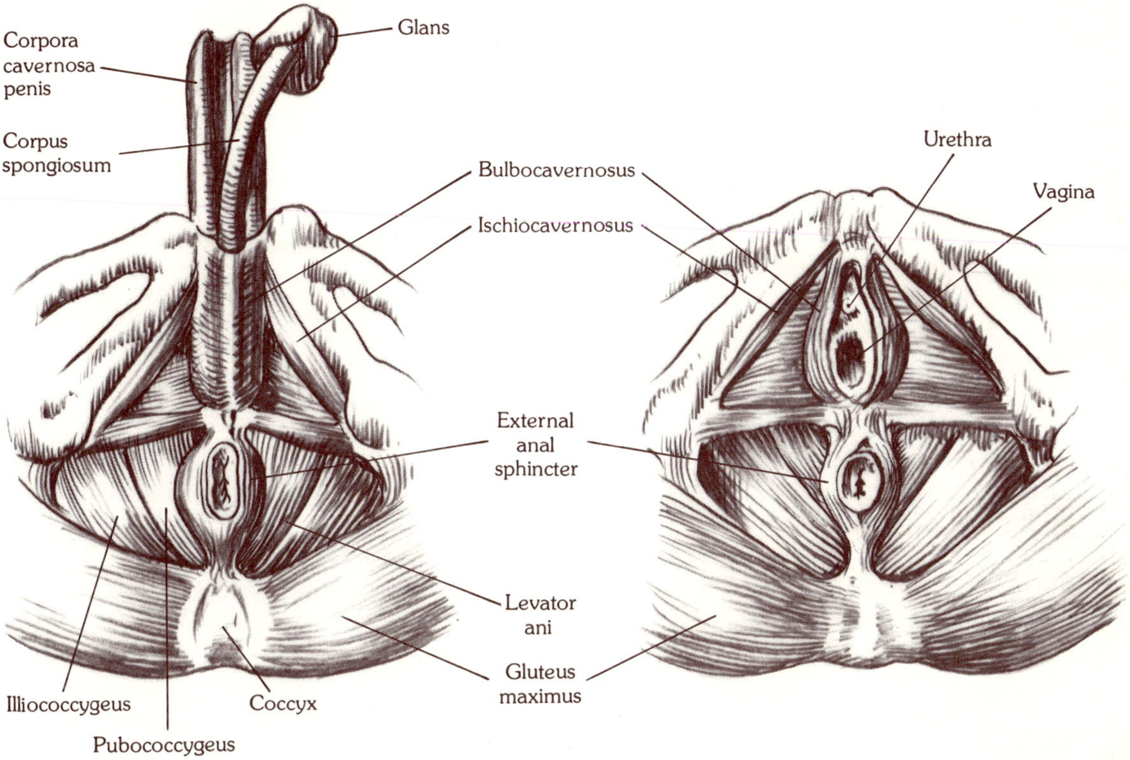

FIGURE 7.9 Muscles on the floor of the pelvis

onds, repeating the exercise twenty to thirty times each day for several weeks. This will improve control over them.

The advantage of improved control over these muscles in sexual relations is the effect they can have on the penis once it is in place in the vagina. The contraction of the external muscles tends to intensify the man's erection and increase his sexual excitement, at the same time creating greater stimulation of the nerve endings around the vaginal opening and adding to the woman's pleasure. By alternately squeezing and relaxing the deeper group of muscles, the woman can squeeze the penis. With the penis deeply inserted in the vagina, the woman can rhythmically massage the penis by squeezing first one set of muscles, then the other set. The sensation is highly pleasing to the man and may be sufficient to bring him to orgasm. Or she may combine the action by squeezing the two groups together or alternately while he gently thrusts the penis in and out of the vagina.

Penile Muscles

Although a man's control over the muscles on the floor of the pelvis is not so dramatic as a woman's, there are a couple of exercises that he can do to improve the sensations of intercourse. The superficial *bulbocavernosus* muscle in the male compresses the erectile tissues of the penis during erection and increases its diameter (Figure 7.9). Although the size increase is temporary (since the muscles cannot be contracted for more than a few seconds at a time), the size increase is distinctly felt by the woman and brings pleasure to her. The man achieves this effect by consciously drawing inward on muscles used for holding his urine back.

By learning to contract the deep, or *levator ani*, group during intercourse, he thrusts the penis forward, creating the effect of increasing its length. If he does this when the penis is already fully into the vagina, the deeper forward motion is pleasurable to the woman. Consciously contracting the muscles used to hold back bowel movements strengthens control of these muscles, just as in the woman.

Sexual Response

8

It was not until Masters and Johnson's landmark report, *Human Sexual Response,* that thorough objective treatment of the male and female sexual response was available. Before that there were only partial descriptions of sexual response, and they were often based on individual self-reports or observations of very limited groups. If you wish more specific information on sexual response, try Masters and Johnson.

Sexual Stimuli

Men and women are sexually aroused by a surprising variety of stimuli. Both tend to be highly responsive to touch, but the vast majority also respond to various forms of nontactile stimulation. Erotic literature and pictures of people of the opposite sex or the same sex clothed or nude will often serve as stimulants, especially to men. So are erotic motion pictures, visual fantasies, sounds of sexual activity, or just thoughts about sexual activity. Any stimulus (such as a perfume or a song) that is associated with past sexual experiences can also produce a sexual response.

The most common form of tactile stimulation is fondling of the body. In addition to fondling, most men and women are stimulated by the kissing, licking, or sucking of the man's penis and of the woman's labia and clitoris. Oral stimulation of the penis is *fellatio;* oral stimulation of the woman's external genitals is *cunnilingus.* Such stimulation may be part of either heterosexual or homosexual sex play. When people know that such stimulation brings pleasure to their partners, they may find themselves stimulated in the process. If such oral-genital stimulation is not pleasurable to one of the partners, they would do better to use other forms of sexual stimulation that are mutually pleasurable.

The couple should experiment with many forms of sexual stimulation. Each person shows greater or lesser response to particular stimuli depending upon cultural expectations, cultural conditioning, and the nature of past sexual experiences. If a person fails to respond to some particular stimulus in the same way and to the same degree as someone else, that person should feel no sense of alarm or apprehension. Learning what arouses sexual responsiveness in a partner is a significant part of the sexual relationship.

Male Sexual Response

Male sexual response is not confined to the genitals; it can be aroused over much of the body. Some reactions are superficial while others are deep within the body; some are general while others affect specific sites.

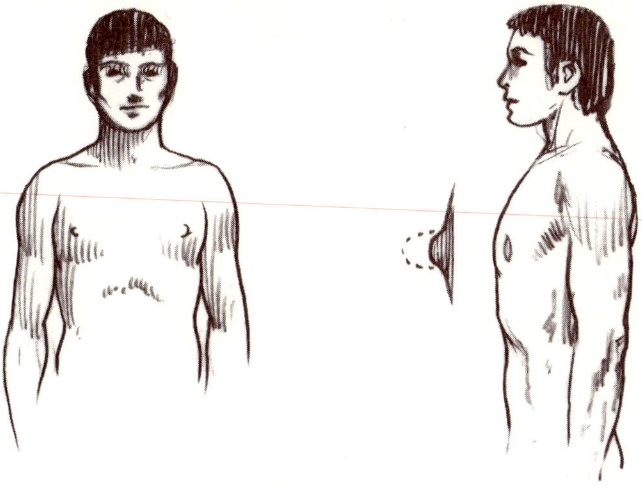

FIGURE 8.1 **(A) Sex flush over chest, neck, face, and forehead. More frequent in warm room and in situations of exteme anticipation. (B) Nipple erection (in about 60% of male subjects, occurring late in excitement phase).**

General Body Responses

The basic sexual responses in the male are widespread vasocongestion and a general increase in muscle tension. Response is highlighted by the appearance of reactions in the skin, muscles, breasts, breathing, heartbeat, and blood pressure.

Sex Flush About 25 percent of men develop a sex flush during sexual excitement. Spreading from the lower center of the chest, it involves much of the front of the chest, neck, face, and forehead (Figure 8.1). Resembling a measles rash, it eventually involves the shoulders, forearms, and thighs. A man may develop sex flush at times of high sexual tension and not at other times when sexual tension is less marked. Both environment and state of mind influence the occurrence of a sex flush. It has been observed to occur more readily in a warm room than in a cool one, and when there is extreme anticipation rather than in a routine sexual situation.

Breasts Many men have nipple erection during sexual excitement, but without the areolar enlargement or venous streaking common in women during sexual excitement (see Figure 8.1). Nipple erection may occur without direct breast caressing. Stimulation of a man's breasts and nipples is often neglected in heterosexual activity, but it is more often considered an important part of male homosexual sex play.

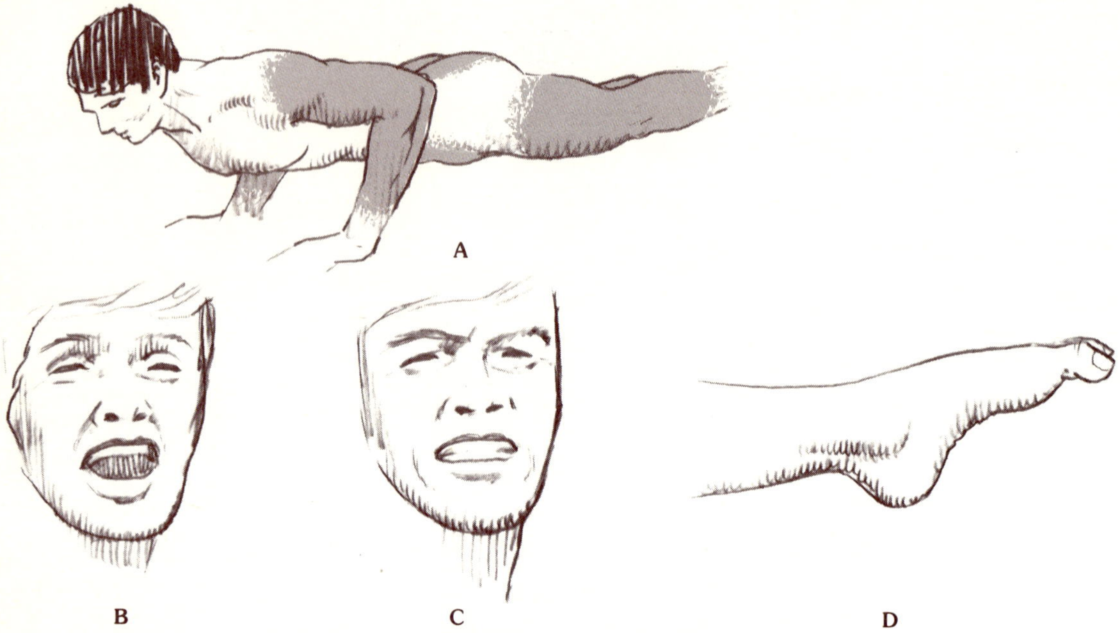

FIGURE 8.2 (A) During orgasm there may be severe spastic contractions of the arms, legs, back, or lower abdomen. (B) The mouth may open involuntarily in a gasping reaction to hyperventilative demand. (C) As facial muscles contract involuntarily, the individual frowns, scowls, or grimaces. (D) Carpopedal spasm—there is hyperextension of the arch of the foot and claw-like contractions of the toes when the male is supine.

Muscular Tension Depending upon coital position, a man's body muscles may contract both voluntarily and involuntarily during intercourse. Initially there is a total-body feeling of restlessness. Then comes an increased tension in the long muscles of both arms and legs, an involuntary tensing of the abdominal muscles, and an increase in the rate of breathing (see Figure 8.2). He may frown, scowl, or grimace, and the mouth often opens involuntarily as he demands more oxygen during orgasm. Neck muscles contract involuntarily. If the man is on his back, he may involuntarily clutch at his partner as sexual demand increases. When he is supporting himself above his partner, the biceps are often in involuntary spasm. An involuntary clawlike contraction of the feet and hands is frequently seen. These contractions may be more pronounced in masturbation than in intercourse.

Early in sexual excitement, the man rhythmically thrusts his pelvis voluntarily, but as he approaches orgasm the rapid forceful pelvic thrusting becomes involuntary and so intense that he rarely withdraws the penis more than halfway from the vagina before again thrusting deeply. During orgasm bodily muscular tension becomes so great that most muscular contraction is involuntary. Muscle strain may be so severe that muscular aches in the arms, legs, back, or lower abdomen may be felt the next day. Once orgasm is complete, muscular tenseness disappears within a few minutes.

Breathing and Heart Rate Just before orgasm the breathing rate increases. The intensity and duration of this hyperventilation is often an indication of the degree of sexual excitement. Breathing rates during orgasm often exceed forty per minute, in contrast to fifteen to twenty per minute in the unstimulated state.

As with breathing, the heart rate of a responding man increases in direct proportion to his rising sexual tensions. Heartbeat rises from the unstimulated state of 70 to 75 per minute to 110 to more than 180 during orgasm. The slower the rate during rest, the lower the rise during sexual stimulation. The type of sexual stimulation appears to have no bearing on the rate of increase. Blood pressure rises during both intercourse and masturbation.

Genital Responses

The man's genital responses can be described as occurring in four phases: excitement, plateau, orgasm, and resolution.

Excitement Phase The man's first physical response to sexual stimulation is rapid erection of the penis (see Figure 8.3). The pelvic arteries dilate to rush the flow of blood into the erectile tissue of the penis. The veins of the penis contain valves that slow the exit of blood. Erection may be partially lost and regained a number of times during prolonged sexual excitement. Distracting noises, thoughts, or conversations during this time may cause partial or complete loss of erection. As an erection occurs, the urethra both elongates and increases in diameter (about two and one-half times). The urethral opening (meatus) at the tip of the penis opens slightly during excitement, even without ejaculation. Masters and Johnson have found that the smaller unstimulated penis enlarges more in erection than a large unstimulated one. Thus in erection there is little or no difference between them. The notion that the larger the unstimulated penis is, the larger it is upon erection is a myth.

The scrotal skin, which in the unstimulated state hangs in many folds or creases, tenses and thickens during erection. The folds are lost as the scrotal sac constricts and elevates. The testes, which may be moved

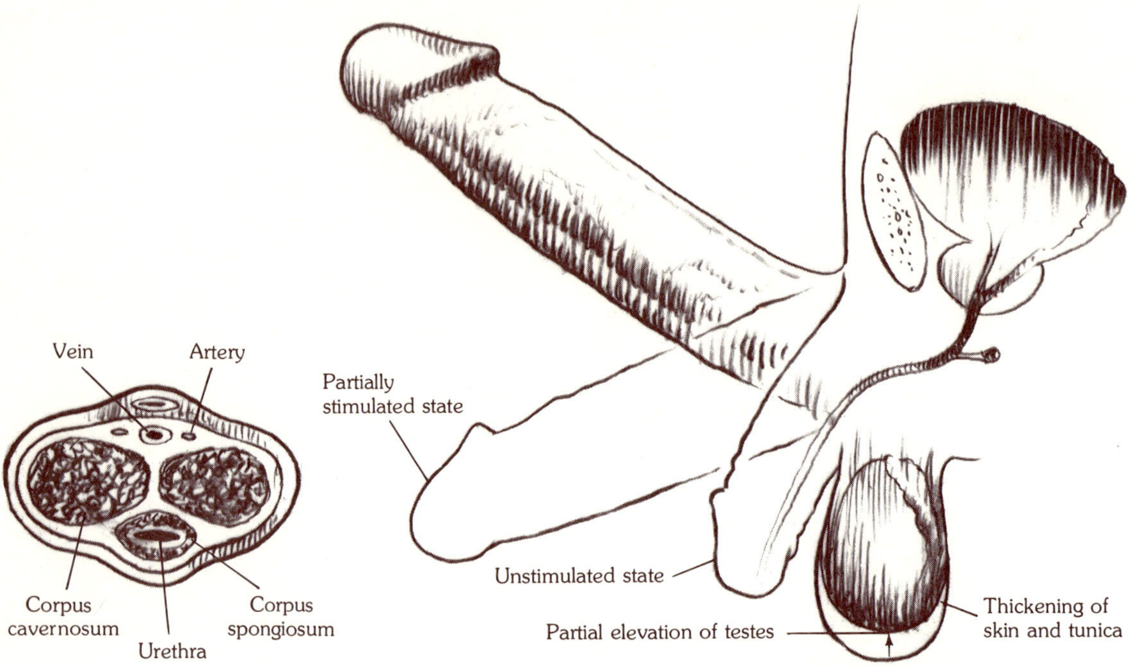

The smaller flaccid penis tends to enlarge proportionately more in erection than the larger flaccid penis, thus decreasing the difference between them.

FIGURE 8.3 Excitement stage

about freely in a relaxed scrotum, move less freely as they elevate toward the body wall.

As excitement mounts there is an increase in muscular tension over the body in general and the pelvis in particular. The rectal sphincter contracts irregularly and nipple erection may occur.

Plateau Phase The fully erect penis increases in diameter, particularly around the ridge of the corona (see Figure 8.4). The color of the corona may deepen to a mottled reddish purple.

The scrotal sac may further thicken and tense as the testes elevate tightly against the body wall. Such testicular elevation is related to ejaculatory pressure; orgasm never occurs without it. The greater the elevation of the testes, the greater the ejaculatory pressure; partial elevation causes a marked reduction in ejaculatory pressure. Some men over fifty tend to experience less elevation, and consequently weaker ejaculation. The left testis (which usually hangs lower in the unstimulated scrotum) may ele-

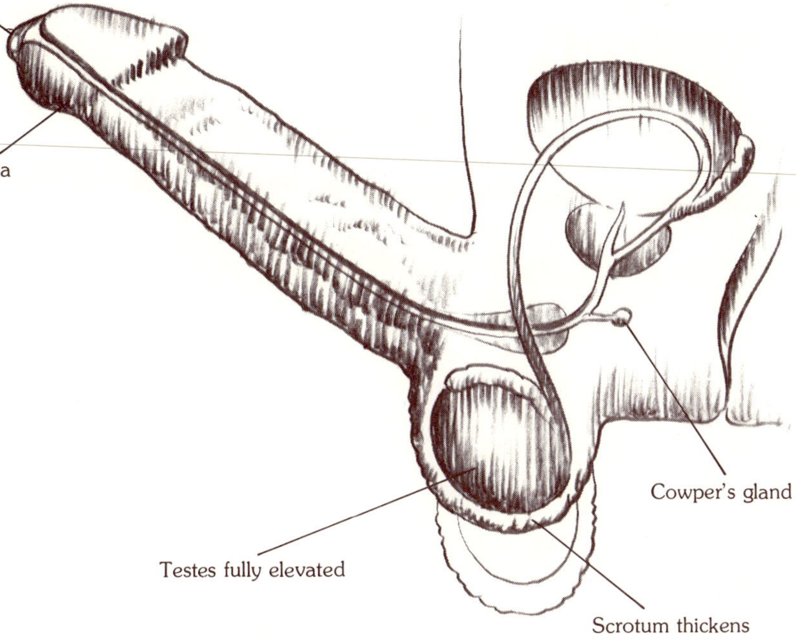

FIGURE 8.4 Plateau stage

vate independently of the right testis; the right may be fully elevated while the left is not. There is an observable increase of up to 50 percent in testicular size. The longer the duration of the plateau phase without orgasm, the more severe is the vasocongestion in the testes and the greater the testicular size increase. The Cowper's glands secrete one to several drops of sticky transparent fluid, which will appear on the tip of the penis. More may be produced if the plateau phase is prolonged. Active sperm are frequently found in this preejaculatory emission.

A sex flush may occur at this time. The rate of breathing increases toward the end of the plateau phase; the intensity and duration of hyperventilation are often indications of the degree of sexual tension. Heart rate increases in direct relation to rising sexual tension. The slower the initial heart rate, the lower the peak rate during sexual stimulation.

Orgasmic Phase The respiratory and heart rates continue to rise during orgasm. There are regular contractions of the urethra, penile tissues,

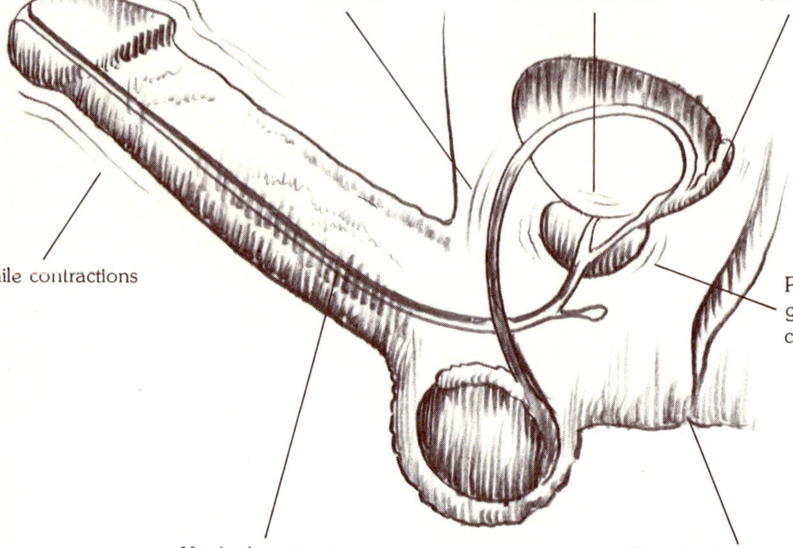

FIGURE 8.5 Orgasmic stage

muscles of the body wall, and rectal sphincter. The penile urethra may enlarge to three times its unstimulated diameter (see Figure 8.5). Ejaculatory contractions occur the entire length of the urethra, forcing the semen out. The intervals between penile contractions are similar to those in the vagina during female orgasm. Initial penile expulsions occur at intervals of less than a second. After the first three or four major expulsions, contractions rapidly reduce both in frequency and in expulsive force. Minor contractions then occur for several seconds. The actual expulsion of seminal fluid from the penis is evidence of orgasm in the male. The ejaculatory process is divided into two separate stages.

In stage 1, contractions begin in the testes and continue through the epididymis, vas deferens, and seminal vesicles, collecting seminal fluid in the ampulla. At the same time the fluid is expelled from the seminal vesicles. All of the fluid collects in the urethra of the prostate gland. The sphincter that controls flow from the urinary bladder closes, preventing both the reverse flow of semen into the bladder and the flow or urine into the urethra.

Immediately before ejaculation, the man can feel it coming. During these two to three seconds he can no longer control or delay the process. This feeling of ejaculatory inevitability develops as seminal fluid begins to collect in the prostatic urethra. The larger the volume collected, the more pleasurable the feeling.

In stage 2 the seminal fluid flows into the urethra of the penis. The muscles of the body wall, the entire penis, and the penile urethra contract rhythmically, propelling semen out through the tip of the penis. If the penis is not in the vagina, the pressure on the ejaculate may propel it twelve to twenty-four inches.

Men in their twenties may ejaculate frequently, with only a short recovery (refractory) period. The volume of semen is progressively reduced with each ejaculation when ejaculation is repeated over a short time. The feeling of pleasurable intensity is also greatest with the first ejaculation. This is in contrast to multiple orgasms in women; they frequently find the second or third or fourth orgasm more satisfying and pleasurable than the first.

Stage 2 of orgasm in the male is roughly comparable to stage 3 in the female. Repeated ejaculation does not strain a healthy male.

The first several forceful contractions provide the male with great pleasure. The final contractions are of lower intensity. Ejaculation after several days of continence results in the expulsion of more fluid as well as a more pleasurable sensation than ejaculation that follows another after only short delay.

Resolution Phase In resolution the penis relaxes in two stages. In the first stage it shrinks from full erection by about 50 percent (see Figure 8.6). Usually occurring quite rapidly, the first stage of resolution may

FIGURE 8.6 Resolution stage

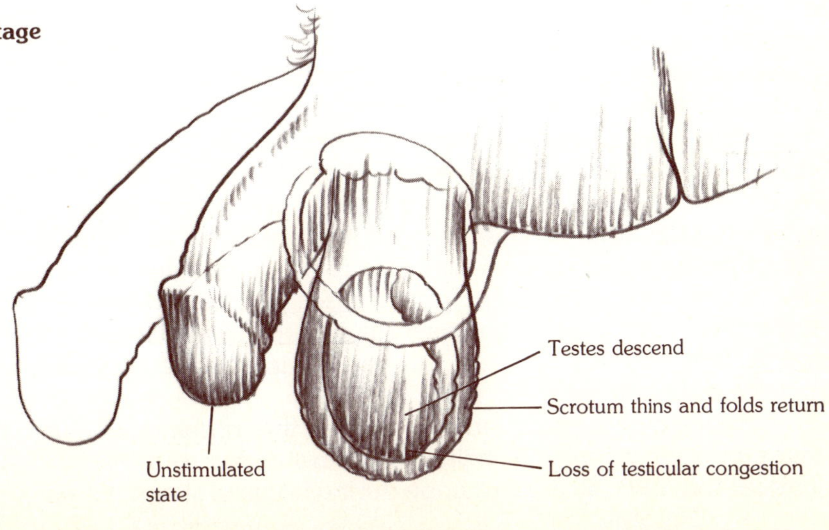

be prolonged when the excitement or plateau phase has been extended. Such extension of plateau usually occurs because the man has learned to delay ejaculation until the woman has been satisfied. When penile erection is maintained for a number of minutes, particularly with longer containment by the vagina, there is more penile vasocongestion even after the actual ejaculation.

The second stage of resolution is slower, but the time may vary. If the penis is removed from the vagina immediately following ejaculation, complete relaxation occurs rapidly. If the penis remains in the vagina or if there is merely close physical contact between the partners, complete relaxation of the penis may not occur for some time. Second-stage resolution occurs more quickly if the man moves around, thinks or talks about nonsexual things, or attempts to urinate (urination is impossible when the penis is fully erect).

The scrotum loses its tenseness and the foldings of the unstimulated state reappear rapidly or slowly, depending on the length of time of earlier stimulation. One or two hours may be required for the wall to lose its thickness. The testicles lose their congestion and redescend into the scrotum rapidly or slowly, depending on the length of the plateau phase.

The sex flush disappears very rapidly, first from the shoulders and extremities, then from the abdomen and front of the chest, and finally from the neck, face, and forehead. The rectal sphincter begins relaxing even before the contractions of ejaculation have subsided.

Some men perspire immediately after ejaculation. This kind of sweating has no particular relation to the amount of physical exertion during the sex act. Most common on the soles of the feet and palms of the hands, it may also appear on the trunk, head, face, and neck.

The minimum time required before repeated male erection and orgasm is highly variable, both among different men and for the same man at different times. It can range from minutes to days. This minimum time increases with the age of the man and with his general physical and emotional fatigue, but it is decreased by the degree of original sexual arousal, the degree of sexual restimulation after ejaculation, and the period of sexual continence before the first ejaculation. If a younger man has been without sexual release for some time, or if he is restimulated shortly after ejaculation, he may be ready for further sexual intercourse within a few minutes after ejaculation. In such cases the penis will not entirely lose its erection, but may still be too sensitive for continued thrusting for a few minutes. Many men, however, are unable to achieve erection again for an hour or more after ejaculation.

Men and boys commonly awaken in the morning with an erection. Many of them mistakenly believe that this is due to a full bladder, distended from the collection of urine during hours of sleep. It is now known to be related to REM sleep. During sleep a person dreams periodically, and during the dreaming state there are mild involuntary muscle jerks and rapid eye movements. Thus this stage of sleep is known as *REM sleep*. REM sleep usually occurs three to four times each night, at intervals of 80 to 120 minutes. Each occurrence of REM sleep lasts from five minutes to more than an hour. About 25 percent of normal sleep is REM sleep. During each REM period males gain partial or full erection and the vaginas of females become lubricated. The degree of erection shows little relation to the occurrence of intercourse. Males who awake and urinate before the last REM period may still experience a morning erection.

Postcoronary Sexual Activity

Sex can be a real problem for people who are recovering from acute coronary episodes: When and how may they resume sexual activity? If the patient has recovered sufficiently to undertake vigorous walking or go bicycling without symptoms of heart distress, an abnormal pulse rate, or changes in blood pressure or electrocardiogram, it is generally safe to resume sexual activity.

Female Sexual Response

Female sexual response is not confined to the genitalia. Physical reactions are both superficial and deep, both general and specific.

General Body Responses

Many of the basic sexual responses of women are similar to men's, differing in certain specifics. Response is highlighted by reactions of the skin, muscles, breasts, breathing, heartbeat, and blood pressure.

Sex Flush While there is variation among individuals, generally the more intense the sexual tensions, the greater the degree of a measles-like rash known as the sex flush. Starting in the center of the chest below the breasts, it rapidly spreads over the breasts to the lower abdomen, shoulders, thighs, buttocks, and back. About 75 percent of all women experience a sex flush.

Breasts The first breast response to sexual arousal is nipple erection (see Figure 8.7). The areola, or ring of darkened tissue surrounding the nipple, enlarges from engorgement with blood. Veins just below the skin surface become visible, especially in larger breasts. The breasts increase in size, most noticeably when the woman is lying on her back. Enlargement of the breasts is most apparent in women who have never suckled a

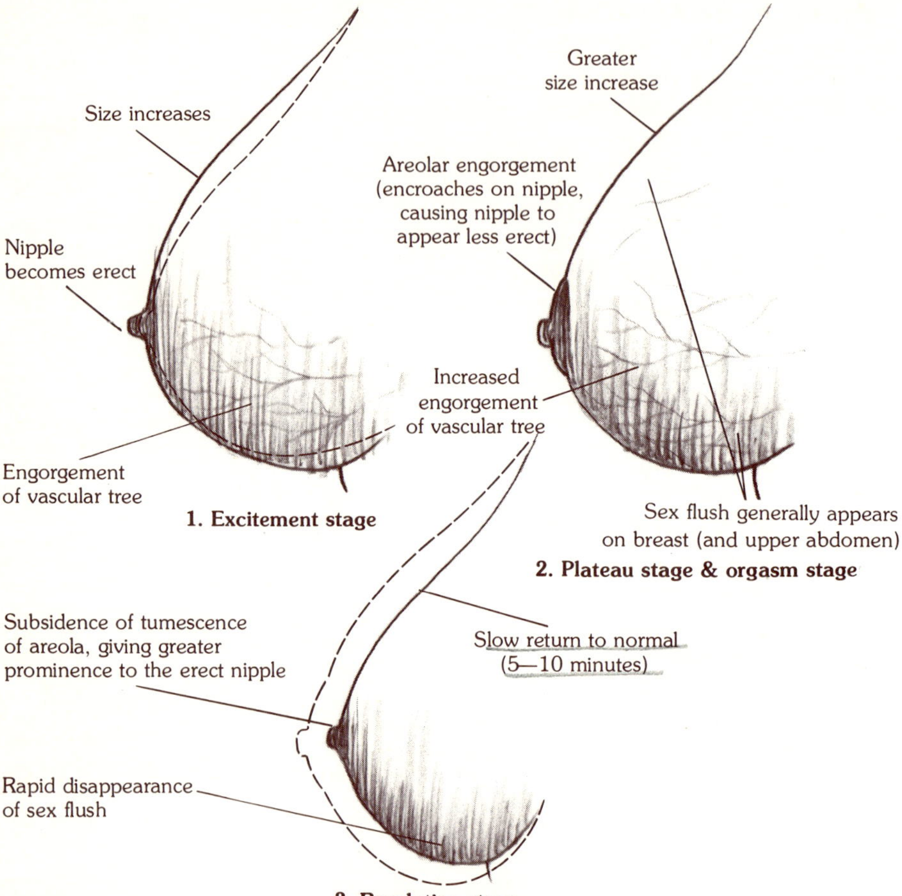

FIGURE 8.7 Breast response to sexual stimulation

child; they become 20 to 25 percent larger than the unstimulated breast. Breasts that have been suckled may show little size increase, since suckling improves drainage of the veins, reducing the vasocongestion that occurs from sexual tension. A bit later, the surface of the breasts may appear mottled.

Muscular Tension A general involuntary tensing occurs in the muscles of the arms and legs, across the abdomen, around the chest, in the face, and along the vaginal barrel (wall of the vagina). The degree of muscle tension increases with sexual response. Upon entry of the penis into the vagina (intromission), the woman's first movements may be slow voluntary pelvic strokings. As arousal mounts, these give way to more forceful movements, becoming involuntary at the peak of orgasm.

Rectum and Urinary Bladder A woman may voluntarily tense the rectal sphincter and the muscles of the buttocks early in sexual response to elevate her sexual tension. During orgasm the rectal sphincter may contract involuntarily. If it does, it indicates the intensity of the orgasm. If the orgasm is intense, the rectal sphincter may contract two to five times, at about the same rhythm as the contractions of the orgasmic platform in the outer third of the vagina. Rectal sphincter contractions occur most consistently in female masturbation, less so in intercourse. Some women feel the urge to void urine either during or just after intercourse.

Breathing and Heart Rates The breathing rate during sexual arousal rises from fifteen to twenty per minute in the resting stage to more than forty per minute at the peak of intense orgasm. Heart rate during arousal increases from 70 to 75 in the resting stage to from 110 to more than 180 beats per minute during orgasm. Levels of heart rate are also related to the degree of orgasmic intensity, and are lighter during masturbation than during intercourse. Blood pressure levels also increase during sexual arousal.

Genital Responses

The woman's body responses can be described as occuring in four phases: excitement, plateau, orgasm, and resolution. Although this section deals primarily with genital response, nongenital responses will be referred to when they closely accompany genital reactions.

Excitement Phase As arousal is initiated, the nipples become erect, surface veining is seen, and breast size begins an expansion that continues into the plateau phase. A sex flush is first seen over the middle chest below the breasts late in the excitement phase, and then spreads rapidly over much of the breasts. Muscles in the arms, legs, abdomen, and chest begin tightening.

Normally rounded and meeting each other at the midline in the unstimulated state, the labia majora flatten out near the vaginal opening with a slight elevation farther away from the vaginal opening (see Figure 8.8). The labia majora may be more elevated and distended in the woman who has had children. The labia minora expand noticeably, pushing out past the flattened labia majora and adding slightly to the length of the vaginal barrel.

The clitoris enlarges along with the vasocongestion of the labia mi-

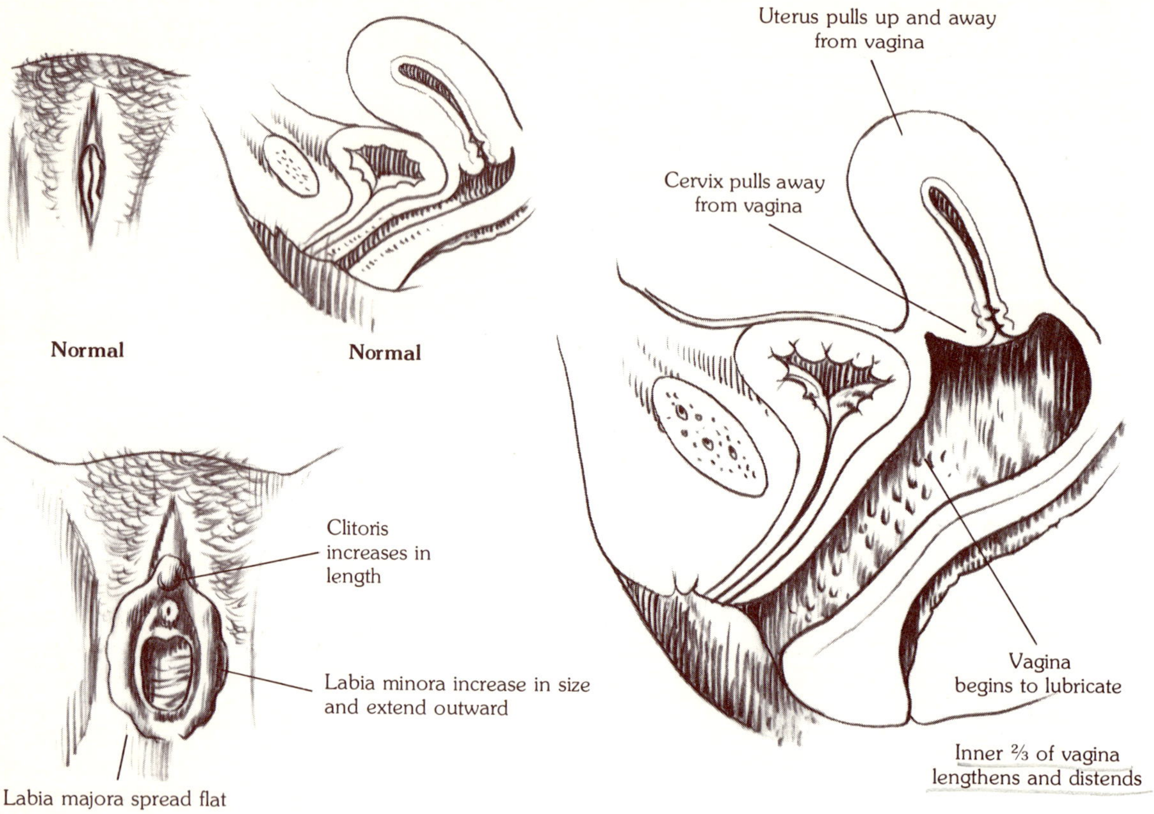

FIGURE 8.8 Excitement stage

nora. The shaft of the clitoris increases in both diameter and length. The head (glans) of the clitoris swells, the enlargement ranging from very slight to as much as double the normal size.

The vagina becomes moistened very early, often within ten to thirty seconds after the beginning of stimulation (see Figure 8.8). The moistening appears as a kind of "sweating" by the vaginal barrel until the entire barrel is coated. This vaginal response may precede other signs of response. Within seconds sufficient moistening may occur to allow for coitus. This moistening occurs even after a woman's uterus has been removed (hysterectomy). At first the inner two-thirds of the vagina both lengthens and distends until it is decidedly expanded with a slight distension of the outer one-third. The color of the vaginal wall slowly changes from purplish red to a darker purple. At first patchy, the coloring soon becomes uniform.

The uterus slowly tilts upward, elevating as sexual tension mounts. The cervix moves from its resting position, and with the expanding front and side walls of the vagina forms a little tent.

Plateau Phase The areola enlarges around the erect nipple. Breasts continue to increase. The sex flush spreads until it may cover much of the body.

The labia minora change from pink to bright red to a deep wine color. When this color change has been achieved, the diameter of the labia minora will have at least doubled. The entire clitoral body retracts against the front of the pelvic bone, withdrawing deeply beneath the foreskin (see Figure 8.9). In this position the length of the clitoris appears

FIGURE 8.9 Plateau stage

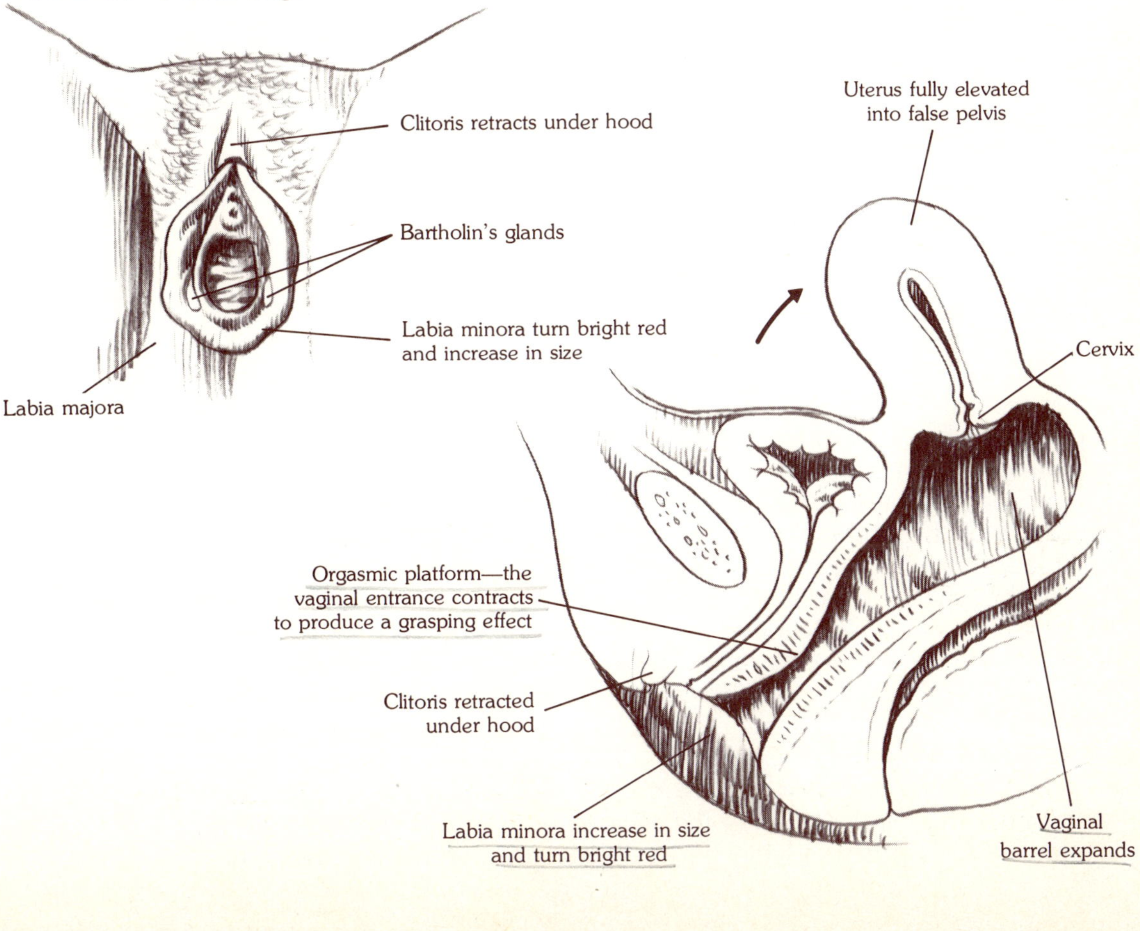

reduced by at least half. Retraction occurs more rapidly with caressing of the mons area and more slowly during breast manipulation and intromission. If stimulation during this phase is reduced, the clitoris returns to its original position, but will retract once again if stimulation is resumed.

The outer third of the vagina becomes quite engorged with blood, reducing the inside diameter (lumen) of this part of the vagina by 50 percent (see Figure 8.9). This tightening is a sure indication that the woman is in the plateau phase. This reaction of the outer third of the vagina, along with the engorged, erect labia minora, is known as the *orgasmic platform.* Vaginal lubrication, so great during the excitement phase, may slow now, particularly if this phase is drawn out. The Bartholin's glands may secrete from one to several drops of mucous material, however, particularly during long-maintained intercourse. As the uterus becomes fully elevated, the cervix and vaginal walls enlarge the tenting effect.

As a woman passes into the orgasmic phase, the orgasmic platform is eventually lost. It is felt that the chances of conception are enhanced if her partner ejaculates during her plateau phase. The ejaculate of the male forms a seminal pool in the upper vagina, and the semen is more apt to be held near the entrance to the uterus if the orgasmic platform is retained for an appreciable time (see Figure 8.10). The orgasmic platform forms a kind of "stopper" effect in this outer third of the vagina, more effectively retaining the semen near the uterus.

Orgasmic Phase Orgasm may be both a psychological and a physiological experience for a woman. Physically, it is release from the peak of muscular tension and vascular congestion built up by her response to sexual stimuli. Psychologically, it may be a peak emotional response to sexual arousal. Orgasm is also a sociological experience; the woman's response is influenced by her cultural background, her expectations, and the immediate environment of the episode. While certain physical responses may tend to occur generally in all women during orgasm, the interrelation of these three factors produce an experience that is highly variable among women and for the same woman at different times.

In this phase no further breast changes occur. The erect nipple is already surrounded by the inflated areola, and the veins are standing out plainly. Sex flush, if it occurs, is widespread over the body. Breathing is heavy and fast. The heart rate increases to the maximum. A few women perspire on their foreheads and upper lips just before orgasm, and about a third perspire over much of the body immediately after orgasm.

The peak of muscular tension is expressed in the contorting and grimacing of the face. Muscles of the neck, arms, and legs contract involuntarily. If the woman is lying on her back, her hands and feet may

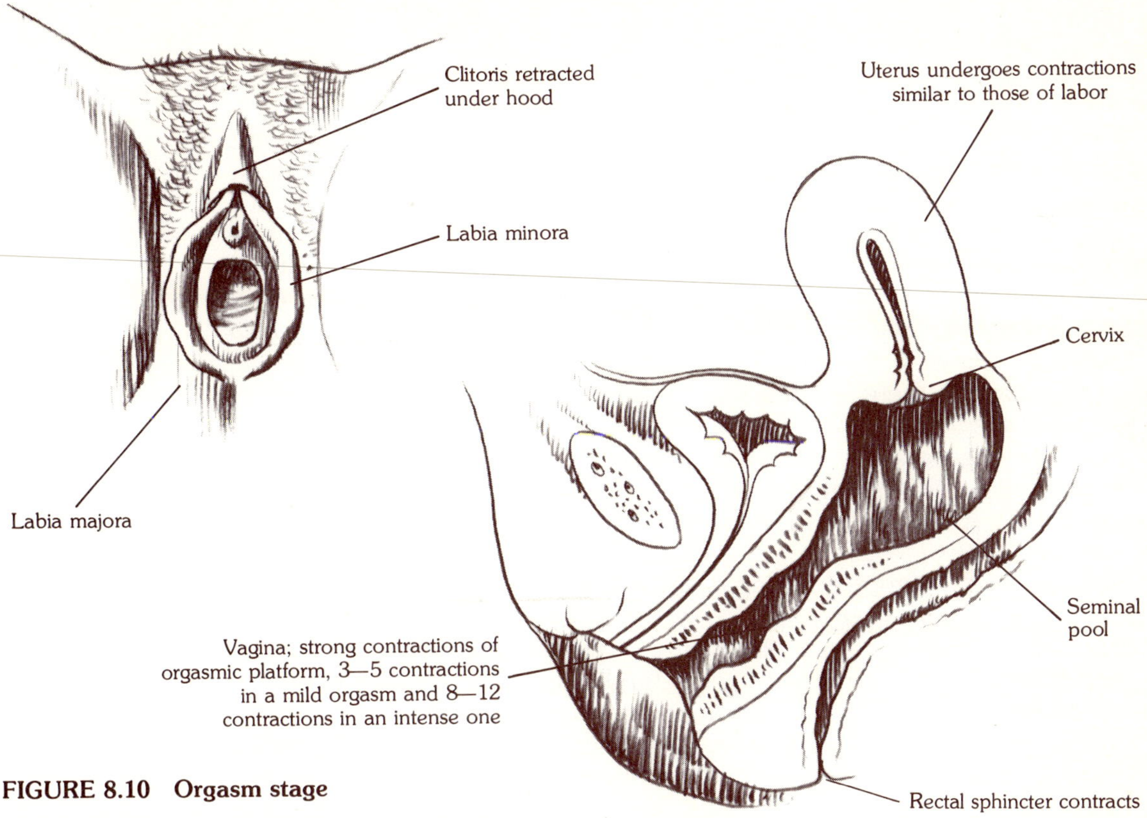

FIGURE 8.10 Orgasm stage

voluntarily grasp her partner. Her fingers and toes may contract in spasm involuntarily when she masturbates to orgasm. Women often produce vocalizations of some sort during orgasm.

The orgasmic platform contracts rhythmically as the tension is released (see Figure 8.10). The first several contractions occur quickly; the late ones occur more slowly and are more extended. The more intense the orgasm, the greater the number and intensity of contractions. The uterus contracts, but more slowly and irregularly than the lower vagina. Contractions begin at the dome, or top, of the uterus and work down to the lower part, resembling contractions of first-stage labor. Although these contractions vary, they tend to be greater in a woman with past experience in both orgasm and pregnancy. The openings to the rectum and urethra may contract involuntarily. Again, the more intense the response, the greater the number of contractions.

Once the female has experienced one orgasm, she is capable of another very quickly if her sexual excitement does not fall below the response levels of the plateau phase. Some women regularly—and many women occasionally—experience a series of rapidly recurring orgasms without (or just barely) returning to the plateau level, in what seems like a single long orgasmic experience. This is known as *status orgasmus*. This series of orgasmic peaks may last from twenty to sixty seconds or more. Heartbeat during status orgasmus may exceed 180 per minute.

The obvious contractions of the orgasmic platform in the outer third of the vagina, along with the noticeable rapid detumescence of the areolae of the breasts, occur only when the woman experiences orgasm.

Psychologically, a woman appears to pass through three distinct stages in orgasm.

In stage 1 there is a feeling of suspension, followed by a sense of intense sensual awareness in the area of the clitoris, which spreads upward into the pelvis. At the same time there may be a sense of bearing down or expelling (some women feel as though they were actually emitting fluid). At this point she tends to become unaware of her environment.

In stage 2 there is a feeling of warmth in the pelvic area and spreading throughout the body.

In stage 3 there is a feeling of involuntary contraction in the vaginal area, described by some as a "pelvic throbbing." The feeling of contraction is perceived as first centering in the vaginal area, followed by a throbbing sensation in the pelvic area which spreads throughout the body. Most women experience from five to eight such strong orgasmic platform contractions, though ordinarily they aren't counting. Eight to twelve such contractions can be viewed as an intense response. Less than five is considered a mild response.

After the first three to six contractions, the interval between them begins to lengthen and they grow weaker. The nature of these contractions not only varies from woman to woman, but may vary from time to time for the same woman. The outer vaginal contractions occur only during the orgasmic phase. Some women feel that orgasmic platform contractions in intercourse during the last third of pregnancy are particularly intense.

Resolution Phase The rapid disappearance of the sex flush signals the arrival of the fourth and final phase of sexual response. At the same time the areolae detumesce, again revealing the full erection of the nipples. The enlargement in unsuckled breasts may last five to ten minutes following the end of the orgasmic phase, with visible surface veining lasting even longer. The nipples may fully return to the unstimulated state before the venous patterning disappears.

The last sites where the sex flush appeared are the first sites from which it disappears. Disappearance is fast from the back, buttocks, lower

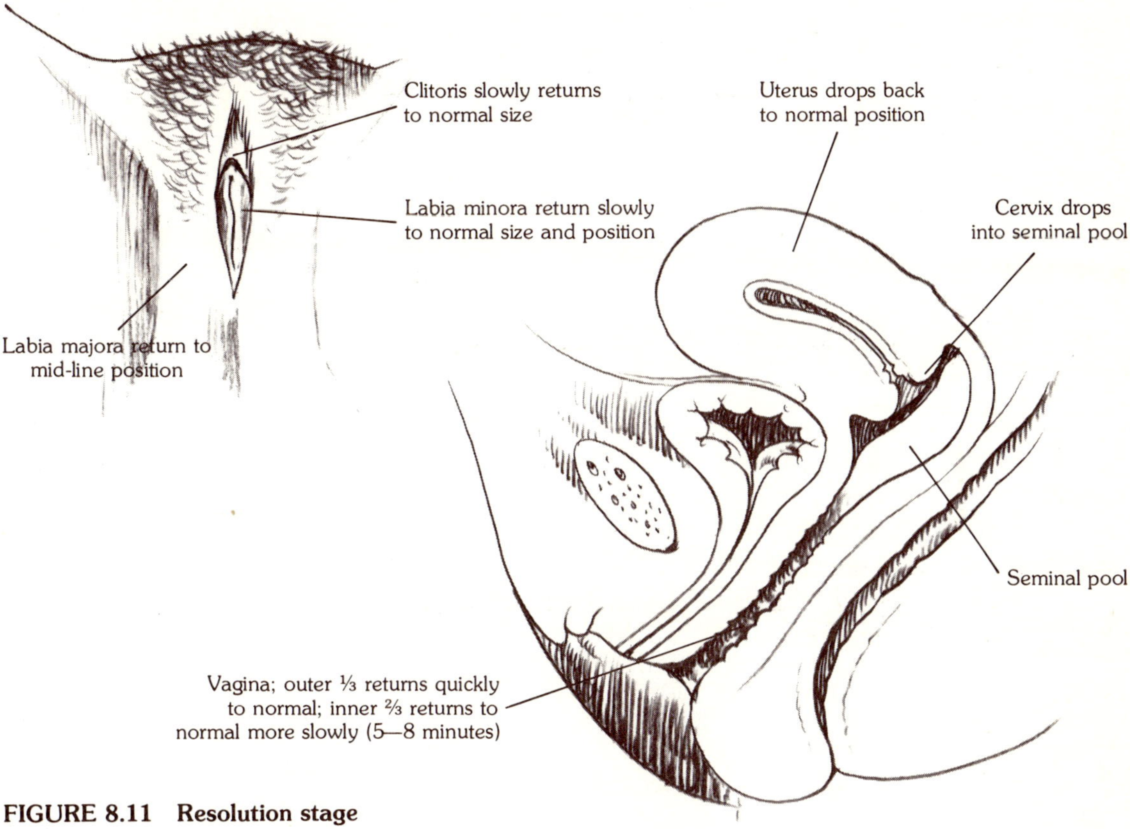

FIGURE 8.11 Resolution stage

abdomen, arms, and thighs, and is slowest from the breasts, neck, face, and central chest.

Often women report changes in feelings of body temperature during resolution. Some feel very warm, others cold. Commonly there is some degree of perspiration, regardless of the amount of activity that has taken place. It may occur over much of the body, including the face, soles of the feet, and palms of the hands. If a woman's sexual response goes only to the plateau level, the sex flush disappears with little or no perspiration evident.

The outer labia return to the unstimulated size quickly if a woman has experienced orgasm, but lose their engorgement slowly if only the plateau phase has been gained (see Figure 8.11). The inner labia change from bright red back to light pink within a few seconds after orgasm, then return to the colorless unstimulated state a bit more slowly.

Following orgasm the clitoris detumesces and returns to its unstimulated position within five to ten seconds after contractions of the orgasmic platform have stopped. Detumescence of the clitoris is as rapid as that of the penis following ejaculation. Relaxation of the glans may come somewhat more slowly if tumescence came early in intercourse and the response was strong and continued. Tumescence sometimes lasts five or more minutes following orgasm. Tumescence of the clitoral shaft and glans may last for hours after the end of sexual activity when the woman has not achieved orgasm.

Because the vasocongestion in the outer third of the vagina is rapidly lost, the inside diameter of the vagina actually increases early in the resolution phase. Then the inner two-thirds of the vagina slowly shrinks back to the unstimulated state. The tenting effect is rapidly lost as the cervix and the front wall of the uterus descend toward the floor of the vagina. The first part of this regression occurs rapidly. The full return of the vagina to its unstimulated size may take five to ten minutes. As the vaginal barrel retrogresses, the deep-purple color and the ridged patterns of the unstimulated vagina return.

As the cervix descends to the floor of the vagina, it becomes immersed in the seminal pool. The ejaculate may remain in the upper uterus for an extended period if the woman remains on her back during the resolution phase. In the vagina of the woman who has never borne a child this may be a matter of hours; owing to the effects of childbirth on the vagina, its outer third will be less constrained and will not hold the ejaculate so easily. If the woman stands, sits, or lies on her side, the ejaculate will be discharged from the vagina more rapidly. Continued penile thrusting after ejaculation will also result in the escape of the ejaculate from the vagina.

The period of sexual stimulation needed to bring a woman to the point of orgasm varies from person to person and from time to time for the same woman. The experience of most couples is that the woman needs a longer period of stimulation to achieve orgasm than does the man. But the Kinsey report of 1953 stated that the average woman can masturbate to orgasm almost as quickly as the average man. They attributed the difference in times to the fact that the masturbating woman can manipulate her sensitive areas more specifically than a man can do it in intercourse. This conclusion seems to have been confirmed by Masters and Johnson, who found that the measurable physiological intensity of female orgasm is greatest in masturbation, moderate in partner manipulation, and lowest in intercourse.

The female orgasm is more variable in intensity and duration than the male orgasm. The physical manifestations of female orgasm include a series of contractions of the vagina and uterus, roughly corresponding in number and interval to the contractions of male ejaculation. There is, of course, no emission of fluid in female orgasm.

Caressing of the clitoris plays an important role in the achievement of orgasm for many women. Yet clitoral stimulation is not essential to orgasm. Sexually responsive women who have undergone removal of the clitoris (vulvectomy) usually continue to achieve orgasm in intercourse following the surgery. Lip or tongue stimulation of the external auditory canal of the ear may of itself induce orgasm. Orgasm has also been induced through stimulation of the anus (such as through the self-administration of enemas, anal coitus, or finger stimulation), through the fondling or kissing of the breasts, or as the result of dreams.

Some couples find appeal in cunnilingus, the oral stimulation of the woman's external genitals, and in fellatio, the oral stimulation of the man's penis. Some women are stimulated by feeling the man's tongue and lips against the genitals and outer parts of the vagina. The man also may be excited by the enjoyment it brings the woman, and by the taste and smell of the vaginal secretions. Some couples engage in fellatio and cunnilingus simultaneously. If both enjoy it, it can be reciprocally reinforcing. Neither fellatio nor cunnilingus is improper or unclean if the partners have bathed properly with soap and water beforehand. It is important though, that such sex play be pleasurable to both partners. If one of you dislikes it, it is wiser to choose some other form of sexual stimulation.

A woman should place as much value on her own attainment of orgasm as she places on the man's attaining his. Aware that she can fully experience orgasm, a woman can enter a sexual relationship without feeling the need to pretend orgasm merely to please her mate. By expecting full sexual pleasure, she can interact with her mate in such a way as to bring both of them a full measure of pleasurable experience.

There are various misconceptions regarding female orgasm. One is that orgasm is centered either around the clitoris or in the vagina. Freud and some of his followers contended that there was a difference between clitoral and vaginal orgasm. The Freudian position was that clitoral orgasm represented an immature, emotionally arrested expression of sexual response, while vaginal orgasm implied a woman's maturity in a sexual relationship. Aware of Freud's notions, many women have tormented themselves with doubts about their own orgasms: Are they occurring in the vagina, or "only" in the clitoris? Masters and Johnson have cleared away this misconception by demonstrating that an orgasm is an orgasm *regardless of the emphasis.* Even when the clitoris is not stimulated directly, it enlarges and participates fully in the total response. A woman's body responds to effective sexual stimulation with consistency regardless of the source of psychic or physical sexual stimulation. The clitoral body responses are identical in all cases and vary only in intensity of one's reaction to the stimulation. There is neither a purely clitoral orgasm nor a purely vaginal one; from the body's point of view there is only one kind, a sexual orgasm.

Another misconception is that large-breasted women are more readily orgasmic than small-breasted women. There is no correlation between breast size and consistency of orgasm or frequency of intercourse. Nor does the age of onset of breast development appear to have any bearing on the matter. In fact, some women attach relatively low value to breast stimulation during arousal. A typical ranking of female genital structures from most to least sensitive to sexual arousal is: clitoris, vagina near the clitoris, labia minora, internal vagina, breasts, and labia majora.

A woman is capable of multiple orgasms (as many as three to five or more within a few minutes) if the man can maintain stimulation long enough. The limit is not the woman's capacity to respond, but the man's capacity for long-sustained erection.

For a woman to fail on occasion to achieve an orgasm does not necessarily mean that she is lacking in sexual responsiveness. Very few women achieve orgasm 100 percent of the time. An orgasm need not be the only goal of sexual activity. Occasionally a woman may feel satisfied by the intromission of the penis into the vagina without orgasm. Yet the attaining of orgasm is often related to sexual foreplay. Intercourse without foreplay rarely results in female orgasm, whereas prolonged foreplay commonly does. It has also been observed that the mental disposition of a woman may be directly affected by the experience of orgasm. Following orgasm there is a feeling of peace and the dissipation of negative feelings. Without orgasm, her sexual tensions unresolved, a woman may tend to be irritable for a time.

Some physical conditions are likely to interfere with orgasmic response in women. These include a heavy, unyielding hymen, acute vaginitis, and vaginal scars. There may be offensive physical disorders in the male (deformities, tumors, conditions with disagreeable body odors) that make coitus distasteful. In such circumstances, entry of the penis into the vagina may not always be necessary for orgasmic response. Finger manipulation of the woman's external genitalia by the male or other types of stimulation may then be utilized to bring her satisfying response.

Pregnancy and Sexual Response

In assessing sexual response during pregnancy, Masters and Johnson found significant response differences in the breasts and in the internal and external genitalia.

Breast Response Early in a pregnancy of a woman who has borne no previous children, rapid increase in size and tenderness of the breasts is common. During the first trimester (first three months) her breasts are more responsive to congestion than they were before she was pregnant. This condition, along with the normal increase in breast size during pregnancy, may lead to severe breast tenderness during later stages of sexual tension. Breast tenderness is reduced during the second and third trimesters of pregnancy.

Following delivery, breast response to sexual stimuli is related to nursing. If milk production is suppressed, the only response is nipple erection. The nursing mother may lose breast milk in involuntary spurts during sexual arousal, and milk may run from both nipples during and immediately after orgasm.

Genital Response During much of pregnancy, women report increased levels of sexual excitement. Some women experience multiple orgasms for the first time when they are pregnant. They may also experience changes in each of the four phases of sexual response.

In the excitement stage the labia majora may not show the elevated and flattened reactions of the nonpregnant woman, while the labia minora may enlarge two to three times their normal size during the first two trimesters. Late in pregnancy the labia minora remain enlarged. Vaginal secretions develop more rapidly and occur more extensively than at other times (more so in women who have had previous pregnancies). The uterus becomes distended and elevated during the first trimester. The vagina expands and distends in response to sexual stimuli as it did when the woman was not pregnant, but with less tenting.

The sex flush continues to occur in the plateau stage. The orgasmic platform becomes quite engorged, so much so that the vaginal passage may appear largely or completely closed in response to sexual tensions. In fact, the more advanced the pregnancy, the more severe the venous engorgement of the vaginal barrel and the development of the orgasmic platform. As the fetus grows, the uterus becomes an enlarged abdominal organ; thus further uterine elevation reactions typical of the plateau phase do not occur.

Vaginal contractions give evidence of orgasm as in the nonpregnant woman, except during the final third of pregnancy, when the venous congestion tends to minimize the effect. Instead of contracting regularly during orgasm, the uterus may go into muscular spasms lasting for as long as a minute. Such uterine contractions have little or no effect on the fetus.

The congestion in the pelvis of the pregnant woman may not be completely relieved by orgasm, and this difficulty may be aggravated as pregnancy progresses. Ten to fifteen minutes may elapse after orgasm before the increased congestion of the labia and vagina subsides during a first pregnancy, and as long as thirty to forty-five minutes during subsequent pregnancies. In the final trimester, pelvic vasocongestion may not be completely lost even though orgasm is intense. The normal pelvic congestion of the third trimester of pregnancy helps to account for this failure in complete resolution of orgasmic congestion. Although orgasm may be intense, the relief of sexual tension may be both slow and temporary, rather than rapid and complete as in the nonpregnant woman.

Sexual performance during first pregnancy is quite variable. Some women reject all forms of sexual activity during the entire pregnancy. Their lack of interest in sex may be due to reduced sexual tensions, fatigue, sleepiness, nausea, or fear of injury to the fetus. Women who have been pregnant before report less change in their levels of sexual interest and performance.

During the second trimester some women may notice an elevation in sexual feelings and performance, whether it is the first pregnancy or the fifth. Sexuality may increase in the second trimester not only in comparison with the first trimester, but also in comparison with the nonpregnant state. By the second trimester feelings of fear are reduced, and social concerns are usually more nearly resolved. And it is at the beginning of the second trimester that the woman begins to feel the movements of her fetus. She can feel the life within her, and the experience is often translated into delight in her sexuality.

In her third trimester a woman may show reduced sexual interest as a result of medical advice to refrain from sexual activity in the weeks immediately preceding the expected delivery date. Some women voice concern over their husbands' apparent loss of sexual interest during late pregnancy, and fear they may turn to slimmer, more active women. It has happened. Most men, however, are proud of their approaching fatherhood and feel particularly tender toward their wives at this time.

Pregnancy is a natural condition, not an illness, and if no complications develop there is usually no need to consider the pregnant woman fragile. But she is uncomfortable during the last few weeks, and nothing is more essential to satisfying sexual activity than physical comfort.

Resumption of intercourse following delivery is of concern to both mother and father. The uterus remains enlarged for about six weeks after delivery. Bleeding from the site of the placenta on the uterine wall may occur for two to four weeks after delivery. Any incisions made to facilitate delivery usually heal within two to three weeks. Tears take longer to heal. Once the bleeding has stopped and incisions or tears have healed, there are usually no anatomical impediments to the resumption of intercourse. Psychological factors, however, may cause a woman to delay. Estrogen and progesterone levels are low and depression is a common result (see chapter 5). A factor favoring early resumption of intercourse may be the effect of long continence on the man. Six weeks before and six weeks after delivery are longer than some men are willing to wait. If early resumption is possible, further delay serves no good purpose to either of the partners. If the mother is suffering from the "baby blues," renewed intimacy may help her through them. If good medical reasons against it remain, the woman can ease her partner's sexual tensions manually or orally, or he can masturbate.

Coitus During Menstruation

There have been many cultural and religious taboos against intercourse during menstruation. While a person may choose to respect such restrictions, there is no physiological basis for them. Some men have believed that intercourse during menstruation creates physical distress for the woman. The clinical research of Masters and Johnson uncovered no such reaction. Quite the contrary, many women actively feel the need for sexual activity at those times, particularly during the last half of the period. While other women do not seek it, neither do they object to intercourse at this time provided they are not at peak flow and feel well. Some women find that masturbation to orgasm at the onset of menstruation serves to increase the rate of flow, reduce pelvic cramping, and relieve menstrual backaches. The release of pelvic vasocongestion following orgasm appears also to relieve the vasocongestion that accompanies menstruation.

If, however, the aesthetics of intercourse, physical discomfort, or a heavy flow distress a woman so that she prefers to wait a few days, this is her option and a man should respect it. At the same time, she may bring pleasure to him and buttress their relationship by voluntarily caressing him to orgasmic release.

Drugs and Sexual Response

Drugs play a major role in modern life. Almost everyone makes some use of drugs—prescription medications of all kinds, nonprescription drugstore remedies, alcohol, tobacco, and street drugs. Many of these drugs have effects on sexual response incidental to the intended effects, either increasing or decreasing sexual desire or capacity. In addition, there are many drugs that are used specifically for their real or imaginary sexual benefits.

Aphrodisiacs and Anaphrodisiacs

An *aphrodisiac* is any drug or substance that can produce in either sex an increased desire for coitus and ability to engage in it. An *anaphrodisiac* is anything that decreases sexual desire and response. Throughout the centuries men have searched for a reliable aphrodisiac—

something to aid in the seduction process, to boost potency, to heighten sexual sensation, and to produce more and better orgasms. Thousands of natural and synthetic drugs have been tried for this purpose. The perfect aphrodisiac—one that is both safe and effective in producing true sexual stimulation—has never been found, but the search goes on.

The most famous and most misunderstood of all aphrodisiacs is cantharidin—"Spanish fly." The drug is extracted from the ground-up bodies of a species of blister beetles, *Cantharis vesicatoria,* an iridescent insect native to southern Europe. The drug is a powerful irritant. Once swallowed, it reaches the bladder and is excreted in the urine. Burning the lining of the bladder and urethra as it passes, it causes a reflex stimulation of the sex organs. In the woman it causes erection of the clitoris, engorgement of the labia, and sensations in the vagina. In the man it causes an immense and painful erection, and may cause priapism. *Priapism* is a persistent (up to several days in duration) erection of the penis without sexual excitement. It is extremely painful. Equally toxic to both sexes, Spanish fly has effects ranging from mild irritation to extensive tissue destruction to death, depending on dosage.

A few years ago there was a flurry of publicity about the aphrodisiac qualities of L-dopa, used in treating Parkinson's disease. Further experience with L-dopa has established that its use may occasionally result in priapism, but very infrequently in true sexual stimulation. A much more common side effect of this drug is mental depression. Thus L-dopa would seem to be a very poor aphrodisiac.

Various chemicals have also been tried in attempts to *decrease* sexual desire—invariably other people's. Decreased sexual drive has been noted by men being treated with the female hormone estrogen. Tranquilizers have had some effectiveness in decreasing sex drive. Saltpeter, or potassium nitrate, although it decreases urine flow, has had little success as an anaphrodisiac, despite its wide reputation.

Alcohol

Despite its reputation as a sexual stimulant and its frequent success as an aid to seduction, alcohol is not really an aphrodisiac. What it may do, however, is diminish the inhibitions (or judgment) that block the sexual drive. Such a disinhibitory effect tends to break down sexual barriers and bring out fundamental traits of the personality. Many psychologists believe that alcohol (and other supposed aphrodisiacs) often stimulate sexuality by providing an excuse for behavior that might otherwise conflict with an individual's moral training or value system. As an ego defense, the guilt-producing behavior can always be blamed on the alcohol.

Heavy drinking causes a decrease in sexual activity by dulling sexual desire and decreasing the man's ability to achieve or sustain an erection. Many men's first episode of impotence is the result of heavy drinking. Alcoholics have the additional problem of physical deterioration, believed to result both from the direct effects of alcohol and from malnutrition, which often produces impotence and reduces interest in sex as well.

Marijuana

Marijuana is often credited with enhancing the pleasure of coitus and especially of orgasm. There are probably several factors working to produce this reputation. First is the general heightening of perception that occurs with social doses of marijuana. The sense of color, sound, and texture may be enhanced. Feelings of general bodily warmth may be experienced, along with a sense of empathy with others. Another factor is the distortion of the time sense, which can cause a sexual experience to seem to last much longer than it really does. Yet another is diminished inhibition, similar to the effect of a moderate amount of alchohol. Marijuana may also be mildly psychedelic, producing euphoria and relief from anxiety. Other users note a feeling of mild anxiety and decreased sexual satisfaction and performance. There is a higher incidence of impotence among marijuana users than among nonusers; thus it fails as a true aphrodisiac.

Amphetamines

Amphetamines, such as Benzedrine, Dexedrine, and Methedrine, are stimulant drugs prescribed for weight reduction, mild emotional depression and delay of sleep. The effects of amphetamines on sexuality related to dosage and are quite inconsistent. In the usual medically prescribed dosages, there is little or no effect on sexuality, though the drug-induced increase in vitality may help a shy or moderately depressed person overcome sexual difficulties.

Higher doses can greatly enhance the intensity of orgasm for some people. Although there is sometimes an ability to prolong erection in the male and pelvic thrusting in the female, however, orgasm may be difficult or impossible. A pleasure-pain correlation is often noted, with prolonged sexual activity leading to muscle spasm and literally raw genitalia (a physiologic effect of amphetamines is a drying of secretions, including vaginal secretions, contributing to pain during prolonged coitus). Some people sense a sudden new confidence, associated with great aggressiveness and increased sex drive, dispelling learned sexual shyness and inhibition (some consider this a true aphrodisiac effect), creating even a fantasy state. When ejaculation does occur, it may be unusually enjoyable. Amphetamine abusers on a "run" report greatest sexual activity at the beginning of the run; after several days, as exhaustion takes over, potency and sexual drive drastically diminish. The accompanying paranoia also lessens sexual interest. Extremely high doses often result in a total loss of interest in sex and impotence in men.

Cocaine

Cocaine, another powerful stimulant, was once used as a local anesthetic, but today it has no legitimate medical use. Cocaine is sought for its general stimulant effect, and in particular for its enhancement of orgasm. It is typically among the most expensive of the street drugs. It is extracted from the leaves of the coca plant and is usually taken by sniffing (snorting) or by injection. The injection of either cocaine or a large dose of an amphetamine often results in an instant orgasm-like "flash," highly prized by users of these drugs. The pleasurable effects of cocaine injection do not last more than five to ten minutes because of rapid elimination. Many men have spontaneous erection on injection. Some men report extremely painful priapism lasting twenty-four hours or longer; a few report multiple orgasm when engaging in intercourse after sniffing "coke." The repeated abuse of either cocaine or amphetamines is quite damaging to many of the vital organs.

Amyl Nitrite

Amyl nitrite has long been used to prevent and relieve heart seizures by quickly dilating the blood vessels leading to the heart. It has also been prized for its effects as a sexual stimulant. Relaxing smooth muscles, it produces a vasodilation of the genitourinary tract, giving a "body trip" with a feeling of warmth rushing to the pelvis and genitals. It also gives a "head trip" similar to the high obtained from sniffing cocaine, with the mind zooming off for three to four minutes. Inhaled from small ampules ("snappers" or "poppers"), it is used to stimulate the sex act either at intromission or just prior to climax. It causes perceptual distortions and may seem to prolong orgasm. Such unpleasant side effects as dizziness, headaches, and fainting may be experienced. It is dangerous unless used under the direction of a physician.

Psychedelics

Among the street drugs tried to improve sexual experiences are such psychedelics as LSD, mescaline, psilocybin, STP, and MDA. Although not true aphrodisiacs, they produce experiences varying all the way from decreased sexual desire and impotence to increased sexual desire and potency. The pleasure of sex under the influence of such drugs is directly related to positive feelings between the sexual partners and an appropriate setting.

LSD is the most commonly used of this group. If the sex act is being performed during the peak of the drug experience, the effects of the drug may be so extreme that the sex act may seem inconsequential. Most users do not engage in sex until the peak feelings have passed and they are returning to normal. During this time, any enhancement will be due mainly to the personal feelings of the individuals and the setting they are in.

Mescaline, psilocybin, and STP seem to produce unsatisfactory sexual experiences, and many who have engaged in sexual acts while under their influence do not feel the drugs enhanced the experiences.

MDA (which is chemically related to the amphetamines) is known as a strong sexual stimulant. It may arouse exotic fantasies and a compelling sex drive leading to prolonged intercourse.

Unfortunately, the psychedelics are not easily managed as sexual stimulants. A few micrograms too much may create physical incoordination and the inability to achieve the concentration necessary to consummate the sex act. When the psyche is soaring the soma is grounded, the pleasure of sex is lost.

Barbiturates

A group of very versatile drugs, barbiturates are widely used in the treatment of epilepsy, high blood pressure, insomnia, and mental disorders; they are also administered before and during surgery. In moderate doses they may stimulate pleasurable sex. Like alcohol, they diminish inhibitions. In higher doses a true sedative/hypnotic effect occurs. As with heavy drinking, physical coordination is directly impaired, reaction time slowed and physical movement awkward. If barbiturates are taken to relieve anxiety (as they sometimes are before engaging in group sex), sexual appetite and ability are invariably diminished. Barbiturates rarely contribute to a satisfactory sex act.

Heroin

Many people quite wrongly associate narcotic addiction with hypersexuality. We have all heard of the "drug-crazed sex maniac," but no one has ever seen one. Actually someone who is addicted to heroin or another true narcotic seldom has any interest in sex. When a person is "on the nod," heroin becomes a substitute for sex, and the heroin addict's sexual relationships dissolve into a nonphysical partnership dedicated to the daily procurement of the drug. Immediately after injection erection is common, but it quickly fades. "Strung out" couples rarely pursue intercourse to orgasm. In fact, little sex can be expected of the heroin addict; he feels the euphoric "total body orgasm" of injected heroin. When strung out, the addict may have intercourse on the average of once a month.

The addict is typically withdrawn from contact with other people, has reduced libido (sex drive), and is often impotent if sex is attempted. Such impotence can result from the depressant action of the drug on the nervous system, the poor physical health of the addict, his emotional state, or a combination of these factors. Female addicts often work as prostitutes, but this activity is favored solely because it is a quick way of getting the money necessary to support a "habit," not because of any great interest in sex. During "kicking" or "coming off" heroin, sexual interest reappears fairly rapidly. Sex is best for the addict when the "junk" wears off. Rather than stimulating pleasurable sex, heroin serves as a *replacement* for sex.

Sexual Dysfunction

9

The preceding chapter considered the usual sequence of events in male and female sexual responses. But many, perhaps most people do not at all times respond "by the book." Few people go through life without experiencing at least some instances of difficulty in their sexual responses. The difficulty may be as minor as that of the man who once in a great while is unable to achieve an erection or to delay ejaculation until his partner is satisfied, or the woman who on rare occasions is aroused but unable to achieve orgasm. Or the difficulty may persist for years.

This chapter has two goals. Its principal goal is reassurance: If you have experienced mild or occasional problems, you should know that most people have similar experiences at times and that most of these experiences are normal and predictable. Such knowledge is important because it can prevent the anxiety that can easily lead to more persistent and severe problems.

For the person who experiences severe problems, it is hoped that this chapter may provide the stimulus to seek professional help. An increasing number of people are seeking such help. It is doubtful that the true incidence of sexual problems has increased significantly, but our expectations and standards for mutually satisfactory sexual relations have definitely been elevated.

In the past, when women were not expected to enjoy sex, orgasmic difficulty or premature ejaculation were not viewed as problems. But today, when a woman hopes to achieve at least one orgasm in a majority of her sexual experiences and is expected by her partner to take an active enthusiastic role in the sexual relationship, such problems may be assigned considerable importance.

A barrier to the treatment of sexual problems is the reluctance of many people to admit that they might have such problems. Since a feeling of sexual adequacy is an important part of a positive self-concept, it is often difficult or impossible to admit to having a sexual problem. Yet whether or not sexual problems are consciously admitted, they act to diminish one's self-esteem. If people realized how common sexual problems really are, they might find it easier to seek help. A sexual problem should receive prompt professional help, just like any other health problem.

The term *dysfunction* is often used to describe sexual problems. (The *dys* means difficult.) This reflects the functional nature of most sexual problems. While some cases of sexual dysfunction do have definite physical or physiological (organic) causes, in the great majority of cases there is nothing basically or organically wrong—just impaired functioning, the result of some psychological factor. When the impediment is eliminated, normal function follows.

Causes of Sexual Dysfunction

Although the exact combinations of factors contributing to sexual dysfunction are as diverse and numerous as the individuals suffering from these problems, we can organize most of the causes into several basic groups. The problems of a particular individual may result from the cumulative effects of many causes. On the other hand, the roots of sexual dysfunction may not lie entirely within the individual; sexual problems very often result from difficulties in the interpersonal relationship of a couple. In the former case, the dysfunction is likely to manifest itself with any of the individual's sexual partners. In the latter case, the affected person may function normally with some partners but be unable to function at all with one or more specific partners.

Physical Causes of Dysfunction

We shall consider organic causes of dysfunction first, not because they are most common, but because anyone suffering sexual dysfunction should have appropriate tests, examinations, and evaluations to detect any physical causes that may exist. Some of these physical problems, in addition to interfering with sexual function, may result in death or disability if they are not corrected. Sexual dysfunction may be the first symptom of some really serious physical problem.

Hormonal Problems and Anemia Diabetes is a prime example of a life-threatening problem that may be signaled by sexual dysfunction. It commonly interferes with both male and female sexual response. Other hormonal problems may also cause dysfunction. There may be insufficient male or female hormones, for example. Or, thyroid hormone or other hormones may be deficient. Most hormonal deficiencies are relatively easy to detect and treat today. So is anemia (inadequate oxygen-carrying capacity of the blood), which also may cause sexual problems.

Fatigue People sometimes associate lovemaking exclusively with bedtime, often late at night when they are tired after a long day's work, and then wonder why they or their partners do not respond well.

Drug Abuse Excessive use of alcohol or other drugs is highly destructive of sexual responses, both as a direct result of the drug and as a result of the physical deterioration and malnutrition that often accompany its abuse. While small amounts of alcohol may facilitate lovemaking for otherwise inhibited persons, larger amounts may have disastrous sexual effects, especially on male potency.

Psychological Causes of Dysfunction

Most of us are to some extent sexually inhibited, and, in view of the antisexual atmosphere in which many of us were raised, it is a wonder we can function sexually at all. It is perhaps a testimonial to the strength of the sex drive and the resilience of the human spirit that we are able to function as well as we do.

Taboos and Inhibitions Every culture has its sexual taboos, which may or may not have valid factual bases. The incest taboo serves to preserve domestic harmony and thus is a strong force for social stability, while the masturbation taboo serves no constructive purpose. Sexual taboos are communicated in many ways, both obvious and subtle. An obvious communication is made when a five-year-old girl and boy are interruped in their perfectly normal and healthy pastime of examining each other's genitals and sternly scolded. A less obvious but equally inhibiting communication of taboo may take place through the tone of inflection used when speaking sexual words (or even through avoidance of discussion of sex). Sexual inhibitions are picked up from many sources. Parents are probably the prime inhibitors, since they usually exert greater influence on their children than any other adults and serve as role models for them. Religious institutions, schools, and peers also play important roles in sexual inhibition.

Excessive inhibition can play havoc with a sexual relationship, especially when one partner is more inhibited than the other, or is inhibited in a different way than the other. There may be serious disagreements regarding oral sex, sex during menstruation, sex in the daytime, in the living room, when the children may be awake, and so on and so on. Some of us are so inhibited that a satisfactory sexual relationship is simply impossible.

A well-qualified counselor can be of much help in overcoming sexual inhibitions. While the specific technique applied varies with the patient, the therapist, and the type of inhibition, there are several general approaches. One is to encourage the patient to verbalize the inhibition, explore its possible sources and its effects on sexual relationships, and then point out its lack of a valid factual basis. It must be emphasized that inhibitions are not easily overcome, since they often date back to early childhood and may be thoroughly integrated into one's personality. Some therapists employ disinhibition techniques that may include role playing, role reversal, and intensive exposure to sexually explicit films, books, and pictures.

Blockage of Sexual Response A major cause of sexual dysfunction is blockage of the sexual response by emotional factors that may themselves have nothing to do with sex. Such emotions as fear, anger, anxiety, and hostility may effectively block normal sexual response. The problem is compounded when initial sexual dysfunction creates fear of further failure, fear that almost ensures further failure. A vicious cycle may be set in motion, spiraling downward to total sexual failure. Often only competent therapy can break this cycle. It is often said that success breeds success and failure breeds failure; nowhere is this saying more valid than in sexual functioning.

Effects of Sexual Dysfunction

Sexual dysfunction may have many effects. In addition to its obvious effects on one's sexual relationships, it may influence one's nonsexual relationships with the opposite sex, especially if the dysfunction is associated with fear of or hostility or resentment toward the other sex. Since a feeling of sexual adequacy is an important part of a positive self-concept, sexual difficulties may have a negative effect on the way one feels about oneself. Low self-esteem is inevitably reflected in behavior patterns. The individual may avoid the other sex, or engage in a round of sexual or nonsexual "proving" of masculinity or femininity.

Sexual dysfunction in marriage may be both the cause and the result of other interpersonal problems between the couple. A vicious cycle is often set up in which sexual dysfunction leads to hostilities that result in even more serious sexual dysfunction. Either partner may feel angry, unloved, rejected, and sexually inadequate, and may, as an ego defense, become involved in extramarital affairs in order to confirm sexual attractiveness or adequacy. The marital relationship may continue to deteriorate until something is done to break the vicious cycle. Professional help (a marriage counselor or other therapist) is often necessary at this point.

The most common physical effect of sexual dysfunction is discomfort resulting from congestion of pelvic blood vessels dilated through sexual arousal but without the relief of orgasm. This problem can occur in either sex. But any physical effects of sexual dysfunction seem minor in comparison with its emotional and interpersonal implications.

Female Sexual Dysfunction

Common forms of female sexual dysfunction include hyporesponsiveness (lack of interest in sex), difficulty in attaining orgasm, and painful coitus (dyspareunia). While these symptoms might seem to indicate totally different types of problems, their underlying causes are often quite similar. Sexual dysfunction is a constant problem for perhaps 15 or 20 percent of women, while transient or situational dysfunction occurs at times during the life of almost every woman.

While the sexual dysfunction of a woman may not be so visible as the flaccid penis of the impotent male, it may be just as destructive to her sense of sexual adequacy and total personal worth and to her relationships with men.

Most problems in sexual response, in either sex, have psychological rather than physical causes. The basic biological drive and capacity for sexual satisfaction are usually present, but blocked by psychological factors that activate the sympathetic nervous system to inhibit sexual response. Since some sexual problems, however, are caused by biological factors, such as diabetes and other hormonal disorders, the first step for any person concerned about sexual response should be a complete physical examination to discover or rule out any possible biological cause.

Many psychological factors have been implicated in female sexual dysfunction. Fear often causes inadequate response. There may be fear of men, fear of the penis, residual fear of punishment from childhood conditioning by overly strict parents, fear of pregnancy, fear of sexually transmitted disease, fear of being physically or emotionally hurt, fear of loss of identity or loss of control, fear of being exploited, or fear of being physically or emotionally close to someone. Hostility is another major obstacle to female response. It may be hostility toward men in general or toward a specific man. Many women who are not sexually aroused by their husbands are highly responsive to other men.

There are many situational conditions or temporary emotional conflicts that may block sexual response: noise, lack of privacy, fatigue, anxiety over problems of any kind.

Sex is the most intimate of human interactions, during which each partner is uniquely vulnerable to the other. To be fully sexually responsive requires total confidence that one will not be physically or emotionally hurt during this time of vulnerability or as a consequence of it. A previously responsive and orgasmic woman may become less responsive after being emotionally hurt a few times in her relationships with men. As an ego defense she begins to avoid full emotional commitment for fear that she may once again be disappointed and hurt. Similarly, a woman who has been emotionally deprived as a child, perhaps raised by cold and unloving parents, may as an adult find herself unable to take the risk of disappointment that is inherent in any close interpersonal relationship. In either case, the woman consciously or unconsciously decides that, rather than love a man and take the chance of being rejected, she will reject him first.

The male's role in causing female dysfunction deserves further emphasis. Many men are really directly responsible for their partners' lack of responsiveness. Some men never display any trace of love or tenderness to a woman, then cannot understand why she is not instantly aroused when they want sex. Other men are themselves so sexually inhibited that they destroy a woman's potential for sexual pleasure. Their inhibition may prevent them from adequately stimulating the woman with precoital sex play and varied sexual techniques. They may approach sex in a serious rather than a joyful manner. They may suffer from frequent premature ejaculation. They may express shock or displeasure at any sexual initiative taken by a woman, or any other form of "immodesty." After enough disappointing and frustrating experiences, a woman often avoids further psychic wounds by becoming sexually unresponsive —at least to that particular man.

Female Orgasmic Dysfunction

The frequency with which a woman may experience orgasm ranges from never in her whole life through any means of stimulation to many times nearly every day through intercourse and/or masturbation. Few women are to be found at either extreme; most are somewhere in between. Very few women achieve orgasm in every single instance of sexual intercourse. To do so a woman would have to be a highly responsive person in perfect health with no emotional problems, no situational difficulties. Her partner would need adequate ejaculatory control, and an excellent relationship would be necessary between the two.

The orgasmic expectations of women likewise vary. One woman might be concerned if she failed to achieve orgasm in 10 percent of her sexual experiences while another might be totally unconcerned though she had never experienced an orgasm. The expectations of men regarding female orgasm also vary. A less enlightened man might not care whether his partner experienced orgasm. Or he might, unrealistically, expect multiple orgasms from his mate every time they made love. The more enlightened male would probably hope that his partner would reach orgasm in most of her sexual experiences, but would also understand that even a highly responsive woman may not always desire orgasm or may not reach orgasm at time because of fatigue or temporary emotional factors.

With the popular media's extreme emphasis on female orgasm during the past few years, many men now judge their own sexual adequacy on the basis of the orgasmic achievement of their sexual partners. While a woman's lack of orgasm may quite truly be the result of her partner's sexual dysfunction (such as his premature ejaculation) or his poor lovemaking technique, it may also be quite unrelated to the sexual adequacy of her lover. Many women, in fact, have orgasmic difficulty with any and all men with whom they engage in sexual intercourse, regardless of each man's sexual adequacy.

Female orgasmic response is a major concern today in many relationships. It may be a realistic concern, based on actual orgasmic difficulty, or an unrealistic concern, based on the undue expectations of either the woman or her lover. Regardless of the legitimacy of the concern, it may be strong enough to be a source of conflict within a relationship, to cause feelings of sexual inadequacy in either or both partners, or to lead either or both partners to seek other sexual outlets.

The question of how often a woman should expect to achieve orgasm is as much an individual matter as that of how often a couple wants to make love. Obviously, no absolute answer is possible or even desirable. Authorities certainly vary in their answers to this question. Though this must not be taken as a performance standard by which sexual adequacy is judged, many sexual behaviorists feel that for most couples a female orgasmic response in at least half of lovemaking sessions helps to assure each partner of feelings of sexual adequacy and to maintain a healthy sexual relationship between the two.

Female orgasmic difficulties may have many sources. Some relevant questions in attempting to determine the cause of a particular woman's problems include: Is she totally *anorgasmic* (without orgasm)? If so, has she always been so? If not, can the onset of the problem be related to any event or change in her life situation? Can she achieve orgasm through masturbation? If she has several sexual partners, is the problem confined to any particular one or more than one? The possibility of a physical cause should be explored. In the absence of such a cause, there should be an examination of the woman's attitude toward herself, toward sex, toward men in general, and toward her particular sexual partner or partners.

Female orgasmic response is to some extent learned and conditioned—more so than male orgasm. Some women, especially those who are more sexually inhibited, have simply never concentrated their attention upon their sexual responses enough to learn their own pattern of orgasmic response. Masturbation often proves useful in such cases as a means of learning one's own responses.

As in all male and female sexual dysfunctions, it seems the more concern one feels over the problem, the worse it becomes. If the lack of female orgasm has become a major issue in a relationship, then the stress associated with this problem almost guarantees its continued existence. It is in a situation such as this that the services of a well-qualified therapist may be essential.

Male Sexual Dysfunctions

The incidence of sexual dysfunction in men is quite high. Since men, perhaps even more frequently than women, often interpret sexual failure as total personal failure, sexual dysfunction may assume great importance to a man.

Impotence

Impotence, also called erectile dysfunction, is defined in many ways. Here are a few: "the inability to achieve and/or maintain an erection of quality sufficient to accomplish coital connection"; "a persistent inability to maintain an erection sufficient to allow orgasm and ejaculation to be accomplished during coitus"; "the inability to sexually satisfy a normally responsive female in coitus." Some authorities thus include premature ejaculation as a form of impotence, while others consider it a separate problem. We prefer to follow the lead of Masters and Johnson in defining impotence in terms of erectile incompetence and in considering premature ejaculation a separate problem. For many men, however, the two problems coexist and are the result of the same cause.

Cases of impotence can be classified as either primary (successful coitus has never been achieved) or secondary (impotence in a previously potent man). The incidence of impotence depends on how the term is defined. Only a few men are totally impotent throughout their lives. Much more common is transient impotence resulting from some temporary emotional problem. On any given day many men are suffering from some degree of temporary impotence. In fact, it would be an unusual man who could go through his entire lifetime without having had at least a few experiences of impotence.

Causes of Impotence Impotence may be caused by physical (biological) or psychological factors, or a combination of the two. The great majority of cases (80 to 90 percent) are mainly psychological in origin, but before automatically treating impotence as a psychological problem, it is important to rule out any possible physical cause. In general, primary impotence is more often associated with biological factors than is secondary impotence, but either can have biological or psychological causes. Much more revealing than coital success in determining the cause of impotence is the incidence of erection. Many men who are impotent when attempting coitus do have erections at other times, such as while asleep or upon awakening in the morning. (As metioned earlier, erection commonly accompanies the rapid-eye-movement [REM] phase of sleep, which often occurs just before awakening in the morning.) Many impotent men are also able to achieve erection and masturbate to orgasm. Such cases of impotence are almost certainly of psychological origin. In contrast, if morning erections seldom or never occur, and if erection through masturbation is impossible, then there is a strong probability that a physical factor is causing the impotence. A very few men go through life without ever experiencing an erection. Such cases, called *absolute impotence*, are almost surely of biological origin.

Many physical factors may cause impotence. Fatigue and heavy use of alcohol or other drugs are prime causes. Many prescribed drugs, such as tranquilizers, may also cause temporary impotence. The possibility of hormonal problems must also be considered. Diabetes is a common cause of impotence. Insufficient hormone secretion by the pituitary gland (gonadotropic hormones) or the testes (testosterone) will also cause impotence. There may be abnormalities in the sex chromosomes. Certain surgical procedures, such as those necessary in cancers of the prostate or colon, are followed by a high incidence of impotence. The normal aging process is usually associated with some decline in potency, though there is great variation among men in this respect. An aging man is likely to feel great concern over declining potency. His concern tends to compound the problem, for the fear of impotence is, ironically, one of the most important psychological causes of impotence.

A multitude of psychological factors can act, either singly or in various combinations, to produce impotence. There is no one underlying psychological conflict present in all cases, nor is there any impotence-causing conflict that is not also present in many normally potent men. In fact, the same case of impotence may be interpreted quite differently by different therapists, depending on the type of training they have had.The Freudian psychoanalyst and the behavior therapist, for example, would almost inevitably come to entirely different conclusions.

Freud believed that some men held their wives in such high esteem (and sex in such low regard) that they could not be potent with them, though thy were fully potent with prostitutes or women who were in some way seen as degraded. He also stressed the unresolved oedipal conflict (sexual attraction to the parent of the opposite sex) as leading to unacceptable incestuous fantasies when a sexual experience with a good mother-like woman is imminent. Another prominent theme in the psychoanalytic literature is castration anxiety, in which the vagina is equated with a "castrating" instrument. The theme of the toothed vagina is found in the myths of primitive people in all parts of the world. (If the vagina were indeed equipped with teeth, the damage it might cause would be amputation, not castration, but the term "castration anxiety" is so firmly entrenched that there seems to be no hope of changing it.) Later psychoanalysts have broadened the concept of castration anxiety to a fear of total obliteration or annihilation of self.

The first instance of impotence for a man often occurs at a time when he has been drinking or using other drugs, is under some great temporary emotional stress, or is fatigued. Perhaps he attains an erection, but loses it halfway through coitus or during the preliminary sex play. You may be sure that the next time he attempts coitus, he is going to be worried about his potency. Remember that erection of the penis is controlled through the parasympathetic branch of the autonomic nervous system. The autonomic nervous system is not under direct conscious control; its actions are greatly influenced by the emotional state of the individual. The parasympathetic branch is stimulated by a feeling of well-being and inhibited by such emotions as fear, anxiety, and anger. It is quite impossible to attain an erection by conscious will if the basic emotional state is such that the parasympathetic nervous system is being inhibited. Thus the fear of failure can set up a cycle in which failure is assured.

Other sources of impotence-causing anxiety include fear of being detected in an extramarital affair (impotence may occur with either woman or with both), fear of premature ejaculation, fear of being judged sexually inferior, fear of causing pregnancy, and fear of sexually transmitted disease.

Other psychological causes of impotence include resentment toward the sexual partner, as in the case of a passive man who is dominated by an aggressive wife, or the converse situation, in which a man feels a woman is overly dependent upon him. Impotence is sometimes seen as an unconscious means of "punishing" a woman by denying the fulfillment of her sexual needs. There may be hostility toward women in general, conscious or unconscious negative feelings or disgust about sex, or a variety of neurotic personality disturbances.

Premature Ejaculation When is ejaculation premature? Anyone would agree that ejaculation before or immediately after vaginal penetration is premature. But what about ejaculation after two minutes? After five minutes? What about ejaculation after the partner has had one orgasm but would like to have several more? What about a man who can maintain erection for fifty minutes, but whose partner needs an hour of intensive coitus to reach orgasm? Obviously there can be no clear-cut definition of premature ejaculation. Masters and Johnson (1966) consider that a man has a problem of premature ejaculation if he cannot delay ejaculation long enough to satisfy his normally responsive partner in at least half of their coital experiences. Perhaps ejaculation is best considered premature if it seems so to either sexual partner.

Indeed, premature ejaculation has not always been recognized as a problem. There was a time when a man might have been proud of the speed with which he ejaculated, as a supposed sign of great virility. As long as women were not really expected to enjoy coitus, it made little difference how long coitus was sustained.

Very few men are likely to get through life without at least a few instances of "premature" ejaculation. In fact, under certain conditions, premature ejaculation must be considered an entirely normal and predictable physiological event. It is unrealistic to expect a young man who has been without any sexual release for many days to withhold his ejaculation while his partner thrusts vigorously and incessantly in her effort to achieve her own orgasm. Similarly, the first act of coitus with a new and highly exciting woman may very well result in premature ejaculation.

How, then, do you distinguish normal premature ejaculation from the problem variety? If a man has regular and frequent intercourse with the same woman, and it often ends in premature ejaculation, it is a problem. In such a case, there may be underlying psychological causes quite similar to those causing impotence: fears and love conflicts; hostility toward the woman (premature ejaculation is a means of denying her sexual satisfaction); guilt about sex (premature ejaculation serves to "get it over with"); feelings of sexual inadequacy (premature ejaculation proves that the penis is still "working").

Ejaculation, like erection, is controlled through the autonomic (involuntary) branch of the nervous system. Thus ejaculation cannot be controlled by direct conscious effort ("willpower"). While erection is inhibited by the sympathetic division, ejaculation is the result of a burst of sympathetic activity. Thus the same emotional stresses that produce impotence can also result in premature ejaculation. In fact, the same man often experiences both problems—erection may be attained with much difficulty, only to be lost with almost immediate ejaculation.

There is no shortage of advice for the man who is bothered by premature ejaculation. If premature ejaculation is persistent, there should be, first of all, a physical examination for such physical causes as urethritis, prostatitis, cystitis (bladder infection), and diabetes. If no physical cause can be found, then psychotherapy is often recommended. As with impotence, if there is a regular sexual partner, it is important that she be included in the therapeutic process. Masters and Johnson, in their book *Human Sexual Inadequacy,* take a directly physical approach, recommending that the woman stimulate the man's penis manually almost to the point of orgasm, then tightly squeeze the base of the glans ("head") of the penis. Practiced repeatedly, as detailed in their book, this technique often solves long-term problems of premature ejaculation.

If premature ejaculation occurs in one of the "normal" situations described earlier, then the male is likely to be highly enough aroused so that a second erection can be attained in a few minutes and, with seminal pressure reduced, prolonged intercourse should be possible. If premature ejaculation occurs repeatedly in second and subsequent erections, then the premature ejaculation is of the problem type and professional counsel should be sought. In many cases, reerection after premature ejaculation is impossible, even in a young man who should be capable of a second erection, illustrating the close relationship between premature ejaculation and impotence.

Many other suggestions are offered for the prevention of premature ejaculation. These are of value only when there is no serious underlying psychological cause. Some physicians prescribe mild tranquilizers for their patients who complain of premature ejaculation. Some recommend that a topical ointment containing a local anesthetic be applied over the glans of the penis to reduce the sensory stimulus. A similar effect can sometimes be obtained by wearing a condom (rubber) over the penis. Regular sex partners can learn to prolong coitus by holding very still for a few seconds whenever ejaculation seems imminent. Some men learn to fantasize about nonsexual objects when ejaculation threatens. Premature ejaculation is sometimes associated with inadequate foreplay and with penetration of the vagina while it is still poorly lubricated and tight; the increased friction makes control difficult. Through experimenting with different coital positions, a couple may find one or more in which ejaculatory control is improved. Positions with the woman lying, sitting, or kneeling over the man are sometimes helpful. There are really very few men in whom premature ejaculation cannot be successfully prevented in some way, though professional help may be necessary.

Retarded Ejaculation Much less common than premature ejaculation, but certainly not rare, is its opposite, retarded ejaculation. In some men ejaculation occurs only with great effort, or not at all. In coitus such a man may struggle to ejaculate until he exhausts himself and his partner. Coitus is usually accompanied by emotional withdrawal and reduced sexual sensations. The man frequently feels emotionally detached from his sexual partner and as if his penis were anesthetized.

Retarded ejaculation may occur when the male is very tired and doesn't have the ready energy required for ejaculation. It may also be due to damage to the nerves controlling ejaculation. Usually, however, it is the result of psychological factors. The personality trait most often associated with this problem is a paranoid tendency. There are two factors characteristic of paranoid males that sometimes act to produce this symptom. One is an excessive concern with masculinity, derived from an everpresent fear of being forced into submission by a more dominant woman. The other is the "paranoid rage," a strong impulse to commit violence. Since ejaculation results in loss of erection, it can be seen as a threat to masculinity. This threat triggers the rage, which acts through the autonomic nervous system to prevent ejaculation.

Persistent retarded ejaculation is usually treated through psychotherapy, in which the goal is to reduce the patient's tremendous concern with his masculinity and his accompanying fear and rage.

Dysfunctions of Either Sex

Dyspareunia

Dyspareunia, or painful coitus, may afflict either sex, though it is a more common complaint among women than among men. It may range from minor irritation to a condition so painful that intercourse is completely avoided.

In either sex, dyspareunia may result from any of a variety of either physical or emotional causes. A physician's careful examination should reveal any possible cause. In the female, dyspareunia may result from any inflammation of the vagina, labia, or clitoris as a result of infection, mechanical or chemical irritation, or allergy. Some women suffer from a "thin" vaginal lining, related to a low estrogen level, an especially common condition following menopause. There may be remnants of an unusually tough hymen, childbirth injuries, or other anatomical abnormalities. All of these physical problems are correctable, either with medications or by minor corrective surgery.

Physical causes of male dyspareunia include a tight foreskin that retracts painfully during erection or coitus, urethritis, or any infection or inflammation of the penis. Herpes simplex virus lesions on the shaft or glans of the penis, for example, may cause extreme pain during coitus. Less commonly, there may be painful downward curvature (chordee) of the penis when it is erect, an impairment frequently resulting from damage occuring in the later stages of untreated gonorrhea.

When physical factors are ruled out, dyspareunia may often be associated with emotional factors. It should be regarded as part of the total complex of sexual dysfunction. In the female, emotional factors may cause the muscles of the vaginal opening to contract tightly (vaginismus), or there may be so little sexual arousal that the production of vaginal lubricant is inadequate to prevent coital pain. The sources of emotionally caused dyspareunia in the male are usually less obvious, but the pain is equally real. The treatment of emotionally caused dyspareunia is usually of the same general nature as that for other forms of sexual dysfunction.

Compulsive Sexuality

Common among both sexes are people whose sex lives consist of an endless series of brief encounters with persons of the opposite sex. Seldom is any level of emotional intimacy established, and there is often a hollow or "something is missing" feeling. Though there may be a high frequency of sexual intercourse, which may seem more than adequate from the "performance" standpoint, there is often no real emotional satisfaction.

In men, this problem is sometimes called the Don Juan complex when the emphasis is on the number of sexual partners, and satyriasis when the emphasis is on the frequency of sexual contact. The term "nymphomania" is sometimes applied to women who seem to have unusually high numbers of heterosexual encounters. (A nymphomaniac has also been described as "a woman who has a higher sex drive than you do.")

Several personality traits are commonly associated with compulsive sexuality. The foremost is probably a feeling (which can be unconscious) of sexual or total personal inadequacy. There is a need for constantly "proving" the ability to attract lovers and function sexually. But regardless of the number of lovers attracted or orgasms reached, the fear of inadequacy remains.

Another commonly associated trait is a fear of intimacy. Many people, perhaps as a result of past emotional hurts or lack of self-esteem, lack the confidence required to establish a close trusting relationship with another person. Lacking intimacy, their sexual relationship always seem incomplete, so the search for satisfaction must continue. Many people have been raised in sexually repressive atmospheres. Sexual guilt or inhibition, perhaps as a result of childhood conditioning, may act to deny one of sexual satisfaction, even though full physiological orgasm may occur.

Finally, compulsive sexuality may be a part of a broader antisocial or sociopathic personality development. Someone with an antisocial personality is unable to postpone immediate pleasure or gratification of an impulse, lacks the capacity for maintaining a close relationship with another person, and feels no guilt or anxiety over antisocial acts. In addition to compulsive sexuality, there may be a history of job problems and perhaps legal difficulties.

Like other forms of sexual dysfunction, compulsive sexuality can often be treated successfully by a qualified therapist. Treatment may involve building a sense of personal or sexual adequacy, developing the ability to establish intimacy with another person, or extinguishing feelings of guilt or inhibition. People with antisocial personalities generally require more basic therapy, since their compulsive sexuality is just one symptom of a total personality disorder.

Body Anxieties

Very few people are entirely satisfied with every aspect of their bodies. The anxieties are especially pronounced in regard to any part of the anatomy that has sexual implications. Many women have anxieties about the appearance of their bodies. While the most common source of anxiety is breast size, women also worry about many other features of their anatomy—waistline, hips, legs, stretch marks from pregnancy. Since the entertainment and advertising media have created an exaggerated and stereotyped concept of the "ideal" figure, many women feel inadequate in comparison with the girl in the centerfold of *Playboy*. A woman may become so obsessed with her "inadequacy" that her sexual pleasure is diminished. She may even be reluctant to engage in sexual relationships or interact with men in any way out of fear of rejection.

In this nation of breast worshipers, the female breast must be considered an organ of much psychological significance. To have physically acceptable breasts is a normal desire, and the emotional implications of this desire must not be underestimated. As a result of the *Playboy* type of publicity, with its emphasis on ample breast development, many attractive women of normal breast size suffer almost paralyzing self-consciousness focused on the feeling that their breasts are too small. At the opposite end of the spectrum are women with extreme breast development, who suffer agonies of embarrassment because their breasts are much larger than average.

In reality, there is no relationship between breast size and sexual adequacy and feminity. The "flat" woman is in no way sexually inferior or inadequate, and the woman with melon-sized breasts is not necessarily more highly sexed than others. Their breast size has no relation to their sexual pleasure or that of their lovers (though their resultant feelings of inferiority may do so). Yet many women are willing to take drastic measures, such as silicone injections or implants, in order to give the appearance of larger breasts, or operations to reduce their size. The injection of silicone into the breasts is very dangerous and should never be done. The surgical implantation of molded silicone presents less physical hazard but is not without some danger. The same is true of breast-reduction operations. The hazards of these procedures must be weighed against their potential value. They can be recommended only in those few cases in which breast anxieties are so severe that they cannot be overcome through psychotherapy. Even then, not every woman will accept silicone implants as "self" to the extent that her feeling of inadequacy is overcome. Most of the other methods promoted for breast enlargement are ineffective but at least relatively harmless. This category includes special diets, development creams, massaging devices, vacuum cups, and so forth. There are exercises that will keep the breasts firm and help to prevent sagging, but they have no effect on size.

Many men suffer needless anxiety regarding the size of the penis. Some worry that it may be too small to satisfy a woman; some fear that it may be too large to be accommodated by the vagina. All of these fears are made needless by the nature of the vagina and of female sexual sensitivity. The size of the penis has little to do with the sexual satisfaction of the man himself or of the woman, and so does circumcision or the lack of it. Sexual technique, experience, and attitude are the important things.

The diameter of the vagina stretches to fit the size of the penis. Even after a woman has had several children, the vagina usually remains small enough in diameter to hold even the smallest penis firmly. On the other hand, the vagina is capable of stretching enough to allow the passage of a baby, so a large penis will certainly create no problem.

As far as length of penis is concerned, there are very few sensory receptors in the deeper part of the vagina. These receptors are concentrated on the clitoris and labia and outer vagina. As a result, it is difficult or impossible for a woman to feel the difference between a long penis and a short one.

Incidentally, when men and women are highly concerned about the body measurements of their sexual partners, it is usually their own sexual adequacy that they are worried about. This may be true, for example, of a man who places great importance on the breast size of his partner, or the woman who searches for a man with an unusually large penis. Sexually adequate and confident men and women are usually more concerned with their partners' personality traits than with their measurements. And certainly the pleasure each partner derives from a sexual relationship is influenced much more by personality traits, a sense of intimacy, sexual technique, and freedom from inhibitions than by body measurements.

Reaction to a Partner's Dysfunction

Of all human interactions, we are the most vulnerable during lovemaking. Either partner has the power to enhance or diminish the other. Those who care at all about the welfare of their sexual partners will want to react to their partners' dysfunctions with the utmost tact and consideration. In such a situation we may feel hurt and rejected, and doubtful about our own sexual adequacy. A partner's sexual dysfunction may threaten our egos. Unconsciously, or perhaps consciously, we think:

Maybe she had no orgasm because my penis is too small. Maybe he can't get an erection because I'm too fat. Maybe he doesn't love me any more. Maybe I just don't turn her on. So to protect our own egos and sense of sexual adequacy we often place the "blame" on the one suffering the dysfunction. Which, of course, doesn't help him or her at all, since any sense of sexual adequacy has already been shattered by the dysfunction.

Another reaction is often retaliation: We have been hurt so we hurt in return. We may resort to name-calling ("frigid"), to ridicule, to unfavorable comparisons with other lovers, to accusations of infidelity. Such reactions will call forth enough anxiety and hostility to practically ensure that our partner's next sexual efforts will again result in dysfunction. Once a person becomes preoccupied with a fear of sexual failure, normal sexual response is almost impossible.

On the other hand, an understanding and reassuring response may prevent the development of a serious sexual dysfunction. It might be as simple as a sincerely felt and expressed "That's all right, we'll have plenty of other chances." It might be an invitation to talk about whatever is bothering the partner (and it may be entirely nonsexual). Or it might be a period of just holding one another with no attempt at intercourse. Above all, open and honest communication of feelings, with no accusations or placing of blame, is the key to a satisfactory sexual relationship.

Treatment of Dysfunction

Since sexual problems most often have psychological causes, their treatment usually involves psychotherapy, counseling, or behavior therapy. Treatment with hormones or other medications is seldom effective. A logical and important first step, is a thorough checkup to detect any possible underlying physical causes.

If no physical problem is apparent, a well-qualified therapist (psychiatrist, clinical psychologist, or marriage counselor) should be consulted. Since the selection of a therapist is critical (there are many poorly qualified individuals in this field), it is advisable to obtain a referral or recommendation from a family physician or other health professional. In many areas there are tax-supported or privately funded family counseling and mental health clinics that treat problems in sexual function.

A traditional approach to treating sexual problems is psychoanalysis (an extensive probing of the unconscious mind), but this process is slow and expensive and the results may be disappointing. The needs of the majority of patients are probably better met through nonpsychoanalytic methods. There are many approaches. One is to attempt to correct faulty attitudes about sexuality by replacing inhibiting attitudes with more positive feelings. Since faulty attitudes may present as great a problem in the partner as in the patient, both partners are often brought into the therapeutic situation. It is important that sex partners learn to communicate openly, for many sexual problems are partly the result of inadequate expression of the feelings of each partner. Behavior therapy, based on the idea that behavior is determined by modifiable stimulus-response patterns, centers around the reconditioning of responses to given stimuli, with the goal of developing more appropriate responses. It is often quite successful. The treatment of sexual dysfunction ideally combines both educational and psychological aspects.

Among the more successful sex therapists are those trained by Masters and Johnson, or whose methods are patterned after theirs. These methods involve a combination of specific coital and noncoital techniques and supportive psychotherapy for the male-female relationship. The relationship and the interaction of the couple are the primary focus of this method. The following aspects of treatment are common to all dysfunctions:

1. The partners are treated together for two weeks. If they are from out of town, they reside at a nearby hotel. Individuals lacking regular sexual partners are sometimes treated through the use of surrogate partners employed by the clinics.

2. A male-female therapy team guides and interprets the experiences of the couple.

3. Extensive history-taking and individual and couple interviews contribute to an understanding of the problem and create a comfortable atmosphere for discussion and treatment.

4. A medical history and examination search for any possible physical causes.

5. During round-table discussions the therapists impart sex information to combat misconceptions.

6. In important *sensate focus* exercises, couples learn to feel and respond pleasureably to simple touching and stroking and to communicate the kind of sensory experiences they find pleasurable.

7. The couple engages in daily discussions with the therapists, during which the next sequence of sexual behavior, to be conducted in private by the couple, is described.

In addition to these general methods, specific modes of therapy are applied to specific problems. In every case it is essential to establish or reestablish verbal communication between the partners in regard to sexual feelings. Every effort is made to remove the burden of performance anxiety through focusing on noncoital sensate pleasures, enabling each partner to think and feel sexually with no thought about performance. The chief goal is to establish communication between the partners and focus their attention on each other rather than on themselves as spectators at their own sexual performances. Sexual response is just like breathing—the less you think about it, the more normally it functions.

Variations in Sexual Behavior

10

Human sexuality is reflected and expressed in an amazing array of behavior patterns. As it is apparently human nature to want to categorize everything, many efforts have been made to determine what constitutes "normal" sexual behavior. There are many approaches from which one might attempt to determine the "normality" of a particular form of sexual behavior. Not surprisingly, the conclusion reached would vary with the approach. Among the points of reference from which behavior may be judged are state laws, religious or other moral codes, prevalent cultural values, the effects of a particular form of behavior upon society, and its effects upon the individual. There is also the rather simplistic approach of defining normal behavior as the most common or "average" behavior.

In the area of sex, the law does not take the lead in suggesting and implementing changes in morality, attitudes, and behavior patterns. Rather the lawmakers usually change the laws when they become aware that social change has already occurred. In other words, the laws are merely a reflection of is already being done. Additionally, laws relating to sexual behavior tend to inflict the values of the majority upon the minority, thus equating "more common" with "more normal." Carried to ridiculous extremes (just for the purpose of illustration), such logic might result in outlawing any sexual behavior other than masturbation (the most universal sexual practice) or make virginity beyond a certain age illegal, since statistically virginity could be considered deviant behavior.

In few areas of social behavior is there such a dichotomy between stated values and actual behavior as in the areas of sex. Many people apparently have one set of standards for everyone else and a somewhat more flexible standard for themselves. While recent years have seen some improvement in this respect, there remains considerable hypocrisy regarding sexual behavior. Further, many sex acts that were culturally prohibited a few years ago as being immoral or sinful are still rejected today, only now we find them unacceptable because they represent deviant behavior. In our enlightenment, we have merely replaced the concept of sin with the concept of illness.

Even the field of psychology is of only limited help in defining normal sexual behavior. The ideas of any professional in this field would depend to a great extent on the school of thought to which he belonged. A behaviorist would probably view a particular form of behavior quite differently than a dynamic or analytic psychologist, who in turn would disagree with each other.

What this all comes down to is that, while some forms of sexual behavior, such as forcible rape, are almost universally condemned as violations of the rights of other people, other forms of behavior, such as homosexuality, meet with a wide range of acceptance, even among mental health professionals. Thus we prefer the term "variation" in behavior to the more judgmental terms "deviation" and "perversion." In the remainder of this chapter, we shall consider some of the more important variations in sexual behavior.

Sexual Orientation

Sexual orientation (or preference) may lie anywhere along a continuum ranging from exclusively *heterosexual* orientation (attraction only to people of the opposite sex) to exclusively *homosexual* orientation (attraction only to people of the same sex). Great numbers of people (some authorities say all of us) fall somewhere between these extremes and are to some degree *bisexually* oriented (feeling sexual attraction to people of both sexes).

Estimates of the number of individuals who have each of these sexual orientations vary considerably, depending on where each authority draws the lines between heterosexuality, bisexuality, and homosexuality. The increase in group sex has further complicated these distinctions, since any voluntary sexual experience involving three or more people almost invariably includes some homosexual contact.

While without doubt many people have always felt some degree of bisexual attraction, recent years have seen a great increase in the number of people who actually experience bisexual activity. This is especially true in the more cosmopolitan areas of the United States and Europe. The reasons for this phenomenon are not yet fully understood.

It appears that somewhere between 4 and 10 percent of our adult population are exclusively or almost exclusively homosexual in orientation. It should be noted that one's choice of sex partners does not always accurately reflect actual sexual orientation, as some people of primarily homosexual orientation marry or date heterosexually for social or professional reasons. Many authorities give higher estimates of the incidence of homosexual orientation for males than for females. This may or may not be the actual case; some authorities estimate the incidence of homosexuality to be about the same in both sexes. In addition to adult homosexual orientation, many young people (estimated at 25 to 40 percent of both males and females) pass through a period of transient homosexual feeling and/or activity during the preadolescent or adolescent years before establishing a heterosexual adult orientation. In a culture that still largely condemns homosexual orientation, this passing homosexual phase causes residual guilt feelings or lingering doubt about sexual orientation in some primarily heterosexual people, but it is a common step in psychosexual development. It should be accepted as such without guilt or anxiety about one's adult sexual orientation.

Homosexual Behavior Patterns

People of primarily homosexual orientation are seldom noticeably different in appearance, style of clothing, speech, or mannerisms from people of more heterosexual orientation. Nor is there any reason to expect such differences. The few males who do make an obvious display of their homosexual orientation may either adopt an effeminate mode of dress and behavior or, to attract other homosexually oriented males, develop a supermasculine image, with strong muscle development, leather clothing, motorcycles, or other symbols of "masculinity." Homosexually oriented females (lesbians) may similarly range in dress and mannerisms from masculine to extremely feminine. However, an effeminate male (even a transvestite) may be exclusively heterosexual, and the same is true of a "masculine" female.

The typical pattern of homosexual relationships differs somewhat between males and females. The male tendency, regardless of sexual orientation, is to seek variety in sexual partners. Long-term exclusive relationships are less common among homosexually oriented men than among women. Some men do establish homosexual relationships that last for many years, but short-term relationships are more common. Some homosexually oriented men engage in a constant search for new sexual encounters, spending a great deal of time cruising "gay" bars and other homosexual gathering places. Actually, this behavior is not too unlike that seen in the heterosexual "singles" bars. Among homosexually oriented women, long-term relationships are quite common, many lasting for years or for a lifetime.

Heterosexuals commonly believe that in homosexual relationships, male or female, one partner will assume a dominant or "masculine" role while the other is passive or "feminine," but this often is not the case. In fact, the "dominant" and "aggressive" male and the "passive" and "submissive" female are totally fallacious concepts, regardless of the sexual orientation of the individual. Any association of sexual aggressiveness with masculinity and of sexual passiveness with feminity is purely cultural; such associations are not part of basic human sexuality. The evidence in comprehensive studies of homosexuality does not support the old concept that homosexually oriented people assume certain specific roles in their sexual relationships. In homosexual relationships, the majority of both men and women freely interchange sexual roles, reciprocating sexual pleasures with their partners.

Among male homosexual practices are mutual hand manipulation of the penis, oral-genital contact, and anal intercourse. Female homosexual techniques include oral and manual stimulation of the breasts and genitals and mutual genital-to-genital stimulation. Contrary to popular belief, dildoes (artificial penises) are seldom used, nor would one logically expect them to be, since the focus of lesbian sexual orientation is not the penis.

As previously mentioned, a few homosexually oriented people enter into heterosexual marriages (actually only about 5 percent of women and 1 percent of men). There are several possible motivations for these marriages. Sometimes the individual is truly bisexual and really enjoys and needs relationships with both sexes. Sometimes marriage is motivated by a desire for children. Marriage may be an attempt to conform to society's expectations, or to one's own. Some homosexuals would prefer to be heterosexual, and hope that with marriage they may change. Others enter into "front" marriages in an attempt to appear socially acceptable while privately engaging in homosexual activities. Much more common is "front" dating. Homosexually oriented people in high-status occupations, such as physicians and attorneys, often date people of the opposite sex to give the impression of heterosexual orientation. And many of them are genuinely fond of the people they date. Most homosexuals enjoy friendships with members of the opposite sex, so long as those friends understand their homosexual orientation and accept it.

Factors Influencing Sexual Orientation

The determination of sexual orientation is not well understood. There is very little evidence to support a biological theory of sexual orientation. While a few studies have shown minor hormonal differences between homosexually and heterosexually oriented men, many other studies have shown no such difference. There is no connection between chromosomal abnormalities and sexual orientation. Most authorities regard sexual orientation as an emotional phenomenon.

It is a mistake to overgeneralize when describing the factors involved in sexual orientation, for there are many, they are psychologically complex, and they vary from person to person. Nevertheless, it does seem probable that the factors determining sexual orientation exert their influence during childhood. Sexual orientation is usually quite definitely established by the end of adolescence, though many people do not act out their sexuality until later.

The relationship between children and their parents is most often singled out as the primary contributing factor in the development of sexual orientation. The role of the father in the establishment of sexual orientation is often stressed. The incidence of homosexuality seems to increase among children of either sex whose fathers are either physically or emotionally absent from the home. The parental combination of an extremely passive father and a dominant, overbearing mother seems to foster homosexual orientation in children of both sexes. The unhappiness of the parents in their marital situation is sometimes a factor. The inability of a child to identify with the parent of the same sex is frequently thought to enter into homosexual orientation. This difficulty may arise when that parent is seen as very unhappy or physically or emotionally abused. The boy whose father is hostile or detached while his mother is excessively close has been considered more likely to develop homosexual orientation. The absence of a satisfactory father-daughter relationship has been thought to be characteristic of the homosexually oriented female. At the same time, all of us know people of unquestionably heterosexual orientation whose fathers were passive or hostile or remote or dead or indeed unknown, whose mothers were domineering or unhappy or overprotective. Clearly these unfortunate circumstances are not in themselves enough to create a homosexual orientation in a growing boy or girl. Something else must enter into it, and we do not yet know what it is.

Opinions on Homosexual Orientation

Authorities on emotional health and sexuality express extremely divergent opinions on homosexual orientation. Some examples: "A stable homosexual orientation is a pathological manifestation of character development"; "It is normal for all individuals to have sexual feelings toward members of their same sex"; "Homosexuality is a symptom of a neurosis"; "Bisexuality is the biological norm and heterosexuality is a culturally imposed restriction." Among psychiatrists and other professionals, homosexual orientation is currently seen variously as an illness, normal, a neurotic behavior pattern, and an alternative life style. This controversy is currently raging in the pages of many medical and psychiatric journals. Significantly, the prestigious American Psychiatric Association no longer lists homosexuality among the mental disturbances.

Many people view their homosexual orientation merely as an alternate lifestyle, presenting them with no more difficulties than the typical heterosexual person encounters. Most of the problems homosexually oriented people experience are not inherent to their sexual orientation, but are the products of a hostile and misunderstanding society. Among the general public, homosexual orientation does meet considerable disapproval. The level of acceptance, however, varies considerably from place to place in the United States. In general, a higher level of acceptance occurs among better educated people and in the larger cities of the east and west coasts, while a lower level is typical of the less educated and rural populations.

The question of the law's response to homosexual activity is now undergoing critical examination. The simplistic assumption that homosexual behavior is strictly a legal question, calling for punishment and imprisonment, is clearly being put aside. In 1972 the National Institute of Mental Health's Task Force on Homosexuality published its final report, concluding that homosexuality is not an emotional illness. The complexity of this issue is revealed in the composition of the commission: It included social historians, sociologists, psychologists, judges, and lawyers. Surely the resolution of the debate about homosexuality will not come from one area of expertise.

Across the United States, larger communities are currently considering legislation that would ban discrimination in housing, employment, and other aspects of civil rights on the basis of sexual orientation.

Transsexuality

Transsexuality is the conscious, compelling desire to change one's sex. It is a feeling that in all but a few anatomical details, one is a member of the opposite sex. A transsexual thinks, feels, and acts like a person of the opposite sex. The individual feels trapped in the wrong body. A transsexual often wears clothing of the opposite sex.

Transsexuality is often confused with *transvestism* (wearing clothing of the opposite sex) and homosexuality. Most transvestites are not transsexual, but most transsexuals wear the clothes of the opposite sex, as do transvestites. Similarly, passive feminine homosexuality in the male transsexual is common, but most homosexuals have a normal gender role (that is, they feel that they are of their own biological sex). A male homosexual feels himself to be male at all times. He enjoys his penis as well as the interest that other homosexuals have in it. He derives genital pleasure from his sexual contacts. The transsexual male, on the contrary, hates his penis and derives no pleasure from it at all. He does not usually experience erection or ejaculation.

The transsexual is usually a biologically normal male or female. With rare exceptions, there are no anatomical, chromosomal, or hormonal abnormalities. Transsexual attitudes can usually be traced back to childhood. There may be a background of parents whose sexual roles were unclear or who were disappointed that the child was not of the opposite sex. A common childhood history includes excessive contact and gratification by a mother figure, ambivalent sexuality on the part of the mother, unusual permissiveness, and a weak or absent father figure —some of which are also said to lead to homosexuality and a wide assortment of neuroses.

In sum, transsexuals are set apart from transvestites and homosexuals by at least part of their childhood histories and, more importantly, by the fact that cross-dressing is only for nonerotic reasons. As love objects or sexual partners, male transsexuals prefer nonhomosexual men who are not interested in their male genitals (as a homosexual would be) but in their acquired feminine characteristics. They want to be loved as women. Interestingly, most male transsexuals consider sexual relationships with females to be homosexual and repulsive.

Psychotherapy has not been highly successful in the treatment of adult transsexuals, though it should definitely be tried before more radical treatment is considered. Many transsexuals have achieved happiness only after surgical and hormonal sex-change procedures. While these are undeniably extreme measures, the alternative for many transsexuals is continued suffering or suicide. Several ethical *gender clinics* have been established within the United States, and the majority of their patients have expressed satisfaction with the results of their sex changes. Those changing from male to female (the more common procedure) may be provided with breasts and a vagina with which they may experience sexual pleasure and even orgasm. In the reverse change, which is much less common, there are several approaches to constructing a penis. One is to include a silicone implant, creating a penis that is firm at all times. Another is to include a balloon-like rubber tube that can be pumped up with fluid from an implanted reservoir. Also, an artificial penis might be worn for coitus. Of course, natural parenthood is impossible after either sex-change procedure.

Transvestism

Transvestism (cross-dressing) is the wearing of clothing of the opposite sex. Cross-dressing may be part of a more basic sexual orientation such as transsexuality or homosexuality, but there are individuals of both sexes (though most of them are males) who are neither transsexuals nor homosexuals, but for whom cross-dressing is in itself a source of sexual or other satisfaction. Transvestite cross-dressing may take place strictly in private, or appearances in public may be essential for satisfaction. Individuals may or may not masturbate while cross-dressed.

Various psychological dynamics may motivate transvestism. A classic Freudian explanation of this behavior in males relates it to an effort to relieve castration anxiety by acting out the fantasy of a woman with a penis, with whom the male then identifies. Other, more behavioristic explanations include (again) the lack during childhood of a strong parent figure of the same sex with whom the individual can identify or the preferential treatment by parents of a sibling (brother or sister) of the opposite sex. There are transvestites, however, to whom none of these factors seem to apply. Transvestites are almost always very harmless people. Their satisfaction is in the cross-dressing itself.

Voyeurism, Exhibitionism, and Obscene Communication

While at first glance voyeurism, exhibitionism, and obscene communication may seem to have little in common, they in fact usually have much the same psychological foundation. The unifying element in the personalities of most voyeurs, exhibitionists, and obscene communicators is an extreme sense of sexual inadequacy—the real or imagined inability to function satisfactorily in a normal sexual relationship. Thus sexual arousal and satisfaction are obtained in very impersonal, indirect, and nonthreatening ways. There is also an element of hostility toward the opposite sex among these individuals, who are almost invariably males.

Voyeurism

Voyeurism is obtaining sexual gratification by looking at sexual objects or situations. Almost all men have some voyeuristic tendencies and are sexually aroused by watching sexually explicit films and stage shows, reading erotic books or looking at erotic pictures, or just watching sexually attractive people. These activities may be accompanied by masturbation and often serve as sources of erotic fantasies for later masturbation or sexual relationships. The point at which voyeurism may be considered variant behavior is quite unclear. An individual could be considered a true voyeur, however, if he obtains his major sexual satisfaction by compulsively and repeatedly observing others, often at great risk or expense. Examples of true voyers include the "peeping Tom" and the person who pays to watch the sexual performances of others without himself participating. Most peeping Toms are quite harmless, though in a very few hostility is strong enough to motivate occasional acts of violence.

Exhibitionism

Exhibitionism is the deliberate and compulsive exposure of the genitals in public, almost always by a male, as a means of achieving sexual gratification. Many women also enjoy displaying their bodies, though seldom the genitals; however, this is generally quite unrelated to true exhibitionism. The typical exhibitionist exposes his penis to an unknown and unsuspecting female, often a young girl, without any intention of further sexual contact. Apparently the exhibitionist's intention is to elicit an emotional reaction in his victim. Because of the underlying sexual inferiority complex associated with exhibitionism, the desired reaction is an expression of shock at the size of the exhibitionist's penis. An amused reaction can be crushing to these pathetic individuals. Most exhibitionists are not harmful and there is seldom any danger of rape.

Obscene Communication

Some men (and extremely few women) are sexually aroused by anonymous obscene communication without any intention of actual sexual contact. In this category belong the obscene phone caller, the sender of obscene letters, and certain writers of obscenity in public places. Like the exhibitionist, the obscene communicator finds sexual release in the act itself or in masturbation accompanying or following the act. The hoped-for reaction is shock and consternation on the part of the victim. The caller or writer is not interested in a real sexual relationship with the victim; he feels far too inadequate for any direct sexual confrontation. The best way to deal with an obscene caller is simply to hang up. The longer one stays on the phone and the more reaction one shows, the more likely the person will feel encouraged to call again. Single women in big cities have been accustomed to having their phone numbers listed under their last names and one or two initials (no first name) as a protection against obscene calls, but now it seems that every obscene communicator is aware of the strategy and it is no longer effective. Many women consider the extra charge for an unlisted number to be money well spent.

Forcible Rape

Psychologically, and often physically, rape is the most traumatic of crimes against women. And for many victims the police investigation that follows is even more shattering. Then, in those few cases in which a suspect is brought to trial, the victim may be subjected to even further indignities. Not surprisingly, rape prevention and the humane treatment of victims have become high-priority items among women's groups.

The Victim

Very simply, the victim of rape could be any female of any age. Neither the very young nor the very old are immune to rape. The psychosexually immature rapist (the pedophile) is attracted to females whose chronological age corresponds to his developmental age, which may be quite young. On the other hand, the hostile, sadistic rapist may select a victim whom he may associate with a hated relative, teacher, or other authority figure, and who thus may be quite elderly. And some seem not to discriminate at all: Babies of two have been raped.

The victim may be a total stranger to the rapist, someone whom he sees for the first time and rapes on impulse. She may be someone whom he has watched for days and who triggers erotic or perhaps sadistic fantasies in him. A common myth, the product of male fantasy, is that a victim often really wants to be raped and provokes her rapist. While this may apply to a very few masochistic women, it is certainly very rarely true, if ever. This myth is just a small part of the total male tendency to treat the victim of rape with contempt rather than understanding.

The Rapist

Most authorities now agree that there is no such thing as a "typical" rapist. A number of classification schemes of various types of rapist have been proposed. Of course, any system of classification is somewhat arbitrary, and many individuals will not neatly fit into any of the categories. One system, for example, proposes five or six categories of rapist, in only one of which is sexual need the primary motivation. These men are criminally oriented sociopaths or amoral delinquents. For them, rape is only one of a variety of antisocial agressive types of behavior. Such men pay little attention to normal social controls and operate purely for their own gratification. They are not sadistic—they simply want to have intercourse and the wishes of the female are of no importance. They are not hostile toward women, but look upon them solely as sexual objects whose role in life is to provide sexual pleasure to men. Though they may use threats of violence, they are less dangerous to their victims than other kinds of rapist because their motivation is strictly sexual and the act does not tap a conflicted reservoir of bizarre aggressive and sexual fantasies.

In the remaining types of rapist the motivation is primarily nonsexual. Of these, the most common type (and possibly the most common of all rapists) is the sadist. He is often a man who routinely uses unnecessary violence in all his activities. He does not commit rape because of a lack of willing sex partners. He *prefers* rape to conventional sex. Sadistic rapists often have underlying inferiority feelings, and a sense of dominance is compulsively important to them. For this type of individual, sexual intercourse is gratifying only if it is accompanied by physical violence or the serious threat of violence. In fact, he may be impotent with a willing partner. This rapist hates women and gains satisfaction from punishing them. Often more violence is used than would be necessary to complete the rape. The dangerous nature of this rapist is obvious.

Other, less common rapists are the psychotic, who are out of touch with reality; those who are under severe though temporary situational stress; those who have masculine identity conflicts; and the drunks. The drunk's aggression ranges from uncoordinated efforts at seduction to hostile and truly vicious behavior released by lowering of inhibitions due to intoxication. Many drunken rapists actually fit into one of the other categories, their behavior being merely released by the alcohol.

Effects on the Victim

Women who have been victims of forcible rape show various types of emotional and physical symptoms. There may be acute (immediate) and/or long-term reactions to rape. The acute reactions include symptoms of physical trauma, skeletal muscle tension, gastrointestinal irritability, urinary and genital disturbances, and a great variety of emotional reactions. Of course, there is the definite possibility of pregnancy and/or sexually transmitted disease resulting from the rape. Long-term effects include increased motor activity, anxiety, nightmares, and the development of phobias to various circumstances surrounding the rape.

Some of the most damaging effects of rape are not inherent in the act itself, but are the result of shabby treatment of the victim by police and the courts. Many police officers take the attitude that the victim is in some way responsible for her own rape and that she must have deserved what she got. Some women report police officers' showing apparent voyeuristic interest in the details of the rape. In court, many women have been made to feel that they were the ones on trial as defense attorneys representing accused rapists have attempted to discredit the victim's testimony through extensively probing her own sexual history, though it has nothing to do with the rape. As a result of these and other problems, only a small percentage of actual rapes are even reported to police, and of accused rapists who are apprehended and brought to trial, only a small percent are convicted. Some states are acting to improve the treatment of rape victims, but this remains a serious problem.

Rape Prevention

There are several aspects to rape prevention. One is apprehension of the rapist and his removal from society until the psychological causes of his violent behavior are determined and adequately treated. This will require vastly improved treatment of rape victims by police and the courts, so that more rapes are reported, more rapists are apprehended and brought to trial, and more convictions are obtained. Further, the convicted rapist must receive psychological evaluation and adequate treatment, rather than just being imprisoned for a time and being turned loose to rape again.

Since none of these things will happen soon, if ever, it is important for a woman actively to prevent her own rape. The best way to reduce the chances of being raped is to avoid those situations that most often lead to rape. Of such situations, visiting bars alone at night is the most frequently mentioned by women who report forcible rape. Going with another woman greatly reduces the chance of rape. Hitching rides is another way to meet a rapist. Among young girls, running away from home often leads to rape. When driving, car doors should be kept locked and the windows up. Be aware of the world around you—watch for suspicious persons. A single woman should never put her first name on her door or mailbox—her last name or last name and first initial is enough.

There is no single best course of action when faced with a rapist. Yet rape can often be prevented by cool-headed resistance. First, the woman should run away if at all possible, preferably toward people. She should also yell; some authorities suggest shouting "fire!" as that often gets a better response than "help!" or "rape!" In any case, yell *loudly*. Many women now carry whistles; to be effective they must be instantly available, not lost at the bottom of a handbag.

More and more rape counselors are advising women to resist physically if only one man is involved and if he is unarmed. Special courses in self-defense are available for women in many areas. If a women has not been trained in self-defense, the automatic responses such as kicking, biting, and clawing should be used, without hesitation and with all one's strength. Make a V with your index and middle fingers and aim for the eyes. A powerful kick in the genitals may disable the attacker long enough to allow escape. Don't be squeamish. A halfhearted struggle is worse than none and will only encourage the sadistic rapist. Some women carry weapons, though certain weapons are illegal and any of them can be turned against the woman. Legal weapons that may distract the rapist long enough to allow escape include aerosol cans of antiperspirant, cologne, and hair spray, which can be sprayed in his eyes. Concentrated ammonia or lemon juice from a plastic lemon can also be used. A lit cigarette can be mashed out on his face or in his eye.

It may or may not be useful to try to talk to the rapist. Sometimes it works and sometimes it only provokes more violent behavior. If a woman decides to talk, she must not show any sign of fear or submissiveness.

Pedophilia

Pedophilia is the sexual involvement of an adult with a child. It may consist of forcible child molestation or the child may be a willing participant. It may take either heterosexual or homosexual forms. With the exception of incest, pedophilia is probably the least acceptable form of sexual behavior in our society. Since the variation lies in the sexual immaturity of the child, the natural break-off point for classifying an act as pedophilia would be the onset of puberty, as determined by the presence or absence of secondary sex characteristics.

Pedophiles are usually characterized psychologically as suffering from arrested development (fixation)—they have never grown psychosexually beyond the immature prepubertal stage—or from a regression back to this stage of development. As a result, the great majority of a pedophile's sexual acts consist of the sort of sex play engaged in by children—looking, showing, fondling, being fondled. The nature of the sexual act usually corresponds to the maturity expected at the age of the child rather than at the age of the pedophile. Research has shown that the social aftereffects of molestation can be much more devastating to the child than the incident itself. Pedophiles may be dangerous, though: They may panic and kill the child to avoid being identified.

In most cases of heterosexual pedophilia, the pedophile is known to the child and the child's family. Most acts of this sort are commited by the victims' neighbors, family friends, or relatives. In contrast, homosexual child molesters are more often strangers.

Parents, police, and the courts can minimize the psychological effects of child molestation by skillful handling. The effect on the child depends greatly on the reaction of parents and other adults upon their discovery of the offense. If the parents react with obvious fear, anger, disgust, or hysteria, then the child is more likely to suffer lasting effects.

Incest

Incest is a sexual relationship between two people too closely related to marry legally. The relationship can be father-daughter, father-stepdaughter, mother-son, mother-stepson, or brother-sister. Incest is the most ancient and widespread of the sexual taboos. Most incidents of incest occur either with a subculture that has become so disorganized that the social structure has collapsed or as a result of the mental incompetence of one of the partners. Even in the contemporary United States, there remain certain subcultures in which incest is thought of as unfortunate, but not a grave or unexpected situation. Incest in this country is most common among impoverished, unintelligent, uneducated individuals living in rural surroundings; in Latin America it is more likely to occur in the squalid shanty towns that grow up on the fringes of the large cities. In these social circumstances sexual morality is publicly emphasized, but privately breached with impunity.

Sadomasochism

Sadism is the attainment of sexual arousal or satisfaction from the infliction of pain upon another person. *Masochism* is the achievement of sexual gratification from the suffering of pain. In many personalities elements of sadism and masochism are combined, as the psychological dynamics of both forms of behavior are the same. The term *sadomasochism* refers to sexual pleasure related to both sadism and masochism. The abuse involved in sadomasochism may be psychological as well as physical. Some masochists, for example, find it sexually stimulating to be dominated and perhaps bound up, even though no actual physical pain is inflicted. The greater the humiliation or degradation, the more intense the sexual arousal. There are even a few masochists who enjoy being urinated or defecated upon. The sadist is often unable to achieve orgasm without some form of violence. There are both male and female, heterosexual and homosexual sadists. As we mentioned earlier, sadism is often a motivating factor in rape. The rapist frequently uses more force than is necessary to complete the rape, and elements of torture are sometimes involved. Many men are sadistically cruel in their relationships with prostitutes and even with their wives, since they are unable to gain satisfaction without this cruelty. Sadism can take forms that have no apparent relationship to its sexual basis. According to some authorities, such forms of violence as child-beating, wife-beating, and professional boxing have a sadistic basis.

There are both male and female masochists who must be punished in order to gain sexual arousal or orgasm. The punishment often involves beating, whipping, biting, pinching, scratching, burning, and similar painful treatments; or it may be entirely mental.

Reading or viewing sadomasochistic pornography while masturbating is very common among people who have sadistic or masochistic inclincations. The voyeuristic use of this material provides sexual stimulation through fantasies of situations that the individual is unable or unwilling to act out in real life.

As in all sexual variations, the causes differ somewhat from person to person. However, certain similarities often appear in the backgrounds of sadists and masochists. They often report childhood difficulties with parental figures that have precluded any normal expression of tenderness or love. Often the only attention given to these children was in the form of whippings or beatings. Thus aggression is linked with attention. There may be feelings of guilt due to anger toward the abusive parent, and also feeling of low self-esteem and poor sexual identity because of frequent punishment. In sadomasochism, the person being abused may represent either the hated parental figure or the guilt-laden self. This is why many people are both sadistic and masochistic.

The sadomasochistic orientation impairs normal relations because of the inhibition of a loving affectionate relationship. The fear and guilt that arise in a nonsadistic affectionate relationship can prevent normal sexual performance. There may also be fear of losing control during orgasm and lapsing into sadomasochistic behavior.

Fetishism

Fetishism is sexual stimulation from perception and handling of inanimate objects. The psychosexual development of the fetishist is generally poor. Fetishism is a displacement reaction, a sexual response not to a living person, but to a symbol of that person. A certain amount of fetishism is entirely normal—certain items of clothing, such as black lace panties, have so universally been equated with sex appeal that some sexual arousal from the sight of them is neither surprising nor abnormal. At what point, then, does a fetish become abnormal? When the sexual arousal from the fetish item is frequently strong enough to cause erection; when the fetish item is often used in masturbation; when the fetish item is necessary for erection for intercourse; when sexual partners are chosen on the basis of possession of the fetish item; when the fetish item is collected (through purchase or theft).

Other Variations

Bestiality is sexual contact with an animal. Though it is one of the most unsanctioned forms of sexual behavior, it is practiced more often than many people think. Bestiality is commonly practiced by farm boys, although detection makes such a boy an object of ridicule. Less commonly, women have sexual contact with male dogs. Bestiality is usually engaged in only as a substitute for other sexual relationships. The animal is used more as an aid to masturbation than as a sexual object in itself.

Human-animal hybrids have been prominent in mythology and folklore, but the gametes (sperm and eggs) of humans and animals are not compatible and fertilization cannot occur.

Necrophilia is a feeling of sexual attraction toward and arousal by the dead, leading to sexual intercourse with a corpse. Persons who feel so totally inadequate that they are not capable of approaching a living person on such a personal basis may resort to sexual relations with the dead. If the defiled body is killed before being sexually assaulted, the act could be considered an extreme form of sadism and probably indicates a psychotic state. This variation is not common.

Urolagnistic acts are those in which sexual pleasure is derived from urine—either urinating on or being urinated on by another person. *Scatological acts* are those in which sexual pleasure is associated with fecal excretory functions. Both of these variations are often of a masochistic or voyeuristic nature.

Sexuality and Aging

11

To young adults reveling in their bountiful capacity for lovemaking, the prospect of waning sexuality seems remote and irrelevant. But for the sixty-five-year-old, entering into those "golden years" of retirement and relaxation, the awareness of waning sexuality may lead to depression and loneliness. Now that people are living longer and remaining healthier later in life, it is important that we not deny, or be unresponsive to, the sexual needs of older people.

It is well established that men and women can be sexually active into their seventies and eighties. But recent research has shown that the prospects for such extended sexual responsiveness are best for those who have established healthy sexual relationships early and have maintained them through their adult lives. It is also known that continued marital happiness is most likely for those who have been happy during the first years of their marriage.

If human sexuality is significant to the whole person, then it is essential that we examine the effects of aging on sexuality.

Sexual Response at Various Ages

Not only does sexual responsiveness vary with age, but the changes are significantly different between men and women. While these changes are a natural result of growth and aging, a lack of preparedness for them may lead to personal and marital distress. Unaccountably to lose one's ability to respond sexually can be devastating to one's self-esteem.

While sexual responsiveness may follow general patterns, like all other physical and psychic processes, there is much variation among normal individuals of the same sex and age. General patterns should not serve as specific expectations for any individual. Varying from them need not cause apprehension or fear of abnormality.

Changes in Male Sexuality

Sexual interest and pleasure begin in infancy and tend to be rather diffuse. With the onset of puberty there is a rapid increase, reaching a lifetime peak of sexual potency at seventeen to eighteen years of age. This peak of sexual interest correlates with maximal testosterone secretion (see Figure 11.1). Thereafter sexual capacity gradually declines. Thus youthful males tend to be intensely sexual, with great urgency for seminal release. Sexual dreams and fantasies are also urgent and frequent. Sexual release is obtained through heterosexual or homosexual intercourse, masturbation, and nocturnal emissions.

As explained earlier, it is not unusual for a man in his twenties to experience orgasm several times a day, with very short recovery periods following an orgasm. Erection comes very quickly in response to psychic or physical stimulation, and the erection is lost slowly. In orgasm the sensations are intense and the ejaculate leaves the body with considerable force.

In his thirties a man typically finds his sex urges less pressing. Although still highly interested in sex, he is satisfied with fewer orgasms. One or two per love session may satisfy him. Although still quick to respond to sexual stimuli and active in seeking out sexual situations, he is less preoccupied with sexual thoughts and fantasies in the absence of such stimuli. He still attains erection quickly and loses it slowly. By his late thirties the recovery period following orgasm may require a minimum of thirty minutes.

Sexual pleasure may change noticeably for the man in his forties. The intense, genitally localized sensations of earlier years become more diffuse. Orgasms may decline to about two per week during the late forties, and recovery following orgasm may require eight to twenty-four hours. Longer and more intense stimulation may be required for the achievement of erection. As a male grows older, other changes can be expected. Some men in their sixties who lose an erection during long love play may need twelve to twenty-four hours to regain erection even

FIGURE 11.1 Rate of testosterone secretion in the male; note peak at ages 17–18

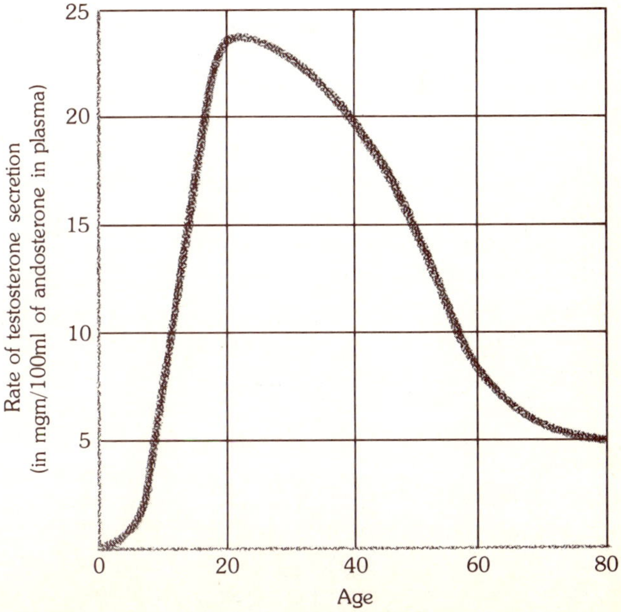

though ejaculation has not occurred. Loss of erection comes rapidly following orgasm and the force of the ejaculate diminishes. During the last decade or two before retirement, a man may be absorbed in his career for weeks without thoughts of sex or without having an erection. Yet even an elderly man may still respond to sexual stimulation with the help of improved sexual techniques, such as more intense stimulation of the genitals and other erogenous areas. The healthy man is able to enjoy sex throughout much or all of his life.

Changes in Female Sexuality

Sexual response in the female is subject to far greater individual variations. In our society it tends to be diffuse during childhood, to awaken more slowly during adolescence and the teens, and to reach peak responsiveness during the late thirties and early forties. Most adolescent American girls are less intensely sexual than boys, less preoccupied with sex, and feel less urgency for orgasmic release. Masturbation to orgasm is less frequent than among boys. No physiological basis for this pattern has been found, and different patterns prevail among women of different societies. Female sexual response is thus greatly influenced by cultural factors.

The Older Man

The major sexual problems faced by the aging man relate to the length of time it takes him to respond to sexual stimulation. While the younger man is well acquainted with prompt erection, rapid intromission, and ejaculation within a few minutes, all of this takes longer in the older man, and he is slow to regain erection.

It is not difficult for the man who has known good sexual adjustment to maintain good response into his fifties. But the man over sixty will probably be satisfied with one or two ejaculations a week. Once erection is lost, as we noted earlier, many of these men are unable to regain erection within twelve to twenty-four hours even though ejaculation may not have occurred, or if they can regain erection promptly, they may be unable to ejaculate. This situation need not be particularly disturbing; many men are happy to have sexual connection with a woman without feeling compelled to experience ejaculation.

Physical Changes in Sexual Response

While the young man may need to try to restrain or delay ejaculation, the older man just wishes he had this sort of problem. There appears to be some uncertainty as to whether this "control" over ejaculation is the culmination of many years of careful practice or whether it is a true reduced intensity of sexual response.

A young man may gain full erection, then partially or completely lose it, only to regain full erection through prolonged lovemaking. But the older man, once he has lost full erection without ejaculation, may not, or only with great difficulty, regain erection until a later occasion. The aging man may attain full erection only immediately before ejaculation.

The propulsive force of the seminal fluid upon ejaculation is also lessened. As we noted earlier, it is not uncommon for semen to be propelled twelve to twenty-four inches by a man in his prime, but six to twelve inches is unusual for the man over fifty years of age. While the spurts of semen are relatively rapid in the younger man, they become progressively further apart in older men.

The period of time until the man can again respond to sexual arousal (refractory period) becomes progressively longer, particularly after sixty. If the man does ejaculate, detumescence is very rapid. Within seconds after ejaculation the sixty-year-old penis is back to normal.

Ejaculation in the young man comes in two stages. In the first the man feels the ejaculation approaching (he can't voluntarily stop it), in the second it occurs. Some older men do not experience this feeling of impending ejaculation or the sense of inevitability. Commonly if the penile erection is maintained for any period at all, the older man expels some semen but without the strong warning feeling. If the older man is fortunate enough to retain the first-stage sense of warning, it lasts longer than it did when he was younger. This feeling may extend from five to six seconds, rather than the two to three seconds experienced by the younger man. Some older men, however, occasionally feel that the ejaculate is coming when it is not. While this experience may be disconcerting, it is usually transitory.

With younger men it is common for the ejaculation to end with a final drop or two seeping from the urethra. With the older man, the entire ejaculation may act this way, without any particular ejaculatory pressure. This is less pleasurable for the older man than the strong pulsations he knew when he was younger. In effect, ejaculation for the older man is resolved into a one- rather than two-stage affair.

Behavioral Changes in Male Sexual Response

As expected, the male's sexual responsiveness diminishes with age. Levels of sexual tension, ability to enter the vagina, ability to ejaculate, and incidence of masturbation and nocturnal emission, all decline for the man over sixty. There may be both physical and psychological factors in the waning of the male's sexual capacity. For some the changes are rapid and final, for others more gradual.

Male Climacteric The time when a person loses the ability to reproduce is known as the *climacteric*. Its unmistakable signal in women is the menopause, or cessation of the menses. Not so well understood or accepted is the male climacteric. When it occurs, the functioning of the gonads diminishes, and eventually they cease functioning altogether. While the climacteric need not interfere with a woman's capacity for orgasmic intercourse, it effectively terminates a man's capacity for orgasm and intercourse.

Caused by a drop in testosterone production, it may occur at any age, but most cases come in late middle age. It is estimated to occur in 20 percent of men aged forty-eight to fifty-eight years, and in 30 to 35 percent of men aged fifty-eight to sixty-eight years. It is not to be confused with emotional sexual dysfunction, which may cause a man to be unable to perform sexually with his wife of many years, while capable of doing so with another woman. Its development is indicated by an inability to achieve erection or ejaculation. If the man does attain erection, it either cannot be maintained for an adequate time or occurs very infrequently. He may report hot flashes (although they tend to be less severe than in women). To other people he may appear to grow less positive, less forceful, more irritable and difficult to live with.

Treatment for affected men may be provided by synthetic testosterone therapy. Without therapy the man's testicular functioning will almost completely disappear. With treatment there should be a return of potency. Treatment may need to be continued indefinitely.

Frequency of Intercourse Sexual functioning in aging men may be influenced by a number of other things, which vary from man to man, and from time to time in the same individual. Masters and Johnson conclude from their research that the most important factor in maintaining effective sexuality is the regularity with which the man achieves orgasm. The man who has high sexual output during his young adult years and on into his thirties and forties has less trouble maintaining sexual response when he is older than one who has been less active sexually. Whether the activity is heterosexual or homosexual or masturbatory seems to have little bearing on the matter.

The incidence of sexual inadequacy increases sharply among men over fifty. Fortunately, many men of this age or younger who have problems of sexual inadequacy can recover through therapy so that they can once again enjoy sexual activity if they are in good health and maintain the proper state of mind.

Boredom Monotony may be the most constant factor in the loss of a man's sexual interest. It may develop from a sexual relationship that has lost its meaning, so that coitus is nothing more than an act of duty or is engaged in largely to relieve sexual tension. The result may be the same if the sexual relationship has failed to mature along with other aspects of the relationship.

Sometimes overfamiliarity may also be a factor. A man may develop sexual restlessness after many years with the same partner. He becomes all too familiar with her sexual wishes and preferences, and sexual response becomes too automatic. Another woman with a different personality, different preferences, and different responses may create renewed sexual tension and capacity in a man.

Preoccupation with One's Career By the forties, fifties, and sixties, a man may be reaching progressively higher ranks in his occupation or profession. Earlier competitive struggles are paying off. Reaching the top in an organization or profession and staying there frequently demand the total or near-total allegiance of a man. This dedication automatically reduces the time he has available for his wife and family. Since he has become so specialized in his interests and devotion to his job, it may happen that he communicates less and less of his professional concerns to his wife. When communication is disrupted a couple's sex life is sure to suffer.

At the same time, some men must guard against allowing their occupational upheavals and disappointments to intrude upon their home lives to the point of being disruptive. Some men are successful in letting sex activity serve as tension relief when things have gone wrong as well as when they have gone well. One should guard against letting a bad day at work inhibit sexual expression at home. Preoccupation with other matters does not make for good sex in either man or woman.

Mental or Physical Fatigue While fatigue may take its toll on the sexual expression of a man of any age, it becomes increasingly important to the older man. Mental fatigue does more than physical fatigue to reduce sexual response in the male.

The middle-aged man with a job that requires any amount of physical output finds that the physical demands of his job have little effect on his sexual interest. The man who suffers more from physical exertion is the one with a physically undemanding job who goes off for some type of weekend recreation that demands excessive physical output. It is not uncommon for men over fifty to suffer partial or complete loss of sexual response for twenty-four to forty-eight hours after such an exhausting weekend.

But the greater villain is mental fatigue. Concerns of a financial, personal, professional, or domestic nature may sharply suppress sexual interest during the time the problem lasts and for an extended period afterward.

Eating or Drinking Excessively Older men fall easy prey to overindulgence in both eating and drinking. They can more easily afford it, may have found the "battle of the bulge" a losing proposition, may feel that their supply of years in which to enjoy the "good things" is running out and they had better enjoy life while they can. Whatever the reason, the effect may be a lessening of sexual responsiveness. Fortunately, the effects tend to be temporary, unless the overindulgence is greatly excessive or more or less constant.

Alcohol is a particular problem. Failure to gain an erection while under its influence is common. While drinking may be the initial cause of impotence, the older man may develop significant concern over his inability to perform sexually without recognizing that the true cause is too much alcohol. So he ends up with a double problem: the drinking and a general fear of impotence. He may try to close his mind to his performance problem by avoiding situations that call for lovemaking. Or he may seek out lovemaking situations with some new companion, feeling that the usual one may be part of the cause. If he is smart enough to avoid alcohol on his first sexual foray with the new partner, he may be pleasantly rewarded with renewed potency. A situation like this puts great strains on a marriage. He may have been unable to gain an erection with his wife, through no fault of hers, but be able to perform admirably with some other sex partner, through no particular ability of hers.

Physical and Mental Infirmities Physical afflictions take a particular toll of an older man's sexual capacity. If the physical problem is temporary, the sexual effect is usually also temporary and easily faced up to. If the problem is long-term, the sexual effect can become long-lasting. Anything that reduces a man's physical stamina tends also to lower his sexual tensions. Some men respond to androgens and related hormones. Some physicians believe that the hormones, rather than being directly responsible for increased capacity for sexual arousal, may improve the general condition, thus giving the man a sense of improved well-being.

Another hazard for the older man is a sex partner who is suffering from some physical infirmity. If she is not feeling well, she probably will not wish sex. Restriction of sexual opportunity can be an important factor in the sexual responsiveness of the older man. With opportunity diminished, his sexual tensions fall rapidly. In our culture the able wife with an infirm husband has less opportunity to find a substitute partner than the able husband whose wife is ill. It is not uncommon for the able husband to seek out other sexual companionship.

Fear of Failure Fear of inability to perform sexually can be devastating to the older male. Impotence may cause him to withdraw from any sexual activity rather than face the devastation of sexual failure. Some turn against their partners, either in anger or in discouragement. Not uncommonly, the vulnerable older man turns to younger sexual companions. Then other problems may arise. A younger woman has far greater sexual capacity than her older male consort. In attempting to meet her sexual needs, the older man may develop even deeper concern about sexual performance than he had before, and he may retire from sexual involvements.

Another problem that can accompany extramarital involvement is its effect on the wife. The man with outside interests seldom tells his wife why he is no longer interested in sex with her. Unless she is extremely perceptive, she will not realize that he is afraid of failure, and may attribute his lack of sexual interest to some inadequacy within herself. If she does know the reason, she may become overly cautious about doing anything that would bring on another episode of impotence, thus losing her spontaneity in sexual interaction. This may lead to reduced sexual arousal on his part and gradual loss of sexual responsiveness.

Adjusting with Age

Once more, the formula for a long and happy sex life for a man includes regular sexual release and a state of physical and mental well-being. These stimulate a vital sexual climate. Sexual tension is maintained, and capacity for sexual performance may be extended into the seventies and eighties.

The older male may enhance his sexual interests by a willingness to explore sensually rather than seek immediate orgasmic release. Ways of doing this are beautifully explained in Alex Comfort's *The Joy of Sex*. The older man needs to have increased interest in himself—projecting his personality, his appearance, the care of his person. He needs to project a love of and a feeling for his sex partner that tells her that he wants to partake of what he reveres. He needs to experience beauty, attractiveness, and goodness. The older man can learn to be more tender and gentle, less demanding in his sexual relationship. With the passing of the urgent need for ejaculatory release, he is in a good situation to explore the pleasures of gentleness. Of course, a man need not wait until he retires to acquire such insight.

The older man tends to be slower, more mellow, but more tolerant of his sexuality than he was in his youth. While a physical slowdown does occur in his response to sexual stimuli, there are few reasons for him to suppress his sexual interests in old age simply because that is what he hears older men are supposed to do.

The Older Woman

Sexual responsiveness shows great variation after menopause. Some women experience a gradual decline in the sex drive and in their capacity for sexual enjoyment; others go right on having multiple orgasms in their seventies and beyond. If a woman believes that her sex life will end with menopause, it very well may; but there is nothing inevitable about it.

Some sexual problems faced by the aging woman are related to the reduced hormone levels that accompany the climacteric she experiences in her forties or fifties. The degree of these changes and the rapidity of their development can have a major bearing on her attitude toward her own sexuality and her sexual relationship with her partner.

Physical Changes in Sexual Response

Nipple erection from sexual arousal occurs in the aging woman just as it does in the young girl, but the breasts show a marked reduction in vasocongestion. The slacker an older woman's breasts and the more they droop, the less their size will increase during sexual arousal. As hormone levels diminish after menopause, there will be less breast enlargement during sexual response, and the breasts will become smaller.

During the plateau phase of arousal there is still engorgement of the areolae of the breasts, although the intensity of the reaction is diminished. Some women over fifty develop areolar tumescence in one breast and not in the other.

The sex flush is seen less frequently with increasing age. After orgasm any sex flush is rapidly lost, followed shortly by the detumescence of the areolae. Nipple erection may be retained for a matter of hours.

Because the lining of the vagina becomes very thin in the postmenopausal woman, it is more sensitive to the irritation of intercourse. There is also more irritation of the urethra and bladder, especially if vaginal secretion is scanty. Thus older women often must contend with a feeling of urinary urgency and the need to urinate immediately after intercourse. Some report urinary burning for two to three days after intercourse, especially following prolonged intercourse.

Clitoral responsiveness continues essentially unchanged into the seventies. In arousal the clitoral shaft enlarges and retracts under the labial hood as in the younger woman, although following orgasm the arousal of the clitoris terminates quite quickly.

The labia majora, which become elevated in the younger woman because of natural depositing of fatty tissue, rise very little in the older woman. The loss of fatty tissue deposits throughout the body are due to lower hormone levels after menopause. The labia minora show little response in the older woman. There is little vasocongestion (thickening and expansion) or color change. Secretory activity of the Bartholin's glands is slowed, but not until the woman is well along in years.

The vagina in the postmenopausal woman has an entirely different appearance from that of the well-stimulated younger woman (see Figure 11.2). As hormone production lessens, the vagina changes from a well-roughened, thickened, reddish-purple barrel to a paper-thin tissue, smoothed and light pinkish. It becomes less expansive under sexual tension, both in length and in diameter. Rather than taking ten to thirty seconds to become lubricated, the woman in her sixties may require one to three minutes for similar lubrication, in spite of the fact that she is undergoing effective arousal and is psychologically responsive. In Masters

FIGURE 11.2 Growth and aging of the female reproductive organs

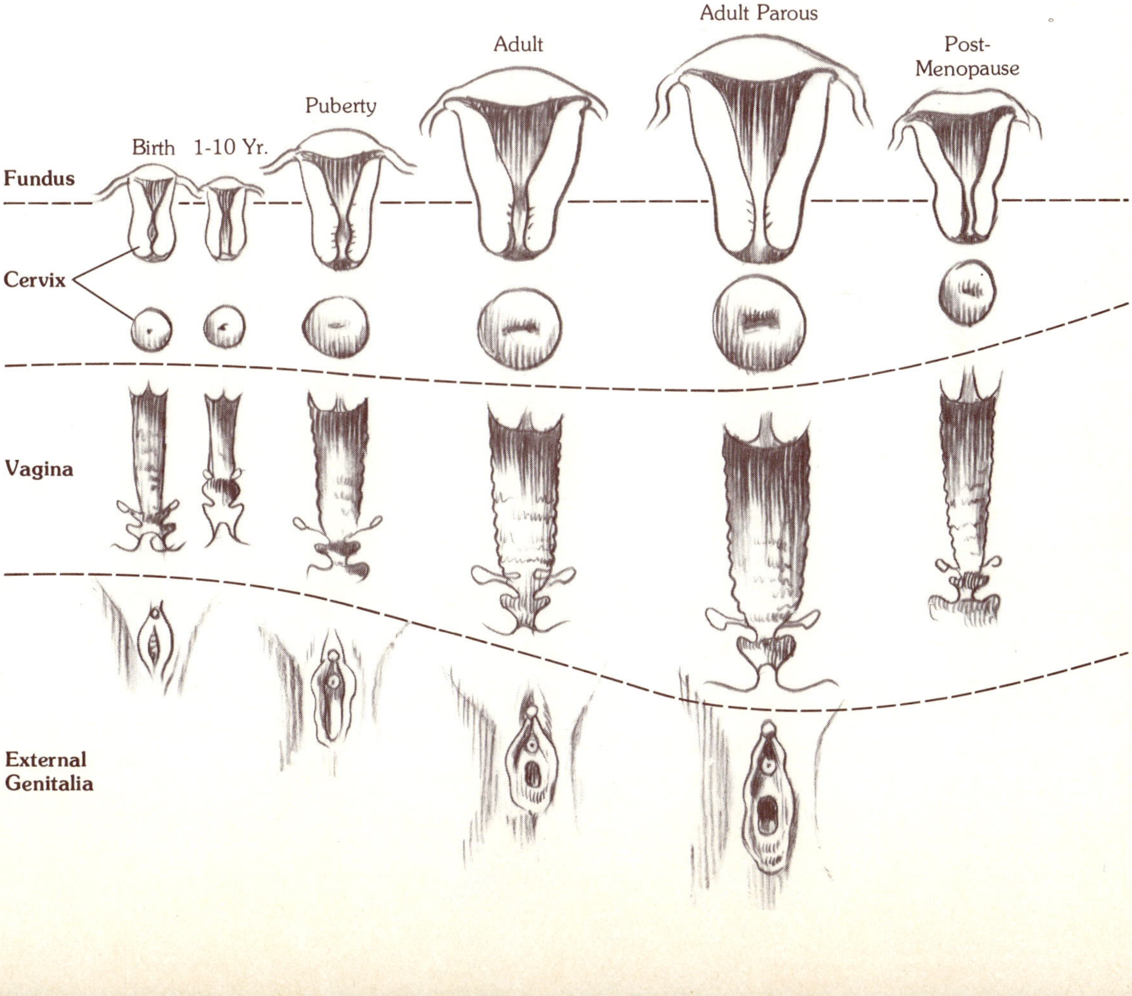

and Johnson's studies, several women who had maintained active sexual relations two to three times a week throughout their adult years retained rapid vaginal lubrication similar to that of the young female. In every case, women who had discontinued frequent sex relations showed the typical reduction in lubrication.

The inner two-thirds of the vaginal barrel expands more slowly as a woman ages, and the rising of the orgasmic platform in the outer third of the vagina is reduced considerably. Yet the inside of the vaginal barrel is quite constricted. The orgasmic phase is shorter, with about half as many orgasmic contractions as in the younger woman. Following orgasm, the expanded vagina shrinks back to its unstimulated state very rapidly.

As hormone reduction sets in, the uterus shrinks dramatically (see Figure 11.2) Within five to ten years following menopause the uterine body and cervix are about equal in length. Lowered hormonal levels reduce fatty deposits in all of the primary sex organs—the breasts, labia, vagina, and uterus. Yet following menopause a woman is still completely capable of sexual performance at orgasmic levels. This is particularly true if she has remained sexually active. The hormone reductions have the primary effect of reducing the rapidity and intensity of physical response in the woman. Loss of psychological tension levels is not due to reduced hormone levels.

Behavioral Changes in Sexual Responsiveness

Many of a woman's psychological adjustments relate to changes in her hormone levels. These may be so disruptive or so little understood as to cause a lessening of sexual response. Behavioral changes may also result from freedom from fear of pregnancy, lessening of family obligations, the effects of advancing age on the sexual capacity of her partner, and the regularity with which coital relations are maintained.

Hormone Changes Because of the hormonal adjustments during the climacteric, sexual complaints by women during the early postmenopausal years are frequent. Intercourse may become very painful during penetration; prolonged intercourse may be followed by pelvic aching, vaginal burning, or general lower abdominal distress. Urination following intercourse may be accompanied by burning and irritation. Distress following intercourse may continue for twenty-four to thirty-six hours. These symptoms usually result from the thinning of the vaginal lining and from the reduced ability of the vaginal barrel to expand during sexual activity. Because of less vaginal lubrication, entry is more difficult and the woman's reaction time is slowed. If the physical changes are too severe, some correction may be made with hormone therapy.

But more important for the older woman in maintaining sexual capacity and effective sexual response is the opportunity for regular sexual intercourse. This has a far greater effect on the sexual response of the older than of the younger woman. Women five to ten years past menopause who experience intercourse as rarely as once a month or less, and who do not masturbate regularly, have particular difficulty in accommodating the penis when intercourse is attempted. Even in younger women vaginal lubrication and expansion are slower during the first lovemaking following a long period of abstinence. But the difficulties of the younger woman are much less significant than those of the older woman in similar circumstances.

Uterine cramping during and following orgasm may be painful as hormone imbalance develops. While such cramping also occurs in younger women during orgasm, younger women rarely find it painful. Distress from such cramping may become so intense that some women avoid orgasm, and even intercourse. Treatment with estrogens and progesterone in combination may relieve such cramping.

A woman who previously demonstrated healthy sexual arousal may become somewhat nonsexual as a result of such menopausal discomforts as severe fatigue, flushing, nervousness, emotional irritability, headaches, and subtle pelvic pain. Sexual responsiveness may be restored to previous levels following the administration of estrogen hormones.

The Last Chance Women respond differently to the climacteric than men. Some experience a return of the reproductive drive—a strong desire to become pregnant once more before it's too late. For many women menopause is a stark reminder that they are getting older, perhaps less attractive, in a culture that is youth-oriented. The reaction to such feelings can be either sexual inhibition or an attempt to reinstate "youthful" sexual vigor by an almost compulsive wish for frequent intercourse. Although a woman may experience the cessation of menses with a sense of relief, there may also be nostalgia for past years.

Relief from Pregnancy For some women the sex drive becomes stronger after they are well into menopause. They may have been burdened with too many children and too little money, and welcome this relief from the burden of pregnancy. Now that they no longer have to worry about becoming pregnant, they can relax and enjoy sex more than they ever could before. Some believe that because of the near absolute reliability of oral contraceptives, fewer women will experience increased enjoyment of sex after menopause than in the past—they will have been enjoying it fully all along.

Reduced Family Responsibilities Another reason for revived postmenopausal sex activity could be the drawing to a close of the demanding physical and mental concerns of raising a family. As the children grow up and move out, the woman is released from these responsibilities and is free to cast about for new interests, new sexual practices, and for some, new sex partners.

The Effect of an Aging Partner It used to be expected that older women would deny interest in sexual activity; sexual intercourse was seen as an activity for younger women. Of little help is the reduced sexual peformance of older men. Further aggravating the problem is the fact that many husbands are several years older than their wives, thus widening the performance gap. Extramarital sex partners of their own age are hard to find for women at this age, and many women are not looking for them in any case: Like men, they prefer younger partners.

Many aging women, however, have long ago become resigned to the old double standard and are afraid of being thought ridiculous if they seek younger partners even after they are widowed. Since men tend to die earlier than women, many older women spend their later years without sexual partners. They make valiant attempts to expend their sexual energy in other physical outlets—grandchildren, business, volunteer work, religion.

Masturbation is of course available to women of all ages when sexual tensions become intolerable and other sexual outlets are simply not available. The frequency of masturbation, however, declines after sixty.

Sex for the Older Single Women Sex may thus be a problem for a single woman in our society. The double standard has been so firmly internalized in many women that they never even consider extramarital sex. Those who do engage in it sometimes find that their feelings of guilt are stronger than any satisfaction they may gain. There is also the problem of finding partners in a culture that is so heavily youth-oriented. It is often assumed that age alone is sufficient to make a person less attractive. For the person of any age to achieve sexual fulfillment it is necessary to have a loving, caring interested partner. The older woman who joins activities that include men and who displays genuine interest in them as individuals has the best chance of developing such a relationship and achieving her goal of sexual fulfillment. She should not worry about the reactions of others if she is attracted to a man who is a few years younger than she if he is also attracted to her. She is far better able to match the responses of a younger partner than most of the men her age, who have no hesitation about seeking out younger women.

At the same time, it is important to realize that continued sexual activity is not needed or essential for all aged persons and should not be over-emphasized. The older woman who has never had or has stopped having sexual relations can still be a completely balanced person. If she is a contented, positive, contributing person, there is no reason for her to feel that her life is lacking in any fundamental way simply because she may not be following the practices of other persons.

Sexual Dysfunctions For the woman who has been plagued with sexual dysfunctions or who has failed to find needed social and emotional reinforcement sexually during her reproductive years, the advent of menopause may only serve to decrease her sexual involvement further. If she has had difficulty in sexual adjustment during her younger years when her hormone balance was optimal, she may find psychic adjustment more difficult when hormone imbalance occurs after menopause. If she has been repelled by sex when her physical potential was high, she will be only further repelled by it when physical potential begins to wane. Such women may use their advancing age as an excuse to avoid painful embarrasment over the inability to perform adequately.

Adjusting with Age

Masters and Johnson found that sex drive in older women is directly related to the sexual habits established during reproductive years. The woman who has known a happy, stimulating sex life before may move into the menopausal and postmenopausal years with little interruption in her interest in and frequency of lovemaking. Her social and economic security at this time of life can also be significant contributors toward her successful sexual adjustment in these later years.

There is little or no physical reason why the frequency of intercourse satisfying to a younger woman cannot be carried into the postmenopausal years. There should be no commanding reason for a particular frequency, however, as long as the women is healthy, active, and well adjusted. If there is an obvious problem of hypersexuality or hyposexuality after menopause, it may respond to treatment. Part of the solution may come in better counseling of women during the premenopausal years. Menopause should not interfere with a woman's sexual drive, performance, or capacity. Her sex drives are normal and deserve attention. These drives are influenced by her conditioning and the effects of the aging process. But age alone does not need to place mandatory limits on the sexual expressions of the older woman.

Differences in Gender Patterns

Part of learning to accept ourselves and our partners for what we are is being aware of why and how the male and female differ.

Sexual behavior is determined by many factors: physical factors (state of the central nervous system, hormone status, and general health); psychological factors (learned patterns of sexual response, presence of conflict about sexuality, and erotic fantasies); and ecological determinants (characteristics of the sexual object, the nature of the environment, sexual mores and taboos of the particular culture). Physical determinants of sex are generally considered more important in males than in females. In females the psychic contributions are more important, thus the greater variability of female sexual response, and the greater vulnerability. Thus the relationship can be enriched by a sensitive and mutually generous adaptation to each other's age related changes in sexual functioning.

Remarriage Among Older People

Today, with people living and remaining healthier longer, there is no reason why sex should stop being an important aspect of life. For many reasons retired people who might otherwise be living alone or in some retirement home may choose to live together, with or without marriage. Some bypass marriage for economic reasons: Were they to marry, the woman might lose pension payments or widow's benefits. If one or both have children, the children may object out of fear of a reduced inheritance if their particular parent dies before the other spouse. Thus some who want love and companionship live together without marriage.

Yet if a couple desires marriage, there may be ways around some of these problems. They may be able to arrange their assets or reinvest them in such a way as to assure adequate financial provision for their needs. They may be able to move to some retirement home and perhaps reduce their living costs. If either or both have separate estates they wish to protect, they can have a prenuptial agreement drawn up by an attorney, clarifying in advance the separation of property. The new marriage will not change such prenuptial agreements. If they depend to any great extent on social security, however, they have a problem unless the woman is receiving benefits on her own account, as a result of covered employment in the past; if she is receiving widow's benefits, they will stop when she remarries, and her benefits as the wife of her new husband will be substantially reduced. This is a most inequitable situation, and unless or until it is changed there seems no good reason why a couple dependent on social security should not live together without marriage if they wish. Love and companionship are too precious to be sacrificed to the arbitrary morality of the Social Security Administration.

Older people have as much right to the fulfillment of human needs as younger adults. If adequate provision can be made for these needs, some of the apprehensions of growing older may be reduced, and elderly people may enjoy the mature years with dignity and reassurance.

Pregnancy and Birth

12

After an egg bursts from its follicle in the ovary, it is soon picked up by the cuplike ending of one of the two fallopian tubes. This cup, with its finger-like *fimbria,* extends toward the ovary; resembling a hand waiting to grasp something, it gently sucks in the egg, which then starts its journey down the fallopian tube. The walls of the tube contain muscles that expand and contract, helping move the egg along. Lining the inside of the tube are tiny hair like protuberances called *cilia* that sway back and forth. Their movement helps clean the *corona radiata* (Figure 12.1) from the newly ruptured egg and also helps move the egg along the tube. It is in the outer half of the tube that the sperm meets the egg. Whether the egg is fertilized or not, it continues its leisurely trip down the three to six inches of tube, taking three to four days to reach the uterus. If the egg has been fertilized, it begins to develop immediately, before reaching the uterus. If it is not fertilized, it is dead by the time it reaches the uterus.

Sperm reach the site of fertilization within fifteen minutes after ejaculation. They are propelled along by both the intrinsic motility of the sperm and the peristaltic movement of the muscles of the female tract. Of the 500 million or so sperm in a single ejaculate, only several hundred

FIGURE 12.1 Human ovum (egg)

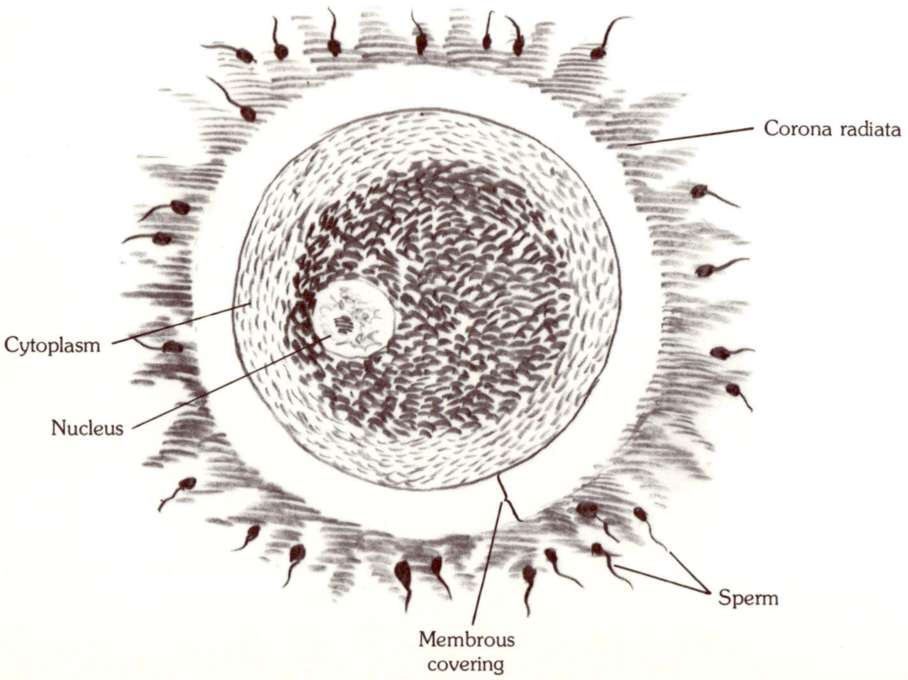

reach the site of fertilization. Most of the loss takes place in the cervix as a result of the action of white blood cells.

Although many sperm surround the egg at the time of fertilization, only one actually penetrates it. The other sperm are believed to assist by secreting an enzyme, *hyaluronidase,* that aids in eliminating the excess cellular material or corona radiata still cliniging to the outside of the egg so that the egg membranes may be penetrated.

As soon as the sperm has entered the egg, the membranes covering the egg thicken and prevent the entry of any other sperm. Following entry, the nucleus in the head of the sperm fuses with the nucleus in the egg, and *fertilization,* or conception, has occurred. The united cell is now referred to as a *zygote* The woman is now pregnant.

Embryology

The fertilized egg immediately begins to divide. From a one-celled zygote it divides to form two cells, four cells, eight cells, and so on (See Figure 12.2). It is now called an *embryo.* By the end of the first week it is a hollow ball of many cells. As cell division speeds up, one side of the ball of cells forms a depression or indentation. This is the first indication that specialized cells, tissues, and organs will be appearing. A fold develops called the *neural groove,* which will later develop into a nervous system. The groove becomes a tube, and the head end of the tube enlarges to become a brain. Blood vessels develop and spread out, and by the twelfth day the primitive beginnings of the head, heart, and limbs are evident.

Implantation

While this development is being initiated, the embryo is being carried down the fallopian tube toward the uterus. The embryo spends about three days within the fallopian tube. By the time it leaves the tube and enters the uterus, the mass of cells looks like a hollow ball, but is actually filled with fluid. Even though the cell mass consists of many cells by this time, the whole mass is no larger than the undivided zygote.

The uterus (womb) is about the size and shape of a pear. Its heavy muscular walls surround a small, narrow cavity. By the time the embryo arrives, the endometrial lining is ready to receive it. Hormones secreted during the past two weeks have made the lining thick, spongy, and engorged with blood.

For the next two or three days the cell mass, now called a *blastocyst,* floats around in the cavity of the uterus. Then, at a random site, the mass attaches itself to the endometrial lining of the uterus. The site of this

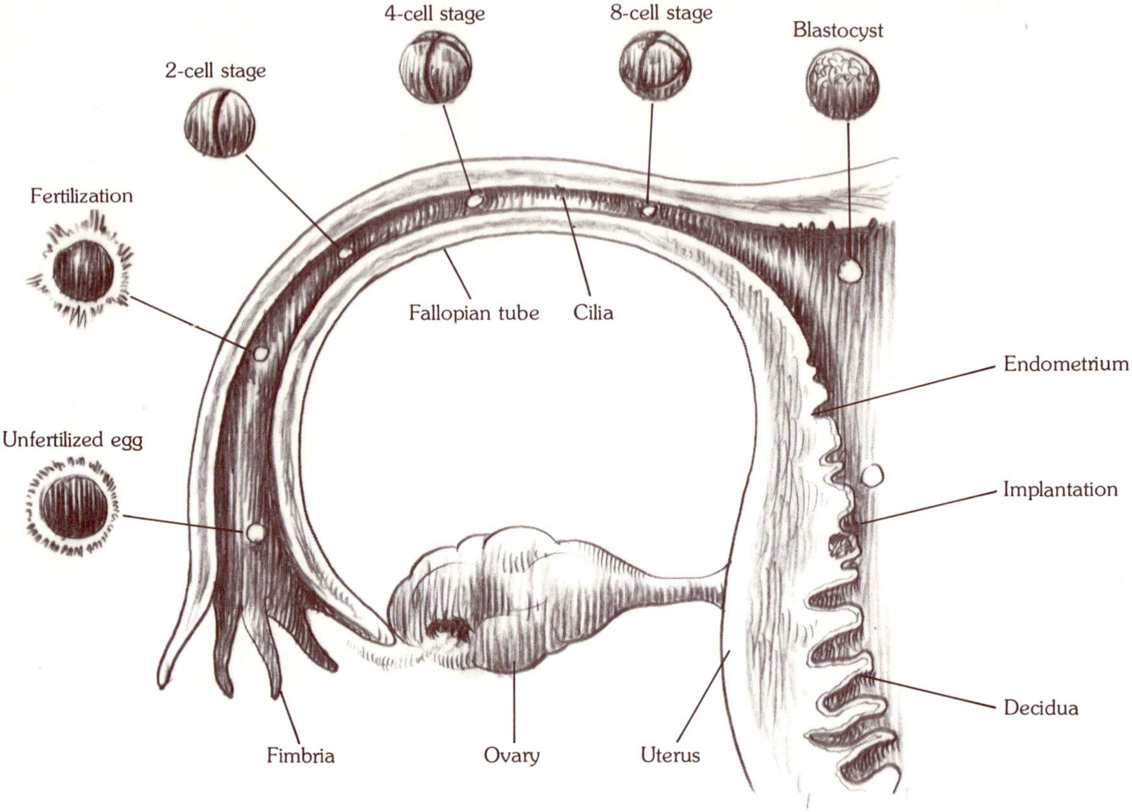

FIGURE 12.2 Stages of development of zygote. The egg escapes from the follicle in the ovary, is picked up by the fallopian tube, and is fertilized by a sperm cell.

attachment, or *implantation*, is usually in the upper half of the uterus. The blastocyst sinks into the spongy endometrium, which encloses over it. Soaking up nourishment from the endometrium, it grows from a dot-sized ball of cells. Increasing in size, it soon bulges into the cavity of the uterus, surrounded with endometrial tissues, now called *decidua.*

Placental Formation

From the outer wall of the blastocyst, small finger-like growths called *chorionic villi* begin to project into the decidua. In the decidua between the blastocyst and the uterine wall, spaces filled with maternal

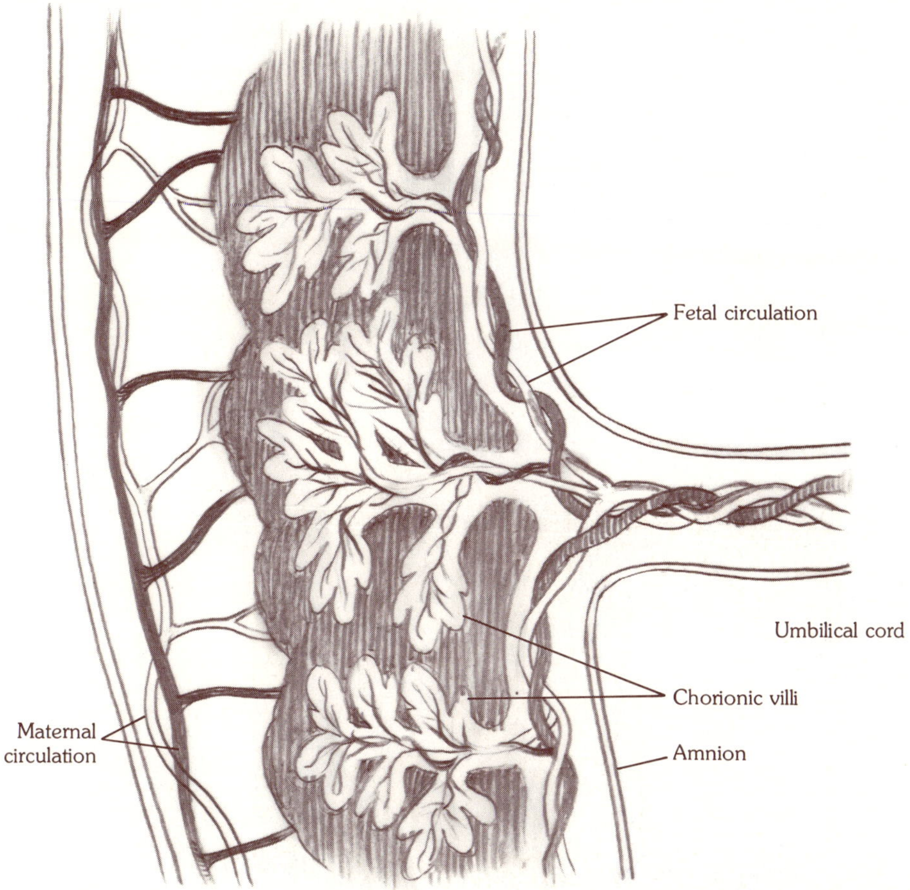

FIGURE 12.3 A portion of the placenta

blood are formed. Here maternal blood surrounds the villi, carrying oxygen and nutrients. Embryonic blood flows into the villi, separate and distinct from the maternal blood (Figure 12.3). This area of special tissue for the transfer of nutrients from the mother to the child and for the transfer of wastes from the child to the mother is the *placenta.* Even though there is a very close relation in the placenta between the villi of the embryo and those of the mother, there is *never* a direct connection between the two circulations. Blood does not cross directly from the mother to the embryo, or vice versa. The placenta actively transfers materials by the beginning of the fourth week after fertilization.

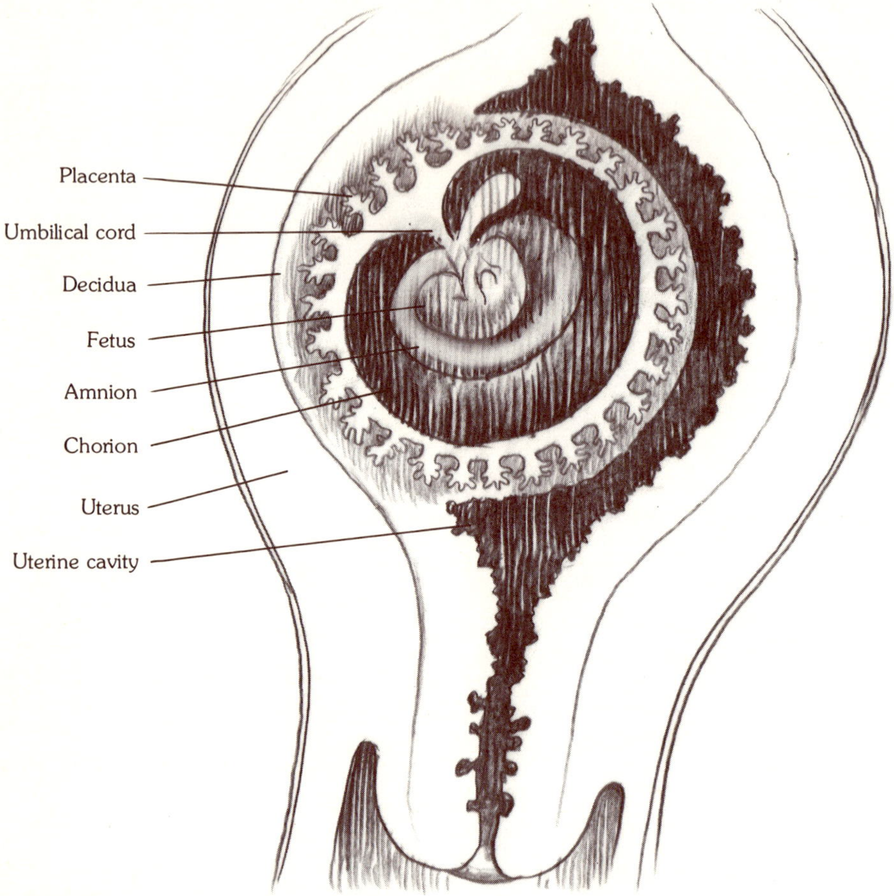

FIGURE 12.4 Fetal development and uterine tissues of early pregnancy

Amniotic Fluid

The embryo is attached to the placenta by the *umbilical cord.* It is surrounded by a double membrane consisting of the *amnion* and *chorion.* The space inside of these layers is the *amniotic cavity,* often called the "bag of waters." The space is filled with *amniotic fluid,* which bathes the developing embryo (see Figure 12.4). This fluid provides the embryo with space in which to develop, protects it against injury, keeps it at a constant temperature, and stores embryonic wastes, which are exchanged with the mother's fluids.

Lunar Months of Pregnancy

During the first eight weeks of pregnancy, the developing child is called an *embryo;* thereafter it is known as a *fetus.* The study of the unborn child is known as *embryology.*

A full-term human pregnancy usually lasts about 266 days from the time of conception, or about 280 days after the beginning of the last menstrual period (if ovulation has occurred about fourteen days after the beginning of menstruation, as it usually has). Pregnancy is commonly divided into ten 28-day periods (lunar months). A full-term pregnancy would be expected to last about forty weeks.

According to the calendar, pregnancy lasts a little over nine and one-third months. These nine calendar months are conveniently divided into three parts of three months each called *trimesters,* lasting about thirteen weeks each. Trimesters serve as landmarks during pregnancy.

First Lunar Month (to End of Fourth Week) The heart of the embryo is already beating and beginnings of the eyes, nose, ears, and brain appear. Arms and legs appear as tiny bumps. Internal organs—lungs, liver, kidneys, intestines—begin to form. The embryo is about five millimeters (less than one-fourth inch) long (see Figure 12.5).

Indications of pregnancy during the first month include cessation of menstruation, increased pressure of the uterus on the bladder, causing the woman to urinate frequently (this may continue until the third or fourth month), and enlargement and tenderness of the breasts. Tests may now be run to help confirm pregnancy. The uterine wall shows no signs of stretching for the first three months (see Figure 12.6).

Second Lunar Month (to End of Eighth Week) The head of the embryo is now as big as the rest of its body. Growing rapidly, the nervous system and the brain begin coordinating body functions. The embryo has started to move its arms and legs, turn its head, open and close its mouth, and swallow. A thin skin covers the body, in which most major structures are already formed. The embryo is 30 millimeters (about one inch) long (see Figure 12.5) and weighs one gram (about one-thirtieth of an ounce). From this point on, the embryo is known as a fetus.

Nausea and vomiting ("morning sickness") may begin by the sixth week and may last into the third or fourth month, occasionally longer. It occurs in about half of all pregnancies and is particularly common with a first pregnancy.

Third Lunar Month (to End of Twelfth Week) Teeth are being formed under the gums. The fingers and toes are evident, complete with tiny nails. Bone tissue is beginning to replace cartilaginous tissue. The

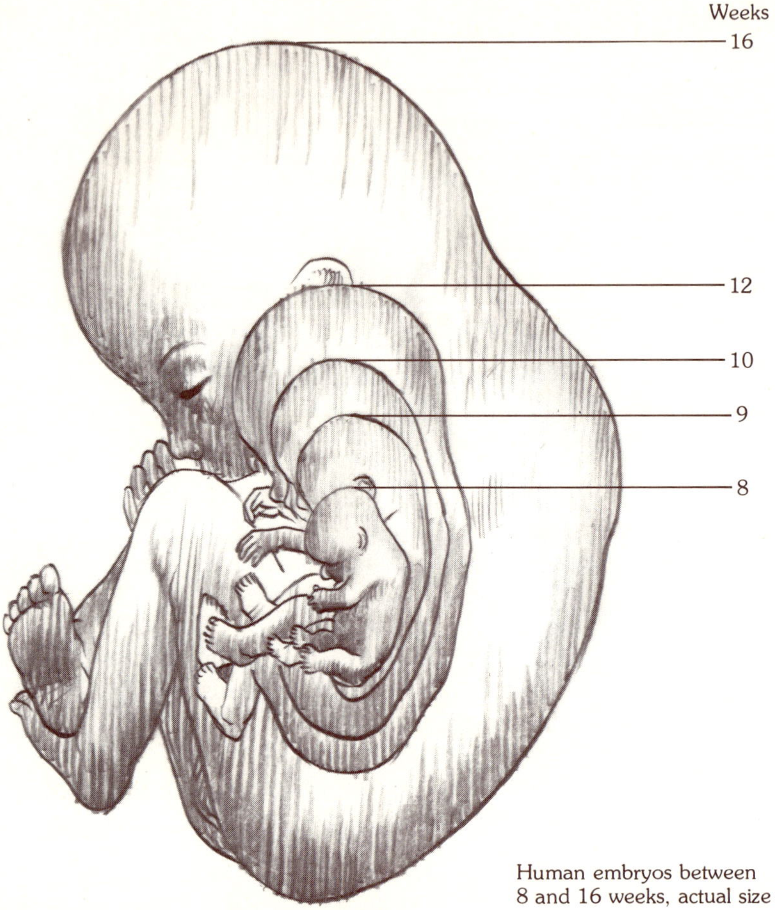

Human embryos between
8 and 16 weeks, actual size

FIGURE 12.5 Growth of the fetus, at natural size

eyes are covered with lids that now fuse and do not reopen until the sixth month. The kidneys begin to excrete wastes. Able to swallow, the fetus begins taking in amniotic fluid. The external genitalia now indicate the sex of the fetus. It may already be moving slightly, although the movement is usually too slight for the mother to feel. The fetus is now seven centimeters (about three inches) long (see Figure 12.5) and weighs about fourteen grams (one-half ounce).

Enlargement of the abdomen begins to become apparent about the third month.

Fourth Lunar Month (to End of Sixteenth Week) Growth is accelerating; the fetus now measures about fifteen centimeters (six inches) long (see Figure 12.5) and weighs about 105 grams (3.5 ounces). The entire body is covered with downy hair, or *lanugo.*

The mother becomes aware of the first movements of the fetus, and her breasts may excrete a yellowish fluid called *colostrum.* The uterus wall continues stretching as the fetus grows.

Fifth Lunar Month (to End of Twentieth Week) The fetus is now about 24 centimeters (9.5 inches) long and weighs about 310 grams (10 ounces). The fetal heartbeats can now be heard through the abdomen of the mother with a fetoscope. Hair begins to appear on its head.

The woman feels stronger fetal movements. Her breasts usually do not enlarge after the fifth month. The uterus is about as high in the abdo-

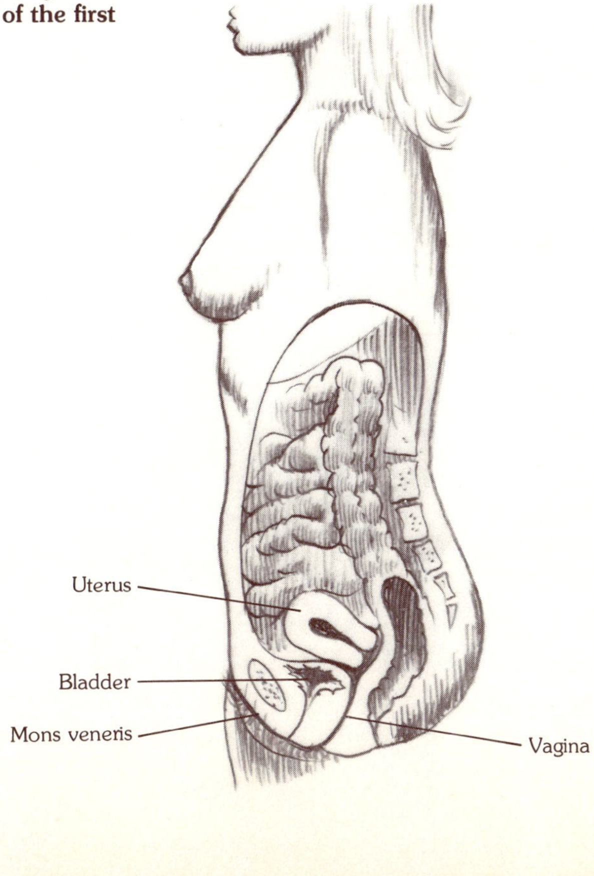

FIGURE 12.6 Abdominal cavity of a pregnant woman at the end of the first lunar month

men as the navel (see Figures 12.7 and 12.8). The end of this month marks the midpoint of pregnancy.

Sixth Lunar Month (to End of Twenty-fourth Week) The fetus is now growing rapidly; it is about 30 centimeters (12 inches) long and weighs about 640 grams (1.5 pounds). The fetal skin appears very wrinkled, the eyebrows and eyelashes have appeared, and the eyelids have reopened. The fetus may suck its thumb and have hiccups. It moves freely in the amniotic fluid and may even turn somersaults. The fetal movements are sharply felt by the mother. If it is born at this time, the fetus may attempt to breathe, but almost always dies shortly after birth.

Seventh Lunar Month (to End of Twenty-eighth Week) The fetus is about 35 centimeters (14 inches) long and weighs about 1080 grams (2.5 pounds). It looks wrinkled and scrawny, and the skin is red-

FIGURE 12.7 Abdominal cavity of a pregnant woman at the end of the fifth lunar month

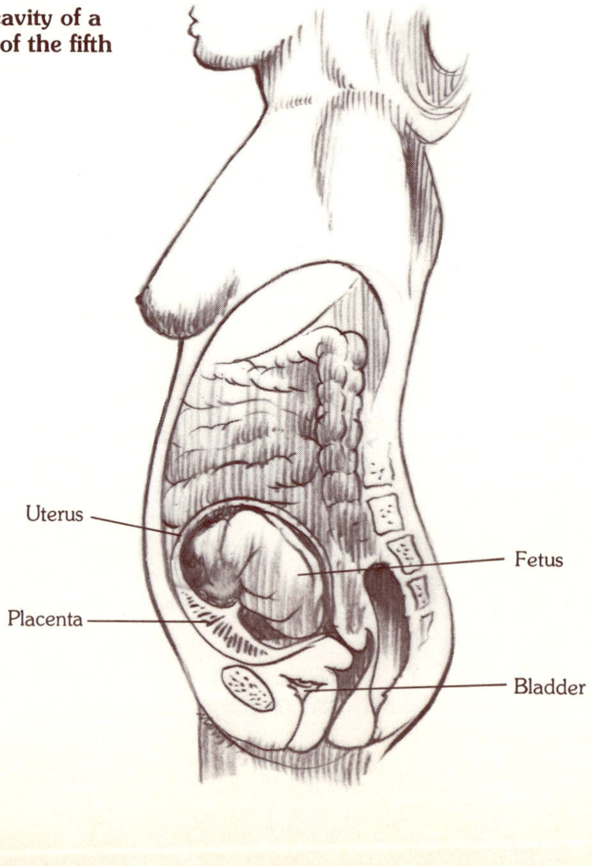

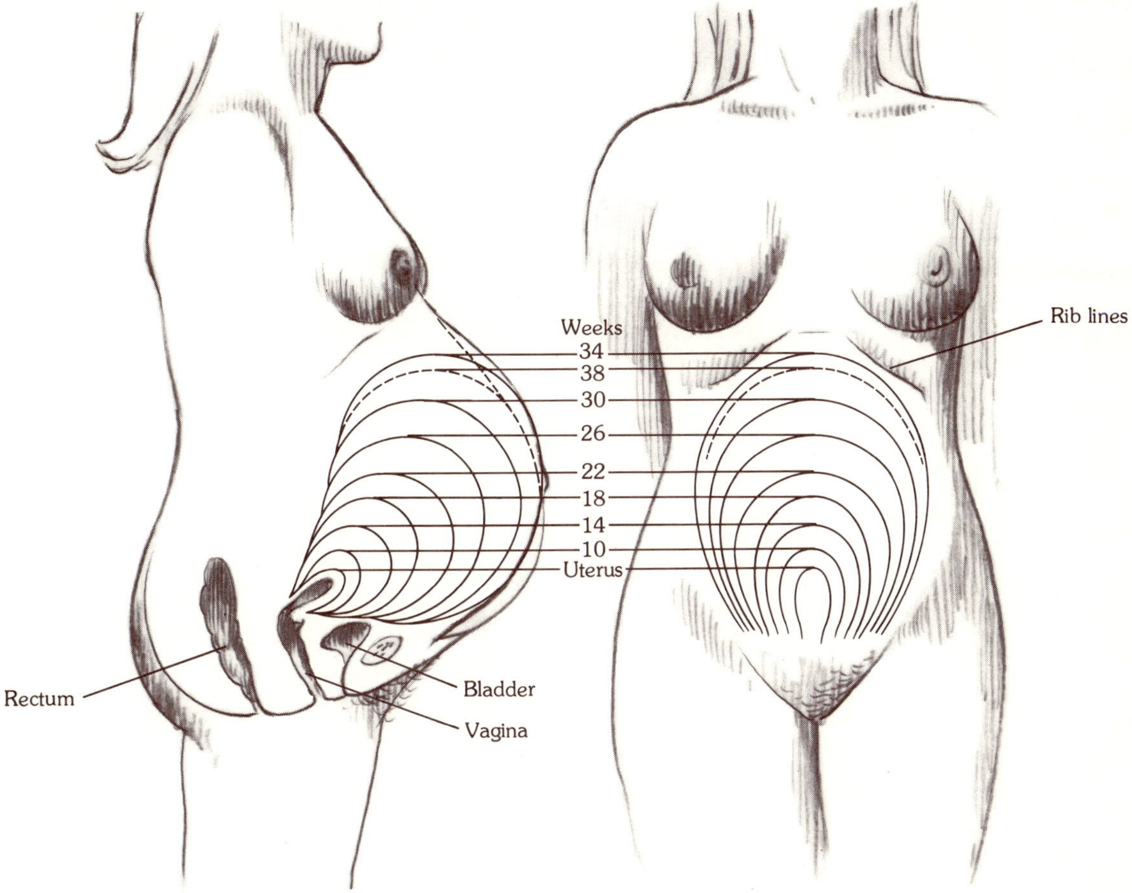

FIGURE 12.8 Enlargement of the uterus and abdomen during the various lunar months of pregnancy

dish. The internal ears are well developed and the fetus *in utero* apparently hears some sounds as early as the twenty-fourth to twenty-sixth week. There is evidence that it is also responsive to variations in taste. If the child is born at this time, it may move and cry. Its organs are sufficiently developed to make survival possible if excellent care is available, but many seven-month babies die.

Eighth Lunar Month (to End of Thirty-second Week) The fetus is about 40 centimeters (15.5 inches) long and weighs about 1670 grams (3.5 pounds). It still appears thin and wrinkled, although hair on its head is more abundant. The lanugo begins to disappear from the face. If the child is born now it has a good chance of survival. There is no truth to the old myth that a baby born in the seventh month is more likely to live than one born in the eighth month; most fetuses delivered after the thirty-second week survive.

Ninth Lunar Month (to End of Thirty-sixth Week) The fetus now weighs about 2400 grams (5.25 pounds) and is about 45 centimeters (18 inches) long. Recent development of fat under the skin gives the fetus a plumper appearance. Much of the wrinkling has disappeared. If the child is born at this time, its chances of survival are excellent.

The top of the uterus is now positioned near the lower tip of the breastbone (see Figures 12.8 and 12.9). The mother may need to urinate often from this time until delivery because the fetal head is pressing against the bladder. She will experience increased difficulty in walking.

FIGURE 12.9 Abdominal cavity of a woman at the end of the ninth lunar month

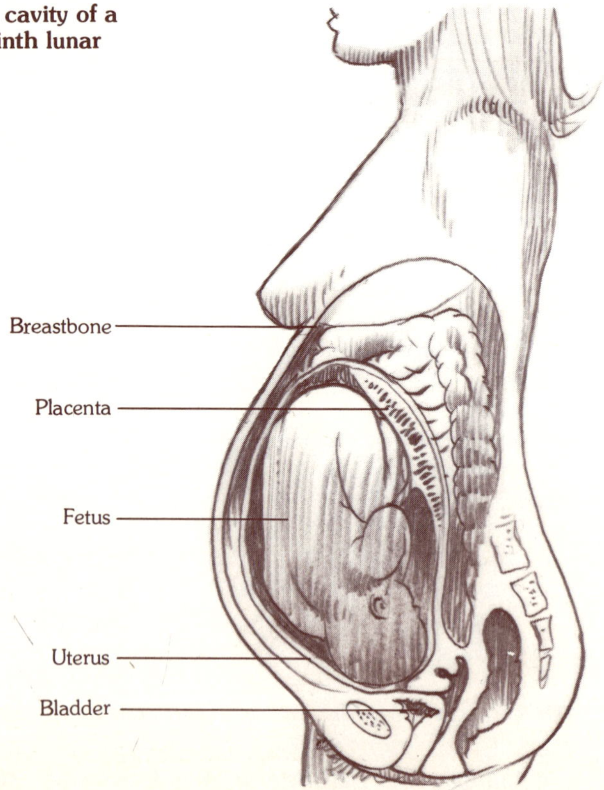

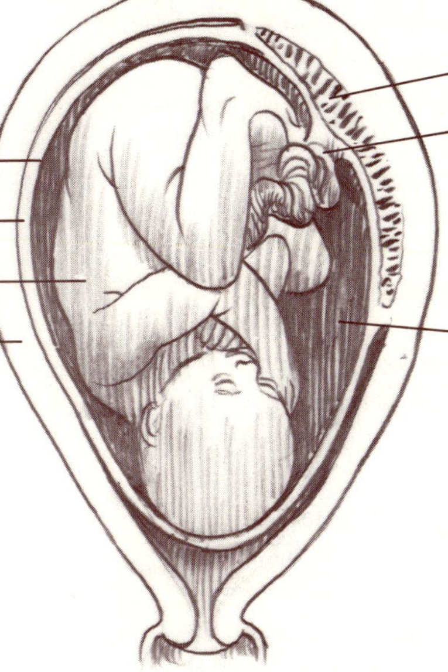

FIGURE 12.10 Fetus at the end of the tenth lunar month (term)

Tenth Lunar Month (to End of Fortieth Week) By this time the fetus has reached *term* (see Figure 12.10). The fetus' skin is smooth, and most lanugo has disappeared. The fingers and toes have well-developed nails and the skull bones are firmer. The average term baby is approximately 50 centimeters (20 inches) long and weighs about 3300 grams (7.25 pounds). A male fetus may be slightly heavier than a female. These weight and length figures are averages; there are considerable variations in both. Normal babies at term commonly vary from 2500 to 5000 grams (5.5 to 11 pounds) or more.

Diagnosis of Pregnancy

The determination of pregnancy can be based on symptoms the patient senses, signs the physician notes from physical examination, and laboratory tests.

Presumptive Signs

Presumptive signs are the least positive evidence of pregnancy. Each of these symptoms may be due to some condition other than pregnancy.

The first symptom is usually a missed menstrual period. One missed period is questionable evidence, but two missed periods in a healthy woman of child-bearing age whose menses have previously been regular is a strong indication of pregnancy. Other early indications of pregnancy may appear in the breasts. They increase in size and firmness, have a throbbing or tingling sensation, and a feeling of tension and fullness. They may be so sensitive that slight pressure is painful. The nipples may become enlarged and the areolae grow darker. Veins under the skin are more apparent.

Chadwick's sign, the darkening of the vulval or vaginal lining, is an early sign of pregnancy. "Quickening" (the mother's perception of movements made by the fetus) may be evident about the sixteenth week of pregnancy.

Probable Signs

The probable signs of pregnancy are usually discovered by a physician. Like presumptive signs, all of them may be simulated by other conditions. Yet two or more probable signs occurring simultaneously are strong evidence of pregnancy.

Near the end of the third lunar month the uterus can be felt through the abdominal wall as an enlargement that gradually increases in size throughout the pregnancy. Besides pregnancy, abdominal enlargement can also be caused by tumors, fluid, or rapid fat increase. Changes in the size, shape, and consistency of the uterus during the first three months of pregnancy are important indications of pregnancy, as is the ability to palpate the outline of the fetus. Sudden pressure against the fetus during the fourth and fifth months, causing it to rebound in a few seconds, is among the most certain of probable signs.

Positive hormonal tests for pregnancy are very reliable. In the event of implantation, the chorion of the embryo gives off a hormone called *chorionic gonadotropin.* Carried by the bloodstream, some of it gets into the urine, and urinalysis may detect its presence about ten to fourteen days after the first missed menstruation or by the end of the first lunar month. There are several other tests for pregnancy.

Immunoassay

Immunoassay tests are based on an antigen-antibody response. The hormones present in a urine sample serve as the antigen and will react with the antibody prepared for use in the test. Absence of agglutination (clumping) is considered a positive test. Results may be obtained in anywhere from a few minutes to two hours (depending on the particular pharmacologic source) and are 99 percent accurate.

Bioassay

Urine from a possibly pregnant woman is injected under the skin of a female animal. If the woman is pregnant, her hormone-laden urine will cause follicular development and ovulation in the animal, which is indicated by the presence of a corpus luteum in the ovary. Rats, frogs, rabbits, and mice may be used for such tests. The rat is the most widely used, provides an answer in sixteen to twenty-four hours, and is accurate 95 percent or more of the time.

Hormone Test

When a woman has missed a menstrual period, estrogen and progesterone may be given to her for two or three days. If she is not pregnant, a normal menstrual flow should occur within the next four to five days. In the nonpregnant woman, the hormones quickly build up the uterine lining; then with their discontinuance this lining is shed with bleeding. If she is pregnant, no bleeding will occur.

None of these test provides positive proof of pregnancy. Many obstetricians use them with reservations.

Positive Tests

There are three positive signs of pregnancy. All three concern the fetus: fetal heartbeat, perception of active movements of the fetus, and ability to see the fetal skeleton by x-ray. Hearing the fetal heartbeat separate from that of the mother is unmistakable evidence of pregnancy. The fetal pulse rate will range from 120 to 140 beats per minute and can be detected by the twentieth to twenty-second week of pregnancy. Fetal movements are commonly felt after the fourth or fifth month of pregnancy by placing the hand over the mother's abdomen. These movements vary from a faint flutter in the early months to brisk motions in later months. The fetal skeletal outline will be visible to x-rays sometime after the sixteenth week of pregnancy. Whenever the fetal skeleton can be distinguished by x-ray, the diagnosis of pregnancy is certain. X-ray is especially useful with obese women or in distinguishing a tumor from a normal pregnancy.

Care of the Pregnant Woman

The care of the mother from conception to the beginning of labor is called *prenatal care.* This care is most important for the good health of both mother and child. Unfortunately, it has been estimated that one-third to one-half of the women delivering children in public tax-supported hospitals in large cities see a physician for the first time when they are in labor.

Because of the demands pregnancy places on the body of the mother, a disorder or disease that might normally have little effect on her can turn into a major complication. A condition affecting the mother can also have a harmful effect on the fetus. Careful medical supervision during this time can avert many damaging conditions.

When a woman suspects that she is pregnant, she should have a complete physical examination, including checking of the uterus, cervix, vagina, bony pelvis, vulva, anus, and rectum. If a Pap smear has not been taken recently, it should be done now. A blood test for blood type, composition, syphilis, and Rh factor should be made. Urine should be examined for glucose and protein, and a chest x-ray is routine. Follow-up examinations should be made periodically upon the physician's suggestion. A woman should also report to her physician immediately in case of:

- any vaginal bleeding
- swelling of the face, fingers, or feet
- severe or continuous headaches
- dimness or blurring of vision
- abdominal pain
- persistent vomiting
- chills or fever
- dysuria (difficulty in urination)
- escape of fluid from the vagina

Factors to be closely watched by the mother during pregnancy include diet and certain disease conditions, some chronic and others infectious. These and other factors known to relate to congenital defects are discussed later in this chapter.

Chronic and Infectious Diseases

Rubella (German measles) and certain other virus diseases during pregnancy can cause abortion or premature labor. German measles in the first twelve weeks of pregnancy may cause congenital malformations (cataracts, deafness, heart ailments, brain damage). The likelihood of major malformations after the first trimester is relatively slight. Rubella is thought to result in the death of the fetus in about one out of every five cases when the mother contracts the disease early in pregnancy. Influenza, mumps, and pneumonia may also have serious effects. If a pregnant woman contracts any infectious disease, she should inform her physician.

Women who have chronic diseases need special attention during pregnancy. Diabetes is harder to control in a pregnant woman; it needs the close attention of a physician. Since the heart must work harder during pregnancy than normally, pregnant women with heart diseases also face possible complications. Special care is also needed for mothers with tuberculosis or kidney disorders.

Sexually Transmitted Diseases

Syphilis and gonorrhea can create serious complications. The spirochetes of syphilis will be transmitted from the mother to the fetus during the last half of pregnancy unless an infected mother receives treatment. Adequate treatment of the mother before the eighteenth week prevents infection of the fetus. But without treatment, syphilis is a frequent cause of fetal damage or death. Gonorrhea often goes unidentified in women. A lack of treatment or inadequate treatment not only allows a woman to infect her sex partners, but at the time of delivery the baby's eyes may become infected. To guard against such a possibility, germicide is commonly dropped into a child's eyes immediately after birth. Both silver nitrate and penicillin are used.

Toxemias

The toxemias of pregnancy are vascular disorders arising either during or immediately following pregnancy. They are characterized by hypertension (high blood pressure) and are sometimes associated with protein in the urine, swelling, convulsions, coma, or other signs, alone or in combination. The term "toxemia" is illogical, since no toxin, or poison, is found in the blood. Acute hypertension may be called *preeclampsia.* Preeclampsia can be considered severe when symptoms include continued high blood pressure, protein in the urine (proteinuria), less than normal urine output (oliguria), cerebral or visual disturbances, blueness (cyanosis), or pulmonary edema. Preeclampsia most commonly occurs during a first pregnancy and then typically during the third trimester. In severe cases, the untreated patient may go into convulsions or coma, and the baby may be stillborn. Treatment includes restriction in dietary salt, complete bed rest, drugs to reduce swelling and to quiet the mother, and prescribed amounts of water.

Vomiting

Pregnant women commonly complain of nausea and vomiting during the first half of pregnancy. Usually worse in the morning, nausea may continue throughout the day. Causes are usually hormonal.

If the vomiting does not disappear during the day, it is known as *pernicious vomiting.* It may become severe enough to interfere with nutrition, leading to dehydration and starvation. A physician can normally control this condition by the use of prescribed foods, fluids, and drugs, effecting a quick recovery without damage to the developing child.

Diet

The mother's diet during pregnancy may have lifelong effects on the physical and mental health of her baby. A pregnant mother is eating both for herself and for her developing child. Proper foods are important in the development of the fetal brain, teeth, bones, and all other tissues. The intake of protein, minerals, and vitamins must be increased.

Of less concern is restricting the weight gain of the mother. There is evidence that the birth weight of an infant is strongly associated with and conditioned by the weight gain of the mother. Excessive restriction of diet during pregnancy may unfavorably affect fetal growth and development. The higher the infant's birth weight, the better his or her growth and performance during the first year of life. Low birth weight (prematurity) is associated with a high incidence of neurological damage and newborn mortality. The incidence of major birth defects is two to four times higher among premature than among full-term babies.

The Committee on Maternal Nutrition of the National Research Council is now recommending an average weight gain of twenty-four pounds, slightly more for the woman whose prepregnancy weight is under 120 pounds. Heavier women should try to restrict their weigh gain to from twenty- to twenty-five pounds.

Termination of Pregnancy

Fetal Position

As shown in Figures 12.8 and 12.9, by the end of pregnancy the upper point of the uterus has risen almost to the breastbone of the mother. As a rule, in the later months of pregnancy the fetus forms a mass roughly similar to the shape of the uterine cavity, folded upon itself so that the chin is almost in contact with the chest, the thighs bent over the abdomen, the legs bent at the knees, and the arms either crossed over the chest or parallel to the sides.

The lowest part of the fetal body or that part first seen in delivery is called the presenting part. The *presentation* is named according to the presenting part. When the head is lowermost, it is a *cephalic presentation;* when the buttocks are lowermost, it is a *breech presentation* (see Figure 12.11). Most babies are born with the back of the head (vertex) appearing first. Much less commonly the part to appear first is the face, buttocks, shoulder, or some other part.

Estimated Date of Delivery

A customary way of estimating the expected day of delivery is to count back three months from the first day of the last menstrual period

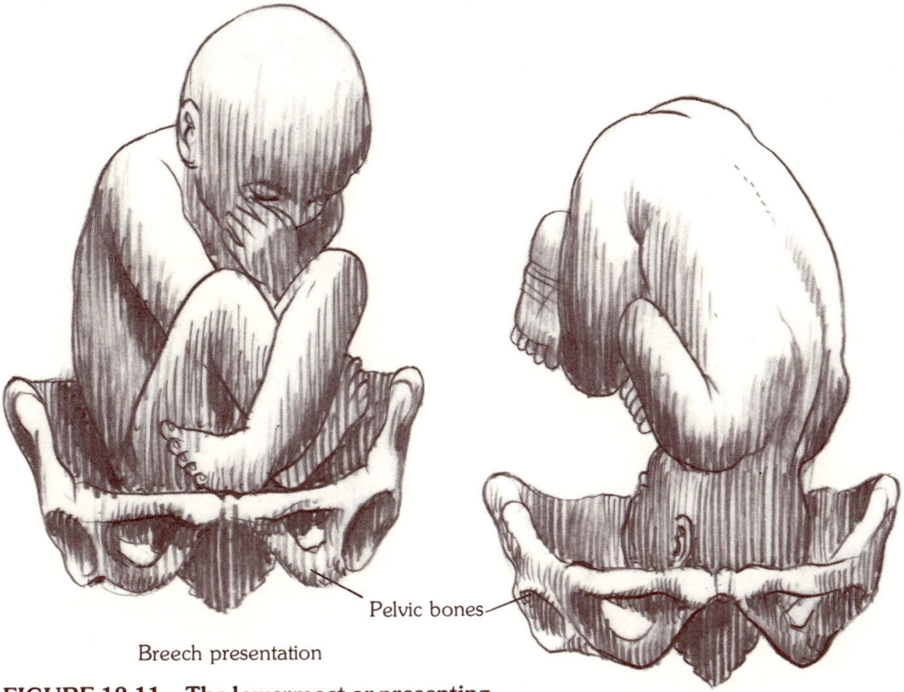

FIGURE 12.11 The lowermost or presenting part of the fetus in delivery

and add seven days (Naegele's rule). For example, if a woman's last menstrual period began on June 10, the expected day of delivery would be March 17. Few mothers deliver on the expected day; deviations of one to two weeks earlier or later than the expected date are common.

False Labor

False labor contractions may occur as early as three or four weeks before the termination of pregnancy. They are nothing more than an exaggeration of the intermittent uterine contractions that occur throughout the entire period of pregnancy.

There are ways of distinguishing them from the contractions of true labor. They occur chiefly in the groin and lower abdomen rather than in the top region of the uterus. Their duration is short and they are rarely intensified by walking about (in fact, walking may even relieve them). They do not increase progressively in intensity, duration, and frequency. True labor contractions cause a dilatation (expansion) of the cervix of the uterus within a few hours, whereas false labor does not.

"Show"

A rather dependable sign of approaching labor is "show" or the discharge from the vagina of a small amount of blood-tinged mucus, that has filled the cervical canal during pregnancy. Labor usually follows within several hours or a few days.

Labor

Labor is the process by which the products of conception are expelled by the mother (also commonly called childbirth, travail, or parturition). The word *delivery* refers to the actual birth of the baby. This is expected to occur at *term*, or the end of the fortieth week.

Labor is conveniently divided into three stages: (1) preparatory state, (2) birth of the baby, and (3) delivery of the afterbirth.

First Stage The first stage starts with the beginning of labor contractions and lasts until the cervix is fully dilated and ready for the passage of the child (see Figure 12.12). The initial contractions are short and mild,

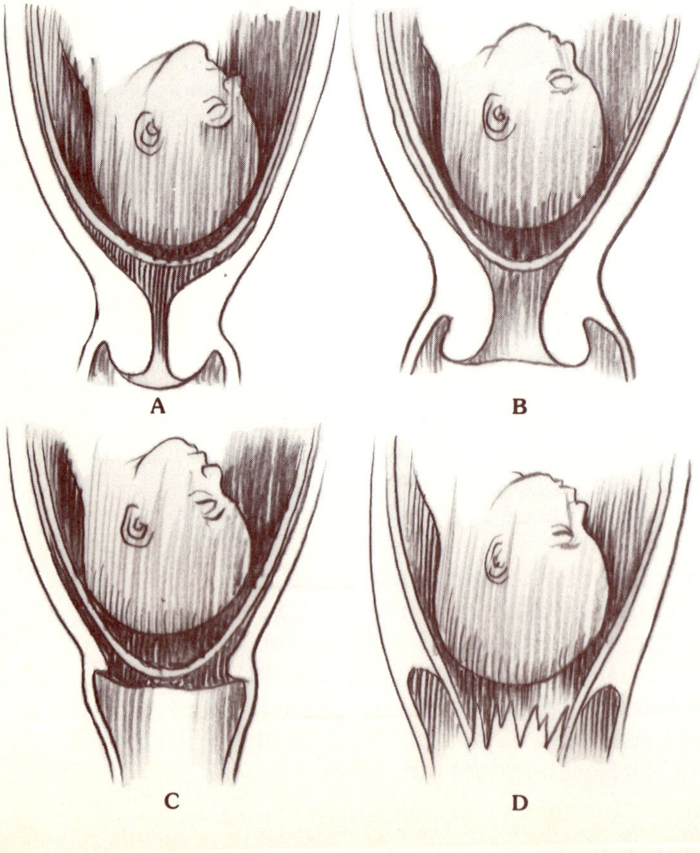

FIGURE 12.12 Labor, first stage: (A) cervix before dilation; (B) beginning of dilation; (C) cervix fully dilated; (D) rupture of the amnion

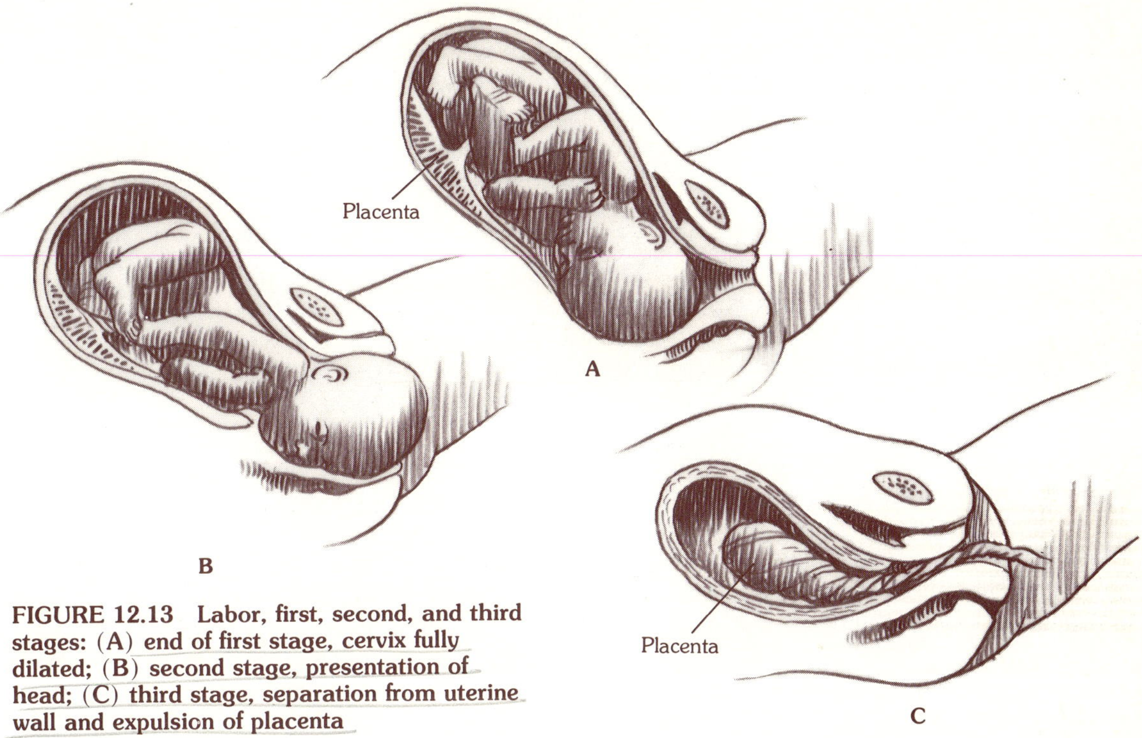

FIGURE 12.13 Labor, first, second, and third stages: (A) end of first stage, cervix fully dilated; (B) second stage, presentation of head; (C) third stage, separation from uterine wall and expulsion of placenta

and usually are separated by intervals of ten to twenty minutes. The woman may walk around between contractions. Discomfort usually starts in the small of the back and then sweeps around to the front of the abdomen. As labor progresses the contractions become more frequent (every three to five minutes), become more intense, and last longer. The contractions preceding full dilation may be quite painful. The average duration of the first stage is about twelve hours for the first child and about seven hours for later children, although there is marked variation.

Second Stage Delivery starts with the full opening of the cervix and ends with the completed birth of the child (see Figure 12.13).

Contractions are severe and may last 50 to 100 seconds, occurring at intervals of two or three minutes. The pressure of the contractions will usually cause the rupture of the amniotic sac ("bag of waters") during the early part of this stage (but sometimes before or during the first stage). During the contractions the mother strains and "bears down" strongly.

When the cervix is open, the child begins to move down into the vagina. Each labor contraction moves the head down farther. With the cessation of each contraction, the head recedes somewhat. Just before the head emerges, it rotates to the side to pass the front part of the pelvic bone. With the next few contractions the neck and shoulders emerge. The body of the child is then quickly expelled and immediately the rest of the amniotic fluid gushes out. As soon as the child has emerged, the physician or midwife ties off the umbilical cord several inches from the navel. Immediately after birth the attending person assists the child to begin breathing by slapping it smartly on the back, if necessary. The child usually begins breathing within one minute and lets out a strong cry.

The average length of the second stage is fifty minutes in the first delivery and twenty minutes in later ones.

Third stage The third stage of labor, often called the placental stage, consists of two phases: placental separation and placental expulsion.

Contractions of the uterine muscle continue at three- to four-minute intervals. With the rapid decrease in uterus size, and since the placenta is not contractible, it is literally squeezed off the uterine wall. As the separation occurs, a bit of the uterine wall is lost and some bleeding occurs. Placental separation takes about two to three minutes.

The expulsion of the uterus may be accomplished by the efforts of the mother or by the attendant manually. Placental expulsion from the uterus takes five to six additional minutes.

Reducing the Pain of Delivery

The delivery of a child is normally painful. The amount of this pain can sometimes be reduced by the methods employed in so-called *natural childbirth.* An instructor, usually nurse, conducts classes in which prospective mothers are taught the physical and emotional aspects of delivery and instructed in controlled relaxation and breathing, which are sometimes helpful in reducing muscle spasm during labor. Most mothers throughout the ages have known little about their anatomy and have not spent months doing breathing exercises; the only "natural" aspect of these methods is the elimination of the anesthetics that have come into wide use to reduce the pain of childbirth (but an anesthetic is administered if the mother asks for it). Some mothers are enthusiastic about natural childbirth; others have found it of some help but still needed an anesthetic; still others would never try it a second time. Natural childbirth had a great vogue some years ago and still has its adherents, but no woman should be made to feel ashamed if she prefers a little unnatural help. This decision is the mother's alone to make. It's her body and her baby.

Some drugs used in childbirth reduce the pain but allow the mother to remain conscious; others act only on selected parts of her body; some cause her to lose consciousness; and some have no effect on the pain but cause partial or complete loss of memory of the pain. Drugs may be injected into the spinal cord to deaden nerves coming from the uterus, but not affect the mother's consciousness. The drugs used depend upon the wishes of the mother and the choice of the physician.

With mothers who are receptive to it, hypnosis has been effective in permitting labor with little or no use of drugs. Although the method is recognized by the American Medical Association, its use is limited. It requires time and patient response.

Handling the Newborn

The moment when the child completely emerges from the mother is the official time of birth. As soon as the baby is delivered, it is grasped by the feet and held head down to drain fluids from the nose and mouth. Excess mucus may be aspirated from the mouth and pharynx. The umbilical cord is clamped and cut, causing a rise in blood pressure, which is considered by some to be important in initiating respiration. (Within a few days the cord stump dries up and drops off.). The baby may, however, breathe before the cutting of the umbilical cord. The baby must breathe almost immediately, because it can no longer obtain oxygen from the mother. Some babies cry and take their first breath before or as soon as they are fully expelled by the mother. In most cases breathing starts within one minute. A strong cry indicates that the respiratory system is functioning well. If there is any delay in breathing, resuscitation must be applied immediately to prevent asphyxiation (suffocation). Delay in breathing can cause damage to the brain cells or death.

A child born in a modern hospital is quickly checked for normal heartbeat, regular breathing, good movement of arms and legs, nervous reflex, and normal color. As already described, the infant's eyes are treated with a germicide to prevent the possibility of gonorrheal infection (this treatment is required by law in most states). The physician inspects the infant for any apparent abnormalities, such as birthmarks, clubfeet, ambiguous genitals, or improperly formed body openings, and also decides whether the infant needs incubator care or not.

Complications of Delivery

Premature Birth

Occasionally a pregnancy ends before the fetus is mature enough to live on its own. Whether or not the fetus survives will depend on the point during pregnancy at which the termination occurs, the causes, and the conditions of the termination.

By definition, a premature infant is one whose birth weight is less than 2500 grams. No fetus weighing less than 400 grams has survived, and only a few weighing less than 500 grams. The less an infant weighs at birth, the less its chance of survival. The survival chances of fetuses at birth are often classified according to the following scale (although exceptions do occur):

1. 499 grams (1 lb., 1 oz.) or less: no chance of survival (abortuses).
2. 500 grams (1 lb., 2 oz.) to 999 grams (2 lb., 2 oz.) poor chance of survival (immature infants).
3. 1000 grams (2 lb., 3 oz.) to 2499 grams (5 lb., 8 oz.): poor to good chances of survival, according to weight (premature infants).
4. 2500 gm. (5 lb., 9 oz.) or more: optimal chances of survival (mature infants).

The fetus may weigh 500 grams (1 lb., 2 oz.) during the sixth lunar month (about twenty-two weeks), 1000 grams (2 lb., 3 oz.) about the end of the twenty-eighth week. Generally the fetus becomes viable (may survive if born) at the beginning of the third trimester.

Known causes of premature birth include multiple pregnancies (twins, triplets, and so on) and maternal disease (toxemia, placental problems, untreated syphilis). As many as half of all premature births, however, occur without known cause. Prematurity is the leading cause of infant mortality (death between the time of birth and one year of age). The death of the infant may often be caused by respiratory difficulties or infections of various kinds.

Cesarean Section

The delivery of the fetus through an incision in the wall of the abdomen and uterus is a *cesarean section* (sometimes spelled "caesarean").

About half of all cesarean sections are performed on women bearing their first child. The most frequent reason for cesarean section for a first delivery is space limitation—too large a child for the birth canal, a birth canal tumor, or pelvic contraction. Other reasons are breech presentation, maternal diabetes, and placental or umbilical cord complications. A cesarean may also be performed in an attempt to save the fetus in the event of the imminent or actual death of the mother late in pregnancy.

The other half of all cesarean sections are performed on women who have had previous cesareans. Once a woman has had a cesarean there is a possibility that the uterine wall, weakened by the previous incision, may rupture during labor. Although it is not necessarily impossible for a woman who has had a cesarean to give birth through natural labor, the risk is usually thought too great to take, and subsequent deliveries are also made by cesarean section. The number of cesareans that a mother may safely have is usually decided by her physician. Usually a mother is counseled to limit her children to two or three, although some women have had more cesarean sections.

A physician will often set a definite date for the operation if the maturity of the fetus can be established with confidence. Otherwise, the physician may wait until the patient goes into labor. In any event, the physician may not want to perform a section more than ten days before the calculated date of delivery owing to the chance of undue prematurity.

Multiple Pregnancies

A *multiple pregnancy* is one in which the uterus contains two or more embryos. Twins occur in about one out of every 89 pregnancies, and triplets in about one out of every 7921 (89 × 89) births. Twins occur more commonly among blacks than among whites.

Twins may result from the fertilization of either two separate eggs or a single egg (see Figure 12.14). Twins that develop from two separate

FIGURE 12.14 Development of twins

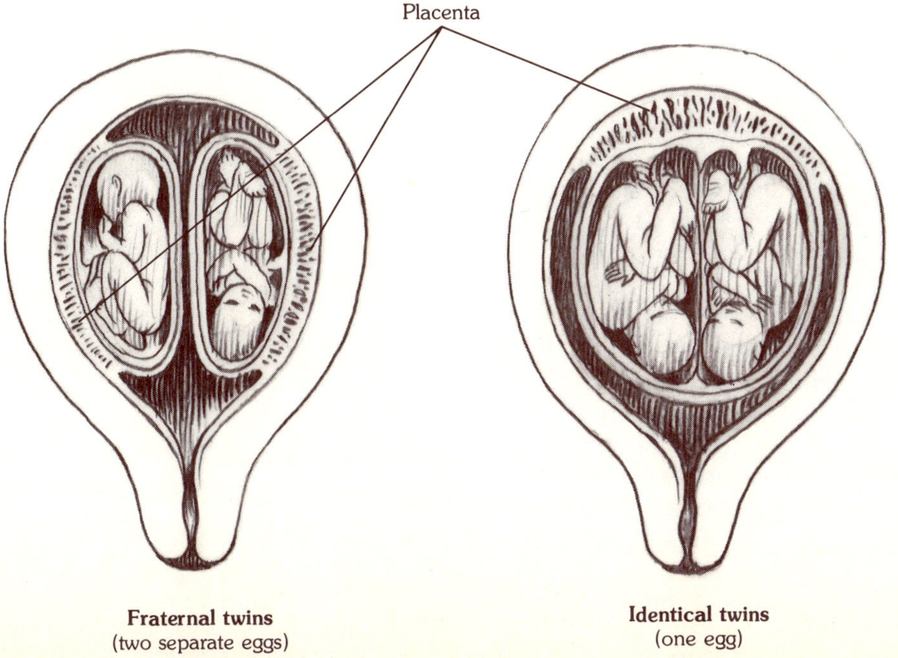

eggs are called *fraternal* twins. Since they come from two separate eggs, fertilized by two separate sperm, they are no more alike than any other siblings. They may be of the same sex or of opposite sexes. They may or may not share the same placenta.

In about one out of every three cases of twins, one mature egg, fertilized by a single sperm, completely divides into two halves. Since both developing embryos are from the same egg and are fertilized by the same sperm, they are *identical,* or alike genetically.

Triplets may arise from one, two, or three eggs. One egg may divide into three parts, in which case the triplets are identical. If they come from two eggs, one of the eggs has divided into two halves, and two of the triplets are identical and the other is fraternal. The same holds true for quadruplets, quintuplets, and all other kinds of multiple pregnancies. In one case (the Dionne quintuplets) it is believed that all five girls developed from a single egg and thus were identical.

Current treatment of sterility due to lack of ovulation, using human gonadotropins, has not only successfully induced ovulation but also produced multiple eggs, often in quite astonishing numbers. The common result has been multiple pregnancies. Efforts are being made to reduce this side effect from the use of such hormones.

Extrauterine Pregnancies

Some pregnancies develop outside the uterus. Implantation anywhere other than in the uterus is an *ectopic* pregnancy. Almost all of these occur in the fallopian tubes. This type of pregnancy is believed to be caused by conditions that prevent or slow the movement of the egg down the tube or by increased receptivity of the tubal lining to the fertilized egg. Regardless of the place the egg lodges, the embryo usually dies. The mother may feel severe abdominal pains and, if hemorrhaging occurs, will show vaginal bleeding. In any event, the affected tube must be removed. This does not preclude later pregnancies, since another fallopian tube is still available for egg transport.

Induction of Labor

Where a pregnancy has developed medical complications, it may be necessary to terminate the pregnancy artificially in order to save the life of the fetus, the mother, or both. Sometimes a physician may decide to terminate a pregnancy for reasons of convenience—a mother who has had a history of rapid deliveries and who might not make it to the hospital in time, or who lives a great distance from a hospital, or who has already had one uneventful delivery, is physically ready to deliver, and wants to get on with it. Physical readiness is defined as dilation of the cervix to a width of at least two centimeters. If the cervix has not yet begun to dilate, labor should not be induced except in unusual circumstances. The incidence of brain-damaged infants is significantly higher when labor is prematurely induced than when it is not. Premature induction is also harder on the mother; contractions are more intense and last longer. Labor should never be induced for the convenience of the obstetrician. But if a qualified physician finds that the mother is ready, induced labor can be a great convenience for everyone concerned, and is no harder on the mother or the child than any other labor.

Changes in the Mother After Delivery

By the end of the first week after delivery, the tissues of the vagina and uterus have greatly contracted. Within six weeks the uterus is virtually back to normal. The abdominal wall should be back to original shape and firmness within two to three months.

Loss of Weight

A mother loses about eleven pounds as soon as the baby is delivered. Within the next several weeks she should lose an additional four and one-half to five and one-half pounds. Unless she has gained excessively during pregnancy, she should return to her nonpregnant weight within six to eight weeks.

Menstruation

Women who do not nurse their babies usually start to menstruate within eight weeks after delivery. If the mother does nurse, menstruation is often delayed until the third or fourth month, although the delay may vary from two to eighteen months. It may return before or after milk production is ended. Although ovulation is normally suspended while milk is produced, a nursing mother may become pregnant even though she has not yet menstruated since delivery. The first few menstrual cycles may be irregular, but the woman will usually return to her regular cycle in time.

Breasts

Breasts begin enlarging early in pregnancy (see Figure 12.15). During pregnancy they may produce small amounts of colostrum, a yellowish fluid. On about the third day after delivery, the breasts become engorged with milk. At first they may feel uncomfortable, but within several days these feelings disappear as milk production becomes regulated. Frequent and complete emptying of the breasts stimulates production. If the baby cannot empty the breasts in the early days of nursing, it is sometimes necessary to empty the breasts artificially. The length of time a

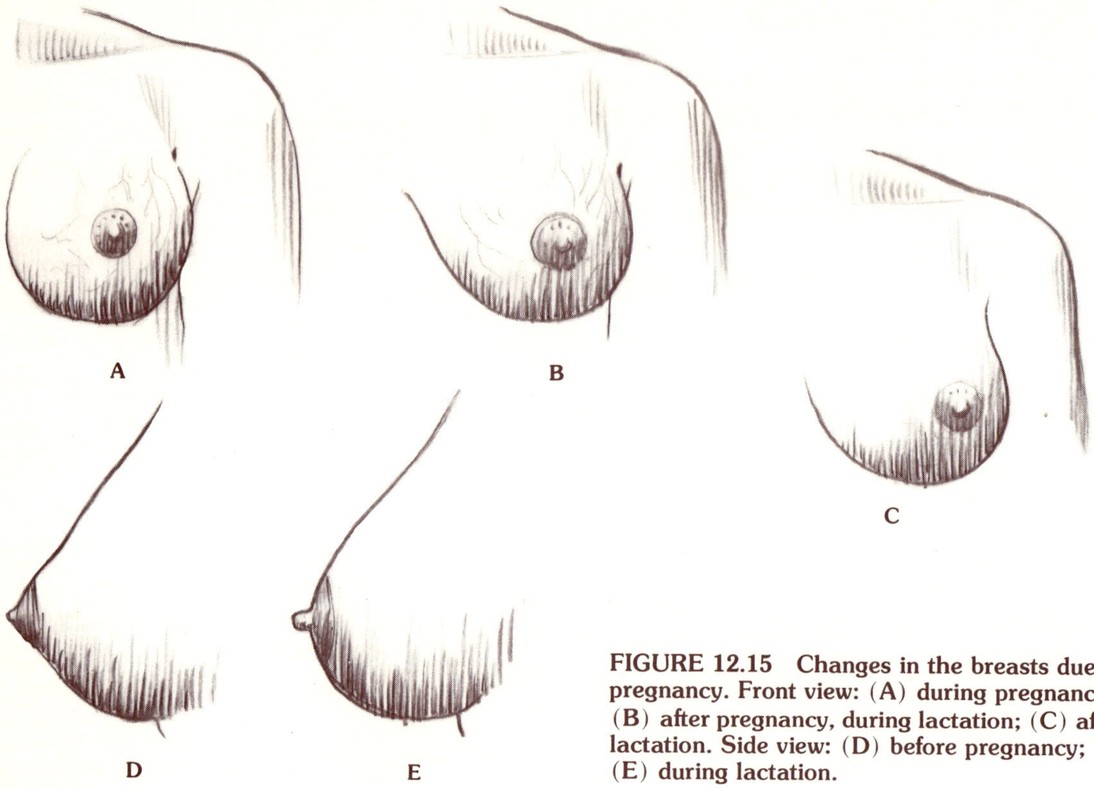

FIGURE 12.15 Changes in the breasts due to pregnancy. Front view: (A) during pregnancy; (B) after pregnancy, during lactation; (C) after lactation. Side view: (D) before pregnancy; (E) during lactation.

mother breast-feeds her child will vary. Discontinuance of nursing should be a gradual process, allowing milk production to decrease.

If a mother chooses not to nurse her baby, milk production can be suppressed by stopping the production of milk-producing hormones. Failure to remove accumulated milk from the breasts will also inhibit further milk production. The breasts will become engorged with milk, however, and the mother will feel some discomfort for several days.

Congenital Defects

Gross structural deformities present at the time of birth are called *congenital defects.* Their incidence is relatively high. About one in every sixteen babies born in this country is born with a serious physical defect. Some defects cause physical and mental handicap, disfigurement, shortened life, or death. Of the nearly 200,000 babies born each year with serious congenital defects, about 16,000 die before they reach their first birthday. Some malformed embryos do not reach full development but are spontaneously aborted. Authorities estimate that about one-third of all "miscarriages" are due to malformed embryos.

Some of the more common congenital defects include birthmarks, cleft lip (harelip), cleft palate, clubfoot, congenital urinary tract defects, diabetes, mongolism (Down's syndrome), hydrocephaly, missing limbs, extra fingers and toes, cystic fibrosis, open spine, sickle-cell anemia, galactosemia, phenylketonuria (PKU), erythroblastosis, and congenital heart disease. We shall discuss two of these.

Erythroblastosis Fetalis

There is a blood factor called the *Rh* (rhesus) *factor* that is found in the blood of about five out of six Americans. Those having it are called *Rh positive;* those lacking it, *Rh negative.* If an Rh-negative woman receives Rh-positive blood by bearing an Rh-positive child, whose Rh factor passes into her bloodstream during the pregnancy, the foreign Rh-positive blood stimulates the production of an antibody, *anti-Rh.* No harm is done to the mother and there may be none to the child; but if she again becomes pregnant with an Rh-positive child, the antibodies produced during her earlier pregnancy pass through the placenta and attack the fetus' red blood cells. Production of antibodies may also be stimulated by the transfusion of Rh-positive blood into an Rh-negative woman.

The Rh factor may be a problem in pregnancy only when the father is Rh-positive and the Rh-negative mother is carrying an Rh-positive fetus (see Figure 12.16). The anti-Rh antibodies produced by the mother's body destroy the fetus' red blood cells, causing a severe type of anemia (inability of the blood to carry oxygen) and jaundice. To compensate, the bone marrow releases erythroblasts (immature red blood cells). In severe cases the infant may be born dead or may die shortly after birth. If he survives, he may be mentally retarded.

Today a physician can test for a dangerous anti-Rh level during pregnancy. Damage can often be prevented by an exchange blood transfusion immediately after birth or even before birth. Vaccines are available for Rh-negative mothers which neutralize any Rh antigen that might enter the maternal blood at the time of delivery of an Rh-positive baby. The vaccine should be injected within seventy-two hours after such a delivery or after any miscarriage or induced abortion of an Rh-negative woman. It is over 90 percent effective in protecting the next Rh-positive child. Also, spacing births sufficiently may allow antibody levels to fall so low that they will not cause trouble for the next fetus.

Congenital Heart Disease

More deaths during the first year of life result from congenital heart disease than from any other cause.

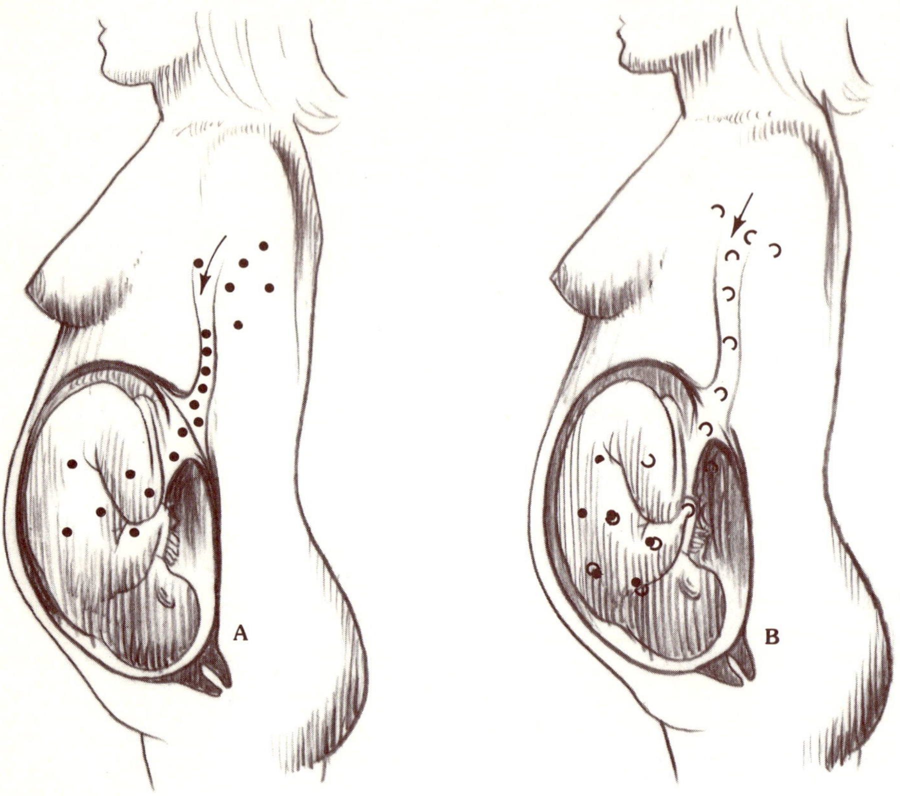

FIGURE 12.16 **The Rh factor. The Rh− mother is carrying an Rh+ child. (A) the Rh antigen, shown by black dots, moves from the child into the mother's blood. This most commonly occurs at the time of delivery. (B) Her body reacts by producing anti-Rh antibodies, shown by black cups, which move into the child's blood, destroying his red blood cells. This usually occurs in the pregnancy following sensitization.**

First a word should be said about a child's fetal circulation. During fetal life the child uses the lungs of the mother for respiration. The fetus' blood travels through the umbilical cord to the placenta, where it exchanges gases and wastes with gases and food in the mother's blood. The blood entering the fetus is rich in oxygen. It passes to the liver, then into the right side of the heart (see Figure 12.17). Since the fetus is not yet breathing, its lungs do not require the great amount of blood that they need after birth. The heart of the fetus therefore has two by-passes, the *foramen ovale* and the *ductus arteriosus*, which allow much of the fetal blood to pass through the heart quickly and out into the body.

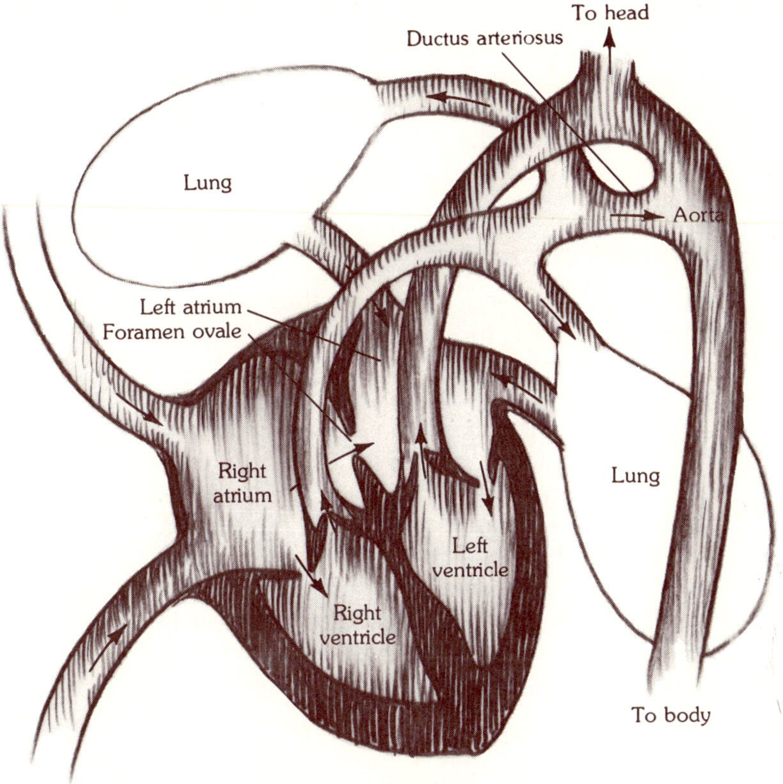

FIGURE 12.17 Fetal heart with two-by-passes, the *foramen ovale* and the *ductus arteriosus*. Both by-passes allow fetal blood to pass into the aorta without first going through the lungs. Both normally close near the time of birth to ensure full pulmonary circulation in the infant.

After birth, when the child starts breathing, these by-passes normally close. But it is estimated that these closures may be incomplete in as many as 20 percent of all children, resulting in congenital heart defects.

Many other types of heart defect may occur. The common symptom of these defects is a blue skin color (cyanosis), due to inadequate oxygen in the blood. A baby with such a condition is often called a "blue baby." Many heart conditions can be surgically repaired during infancy.

Causes of Congenital Defects

Faulty genes cause about 20 percent of all birth defects, a faulty environment in the uterus another 20 percent; and combinations of the two 60 percent. Hereditary defects may cause chemical disturbances in the fetus that may result in such conditions as PKU, galactosemia, and cystic fibrosis.

The uterine environment includes those things that happen to the mother during pregnancy as well as the things that take place in the uterus around the fetus. Virus infections in the mother, particularly during the first three months of pregnancy, may cause defects. One such harmful infection is rubella (German measles).

Drugs the mother takes during pregnancy may cause abnormalities. Thalidomide, a tranquilizer-sedative that was available in Europe during the early 1960s, caused deformity of the long bones, so that children were born with defective arms and legs or, in severe cases, with both arms and legs missing. The deformity occurred when mothers took the medication during the important second month of pregnancy.

Most defects start during the first ninety days of pregnancy. Drugs (alcohol, sedatives, tranquilizers, and others) that might be safe to take under most circumstances may be dangerous in the context of the rigorous demands of early pregnancy. The danger is especially great in an unplanned pregnancy, as damage may be done before the woman even knows she is pregnant. Knowing that there may be other causes for a missed menstrual period, a woman may exercise insufficient caution in her exposure to x-rays, virus infections, or drugs. She may not see a physician for several months, and by then she has already passed the period of greatest fetal damage.

Prevention of Congenital Defects

Here are some simple suggestions on ways in which prospective parents may reduce the chances of birth defects in their children.

1. Do not marry a close relative unless both of you are unusually brilliant and talented, and have numerous brilliant and talented relatives. Charles Darwin, grandson of the illustrious philologist Erasmus Darwin, married his cousin Emma Wedgwood, of the pottery Wedgwoods, and together they produced five sons, of whom four were eminent scientists; three of them were knighted. Most of us, however, have a greater share of genetic weaknesses, and marriage to a near relative increases the risk of producing a defective child. This increased risk is the basis for state laws prohibiting the marriage of close relatives.

2. All married couples should have a family physician. He should be made aware of any known history of family defects or sources of complication such as an Rh incompatibility, so he can correctly counsel the couple. Both husband and wife should seek his counsel before planning a pregnancy, and then the woman should see him at regular intervals during pregnancy. Since premature babies are more likely to be defective than full-term babies, medical care during pregnancy is essential to reduce the chances of premature delivery.

3. A physician consulted for reasons other than pregnancy should be told of any suspected pregnancy, even though the woman may not be absolutely sure of it herself. A woman who either is pregnant or apt to become pregnant should take *only* those medications prescribed by her physician.

4. The pregnant woman should try to avoid contact with persons suffering from communicable diseases. If there has been known contact, she should inform her physician.

5. Except in emergency, x-rays should be avoided during the first ninety days of pregnancy.

6. Smoking and drinking alcoholic beverages should be avoided during pregnancy. Statistically, the more a mother smokes during pregnancy, the less her baby is likely to weigh at birth. As we have already pointed out, the weight of a baby at birth is positively correlated with his chances of survival, especially if he is exceptionally small. Alcohol has also been shown to be damaging to a fetus.

7. The age of the mother must be considered. A high correlation exists between birth defects and the age of the mother, and in some cases of the father. Mothers under eighteen and over forty produce a greater percentage of defective children than those between the ages of eighteen and forty. Many physicians recommend that a woman have her pregnancies by the age of thirty or thirty-five.

8. Since diet affects growth, women should be careful to eat properly. Diet affects not only a woman's own health, but also the future growth and development of her children. The fetus depends entirely on the diet of its mother.

Much is being done to cope with nature's errors. Some chemical defects can be detected early and treated with special diets. Others can be treated with specific drugs. When the defect is structural, surgeons can perform remarkable repairs. Sometimes the results are perfect. When they are not, other rehabilitation therapy often can make possible an almost normal life.

Fertility Control

13

Beyond question, love and/or the need for the release of sexual tension, rather than a desire for pregnancy, is the basis of most sexual intercourse. It has been estimated (Connell, 1972) that in only about one in a thousand acts of sexual intercourse is pregnancy the desired goal. Some couples, not necessarily choosing pregnancy, will accept it gladly or at least philosophically if and when it occurs. Others may choose to abort the pregnancy.

Two people reach out to each other for love and fulfillment. Their desire for children (if indeed they want them), the number they will have, and the time they will have them are all-important in the attainment of these goals. The thoughtful man and woman who desire children want the assurance that they will be ready for them in terms of family stability, personal contentment, physical health, finances, and living conditions. For the couple that does not want children, the prevention of pregnancy is no less important. The ideal in family planning is parenthood by choice rather than by chance.

Methods of controlling birth fall into four general categories: sexual abstinence, contraception, sterilization, and abortion. Within each of these broad categories there are various methods commonly in use today. Each method has its advantages and disadvantages, its benefits and risks.

Sexual Abstinence

Abstinence requires that a couple refrain from sexual intercourse either completely or during those days, or at least those moments, when fertilization is most apt to occur. This simply prevents the sperm from fertilizing the egg.

Withdrawal (Coitus Interruptus)

Coitus interruptus, without doubt the most ancient form of birth control, consists of withdrawing the penis from the vagina just before ejaculation occurs. It was a common method before the development of mechanical and chemical contraceptives, and is still widely used.

The effectiveness of the technique depends on the man's alertness to the first signs of orgasm. He must be prepared to terminate intercourse at any moment. In the withdrawal both distance and speed are crucial. Even before ejaculation, the drops of clear Cowper's fluid found at the end of the penis are carrying sperm (in fact, about 50,000 sperm per drop). If these drops get into the vagina there is a possibility of pregnancy. Any sperm left in the vagina stand a chance of making it the rest of the way to the egg. Any misjudging of the ejaculatory reflexes and mistiming

TABLE 13.1 Effectiveness of Fertility Control Methods When Properly and Consistently Used

Method	*Pregnancy Rate**
No attempt to avert pregnancy	70
Rhythm	38
Withdrawal	23
Condom	14
Diaphragm	9
Sequential pills	5
Foam (double application)	5
IUD	3
Minipill	3
Condom with foam	1
Combination pills	0.1
Sterilization	0.003

*Based on the number of pregnancies per hundred woman-years of exposure. In other words, for every one hundred couples practicing each of the listed methods for a full year, this is the number of women who can be expected to become pregnant.

Source: World Planned Parenthood Council.

of withdrawal may permit semen to be deposited in the vagina. One drop is more than enough to cause pregnancy. The first drops of discharged semen contain a higher concentration of sperm than later drops.

The disadvantages of this method are numerous. For every hundred couples that practice withdrawal for one year, twenty-three women become pregnant. As shown in Table 13.1, its effectiveness is low in comparison with other methods (although better than the douche or the rhythm technique). Equally important, stopping intercourse just before the peak of ecstasy greatly interferes with the enjoyment of intercourse for many people. Orgasm *after* withdrawal may seem less pleasurable. Unless the woman reaches orgasm before the man, she may be left with unresolved sexual tensions. Even is she does, she may be left with a feeling of incompleteness. On the positive side, it takes no preparation, no equipment is necessary, no medical supervision is required, and it costs nothing.

The Rhythm Method

The rhythm method is based on the fact that there is a fertile period of a few days each month when a woman can become pregnant. These fertile days are the several days before and after ovulation, the release of a ripe egg. Ovulation generally occurs at about the midpoint in the menstrual cycle, and if intercourse is avoided during this time, pregnancy can be prevented. This is all very fine *if* ovulation occurs at midmonth.

The rhythm method is based on several physiological facts: The egg is fertilizable in the tubes for about twenty-four hours after ovulation; sperm cells ejaculated into a woman's body are able to fertilize an egg for about seventy-two hours (three days) after they have been ejaculated; and the next menstrual bleeding occurs between twelve and sixteen days after ovulation. In other words, ovulation is tied more closely to the next onset of menstruation than to the last one. But even assuming that a woman has menstrual periods that are invariably twenty-eight days apart (see Figure 13.1), there is no way of predicting in any given month exactly when ovulation will occur. To be "safe," a woman must avoid intercourse during these five days (between days twelve and sixteen before the next expected period). In addition, sperm can live in a woman for three days, so intercourse two days before the earliest expected day of

FIGURE 13.1 Theory of the rhythm method. The shaded sections indicate days of greatest chance of pregnancy (the greater the shading, the greater the chance). This chart is based on an average 28-day menstrual cycle.

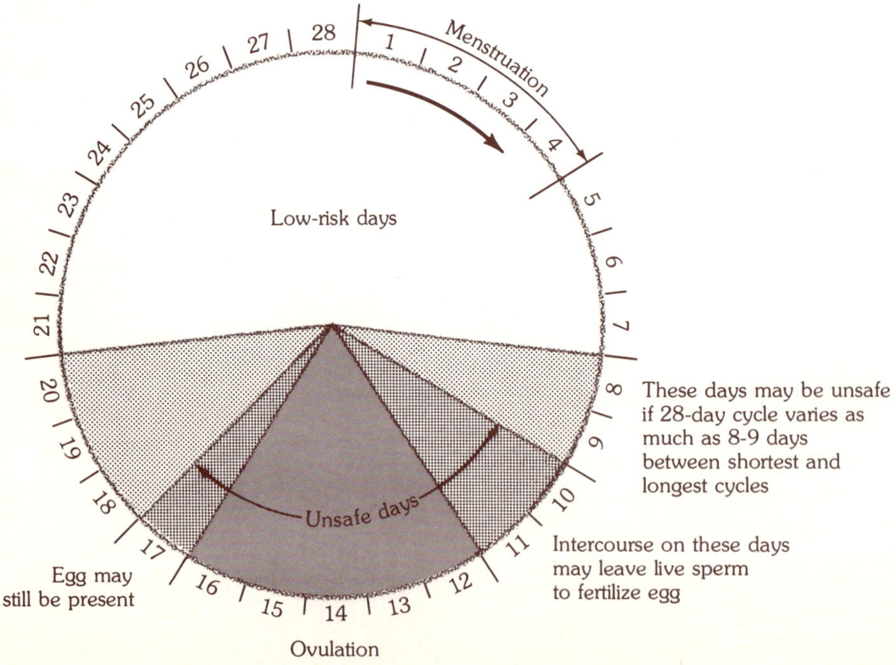

ovulation could still leave live sperm to fertilize the egg. Since an egg can live in a woman for one day, intercourse a day after the latest expected day of ovulation could mean an egg still present to be fertilized. Just for insurance it is recommended that she refrain from intercourse from the nineteenth to the twelfth day before her next menstrual discharge, or from day ten to day seventeen after the beginning of her last discharge. For a period of eight days each month she must not have intercourse.

Unfortunately, most women do not have predictably regular menstrual cycles. Some women have menstrual cycles as short as twenty-one days, others as long as thirty-eight days. The average woman may vary as much as eight to nine days between her shortest and longest cycles.

Determining Safe Days To use the rhythm method effectively a woman must make allowance for these irregularities. She should determine the exact length of each cycle for a year by keeping an accurate written record of the dates of onset of each menstrual period. After twelve or thirteen such cycles within a full year, she will know the length of her shortest and longest cycles. Subtracting eighteen days from the number of days of the shortest cycle gives the first day on which intercourse might result in pregnancy. Eleven days subtracted from the number of days in the longest cycle gives the last day of the cycle on which sexual intercourse might result in pregnancy (see Figure 13.1).Figure 13.2 is the standard chart for the rhythm method used by physicians.

This method of calculating days for sexual intercourse each month is a major drawback to many couples. Regulating lovemaking according to the calendar rather than by the way a person feels isn't the most exciting prospect for sexually healthy persons. Some women, perhaps as many as fifteen out of every hundred, have menstrual cycles so irregular they cannot use the rhythm method at all. Even a woman who normally has very regular cycles may ovulate at an odd time as a result of physical or emotional stress, travel, illness, or any number of other things. Following childbirth the cycles may be upset for several months, with ovulation unpredictable. Even faithful adherence to the chart is not totally effective in preventing pregnancy. According to Table 13.1, 38 out of 100 women practicing this method for a year can expect to become pregnant.

Signs of Ovulation The major drawback of the rhythm method is detecting the day of ovulation. Some women practice the rhythm method by relying on physical signs to indicate when ovulation occurs.

On or about the day of ovulation, roughly 25 percent of women may experience a dull pain in the back or lower abdomen. Or it may be sharper and localized in either side of the lower abdomen. Called *mittelschmerz,* it occurs as a result of irritation from the ruptured follicle.

THE RHYTHM METHOD How to Figure the "Safe" and "Unsafe" Days

Length of Shortest Period	*First Unsafe Day After Start of Any Period*	*Length of Longest Period*	*Last Unsafe Day After Start of Any Period*
21 DAYS	3RD DAY	21 DAYS	10TH DAY
22 DAYS	4TH DAY	22 DAYS	11TH DAY
23 DAYS	5TH DAY	23 DAYS	12TH DAY
24 DAYS	6TH DAY	24 DAYS	13TH DAY
25 DAYS	7TH DAY	25 DAYS	14TH DAY
26 DAYS	8TH DAY	26 DAYS	15TH DAY
27 DAYS	9TH DAY	27 DAYS	16TH DAY
28 DAYS	10TH DAY	28 DAYS	17TH DAY
29 DAYS	11TH DAY	29 DAYS	18TH DAY
30 DAYS	12TH DAY	30 DAYS	19TH DAY
31 DAYS	13TH DAY	31 DAYS	20TH DAY
32 DAYS	14TH DAY	33 DAYS	21ST DAY
33 DAYS	15TH DAY	33 DAYS	22ND DAY
34 DAYS	16TH DAY	34 DAYS	23RD DAY
35 DAYS	17TH DAY	35 DAYS	24TH DAY
36 DAYS	18TH DAY	36 DAYS	25TH DAY
37 DAYS	19TH DAY	37 DAYS	26TH DAY
38 DAYS	20TH DAY	38 DAYS	27TH DAY

FIGURE 13.2 The "safe" and "unsafe" days of a menstrual cycle may be figured by using this chart. In using this chart, a woman should keep a record of her menstrual cycles for a year, counting the day on which menstruation begins as the first day of each period. Knowing the number of days in her shortest and longest cycles, she can find her first and last unsafe days from the chart. For instance, if a woman's shortest period on record was 26 days, she is safe until the 8th day of her new period; if her longest period on record during the past year has been 30 days, she is again safe after the 19th day of each new period.

Immediately after menstrual bleeding, the body temperature falls, then falls even lower on the fertile days. When ovulation is over, the temperature rises (see Figure 13.3). The temperature must be taken carefully each morning before rising or eating or drinking. Even if the woman has been up during the night, she must take her temperature in the morning. The temperature is taken by putting a clinical thermometer (marked in tenth-of-degree graduations) about two inches into the vagina, moving it sideways to assure good contact, then leaving it in position for about five minutes.

The woman has to keep a careful record each day to determine her pattern. The temperature must be recorded and charted each day in graph form. Some precautions: The couple should abstain from inter-

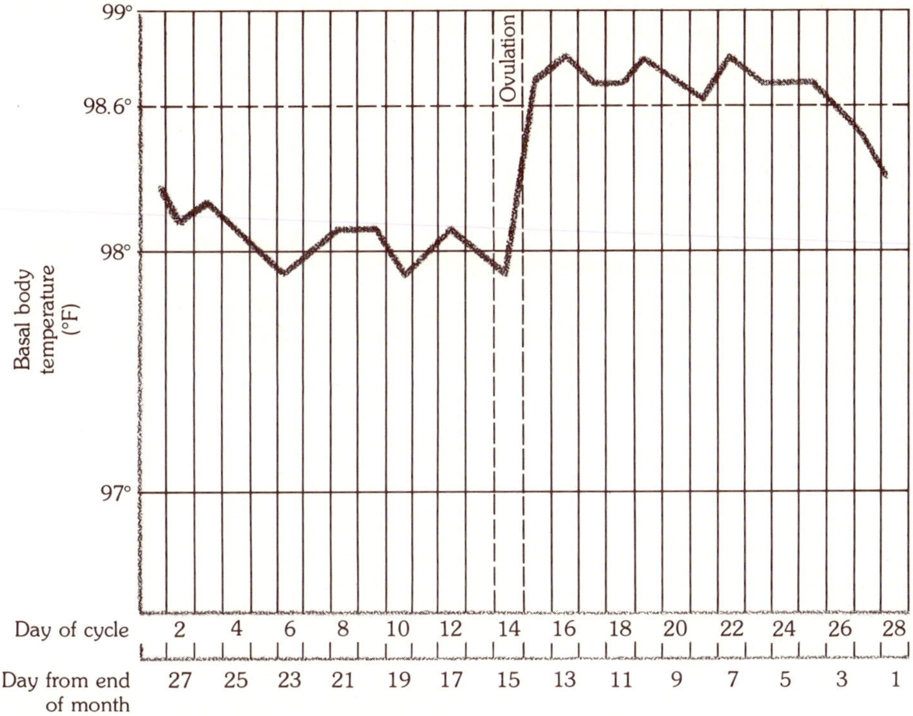

FIGURE 13.3 Basal body temperature (BBT) during typical menstrual cycle. Ovulation most commonly occurs 14 days before the end of the cycle. Since length of menstrual cycles vary, the days of the chart are listed in reverse order.

course until forty-eight hours after the temperature shift. But only about 25 percent of all women exhibit a midcycle temperature rise as clear-cut as that shown in Figure 13.3. And any kind of illness, distress, or activity may throw off the reading.

Contraception

Contraception, by past definition, has amounted to one of two things: the prevention of fertilization (union of sperm and egg) or the prevention of ovulation (release of the egg by the ovary). Many authorities also feel that true pregnancy does not exist before the implantation of a fertilized ovum in the uterine wall. The types of contraceptive methods fall into three categories: mechanical, chemical, and hormonal.

Mechanical Contraceptives

Condom ("Rubber") The condom is a synthetic rubber or animal-skin sheath that fits snugly over the erect penis (see Figure 13.4). There is a rubber ring at the open end to help hold it in place, and some are equipped with a small nipple or reservoir at the end to hold the ejaculate. Some condoms are prelubricated with various lubricants, while others are unlubricated. The function of the condom is to prevent the sperm from reaching the vagina. It is almost as effective as the diaphragm in preventing pregnancy, and its effectiveness can be increased if it is used in conjunction with a contraceptive jelly applied to the outside of the condom or foam inserted into the vagina before intercourse.

The condom is used widely around the world both for the prevention of sexually transmitted diseases and the control of pregnancy. Its use also combats *Trichomonas* infection and reduces the chances of transmission of *Herpes simplex* virus. It is sometimes useful to men bothered by premature ejaculation, since it reduces penile sensations. It is one of the handiest methods to use and can be purchased almost anywhere for from ten cents to $1.50 per condom. It has no side effects and no aftereffects. Pregnancy can be expected in about fourteen women

FIGURE 13.4 Condoms

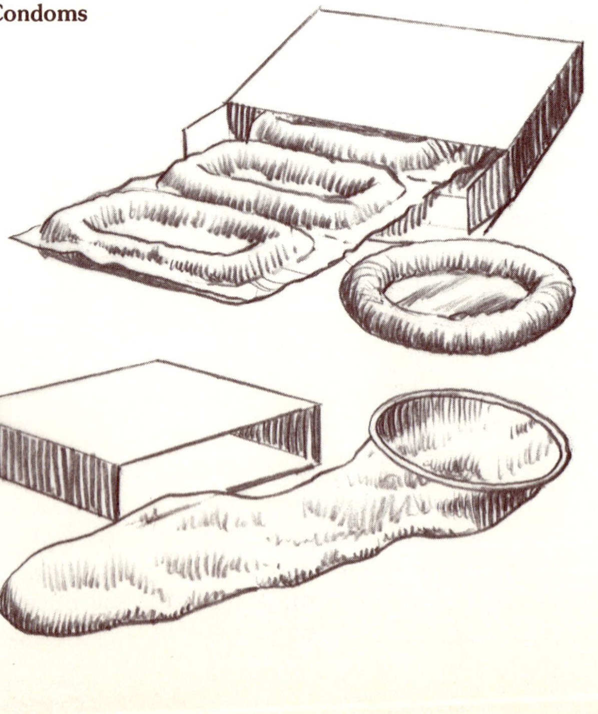

per year out of every hundred whose partners use the condom as recommended. When it is used with foam its effectiveness is very good.

Among its disadvantages is the fact that the condom may interfere with the man's full enjoyment of intercourse by dulling his sensations. It requires interruption of the act to put it in place, although a woman can make putting it on a part of foreplay since she is in that area anyway. Condoms are subject to a break or tear, and they can come off during intercourse. Some men are allergic to rubber, but condoms made of plastic or lamb intestines ("skin") are available.

In using a condom, a man should remember:

- that breakage or tearing is usually due to friction or lack of lubrication. Lubricating the condom with a spermicide is better than using prelubricated condoms. Petroleum jelly (e.g., Vasaline) may react with the condom and damage it, so it should not be used as a lubricant.
- that the failure rate can be reduced by using only high-quality condoms (less expensive brands are more apt to contain holes).
- to leave at least one-half inch of space at the end of the condom to contain the ejaculate if it lacks a nipple or reservoir.
- to remove the penis promptly after ejaculation to prevent sperm from escaping out over the top of the condom into the vagina (the top of the condom should be held in place as the penis is withdrawn).
- to wear the condom throughout intercourse in order to catch sperm that may be expelled before orgasm.
- to use condoms throughout the menstrual cycle, not just when fertility seems most likely.
- never to reuse a condom.

Diaphragm The vaginal diaphragm is a shallow rubber or synthetic rubber cup designed to cover the cervix and thus prevent sperm from entering the uterus. Two to three inches in diameter, it has a flexible metal spring or coil within the rim to hold it in place (see Figure 13.5). The rim is squeezed together and the device is slipped into the vagina, where it springs back into shape. In place, it fits between the back wall of the vagina and the pubic bone. To test for correct fitting, the woman should run a finger over the diaphragm's dome. If it is covering the cervix, it may feel like the end of the nose.

The size of the vagina is as variable as the size of the penis. Since a diaphragm of the wrong size may slip out of place or be displaced during intercourse, a woman must be measured for a diaphragm by a physician. She then purchases the diaphragm by prescription at a drugstore. The physician will provide her with instructions in its proper insertion and removal. Since a woman's vagina is stretched by childbirth, her vaginal dimensions should be rechecked after delivery. No woman should ever

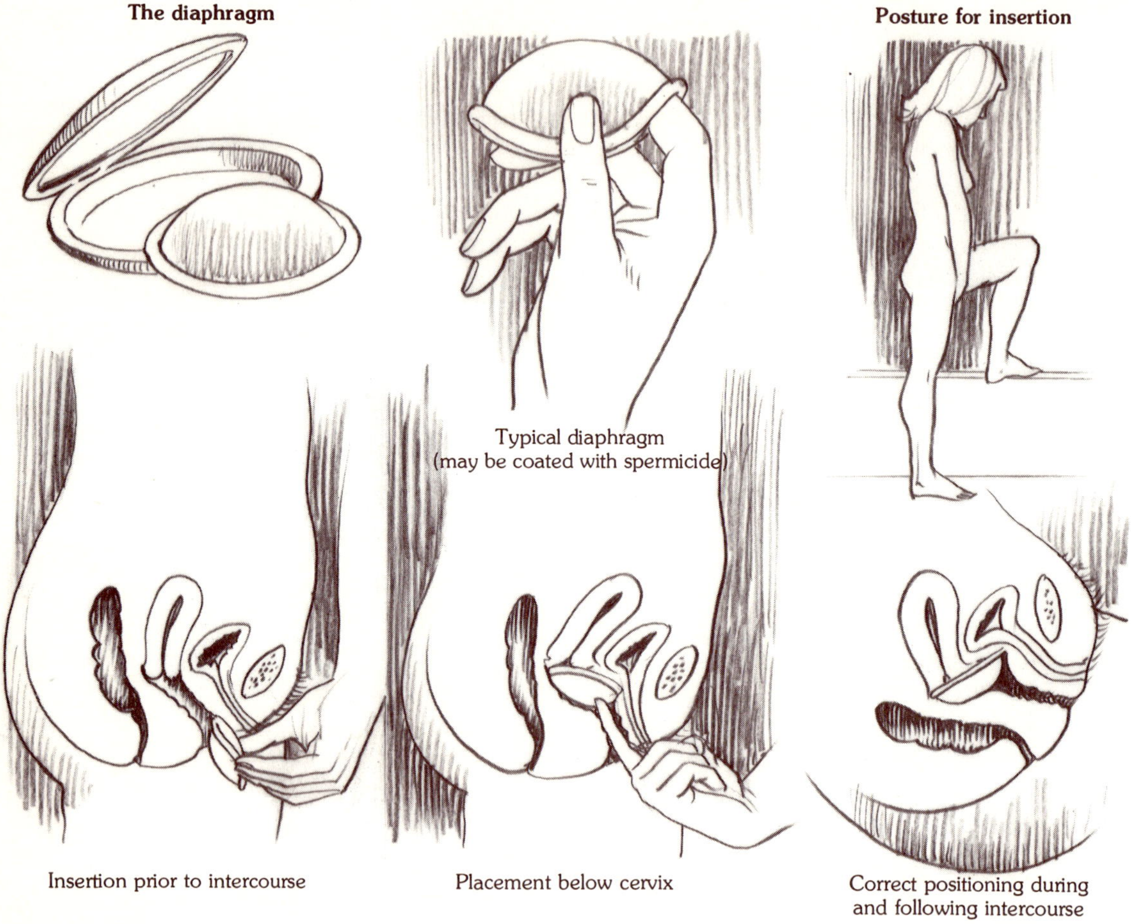

FIGURE 13.5 Diaphragm

borrow a friend's diaphragm. Two women of similar stature may have very different vaginal dimensions.

A contraceptive jelly containing a *spermicide* (material that kills sperm on contact) should always be used with the diaphragm. Jelly or cream should be applied around the edge and on both sides of the diaphragm before it is inserted. Masters and Johnson have shown that the vagina widens and elongates during sexual excitement (see Figure 13.6) and that even the best fitting diaphragm moves quite freely in the vagina. Jelly on the inner side of the diaphragm serves to protect the cervix from wandering sperm.

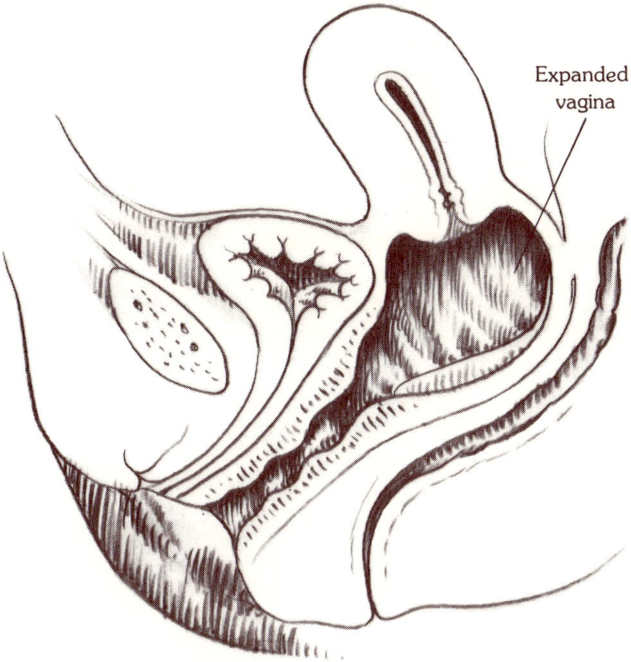

FIGURE 13.6 Elongation and widening of the vaginal barrel during orgasm. Even the well-fitted diaphragm may "float" with such expansion of the vagina.

Before inserting a diaphragm the woman should hold it up to a light to make sure there are no pinpoint holes. The diaphragm can be inserted up to two hours in advance and must be left in place for eight hours after intercourse. If intercourse occurs a second time within the eight-hour period, another application of spermicide should be placed in the vagina. This can be done with an applicator without disturbing the diaphragm. The diaphragm may be displaced when the vaginal canal expands during intercourse, causing the device so properly fitted by a physician to become almost free-floating. It may also be displaced by violent thrusting accompanying the plateau phase of intercourse, when the vagina is enlarged, or when the woman is atop the man during sexual intercourse.

A diaphragm properly fitted and inserted should not be felt by either partner and should not impair sexual sensation for either of them. It may be left in position for twenty-four hours without any harm or discomfort. After removal, the diaphragm should be washed, patted dry with a towel, and dusted with talcum powder to keep it soft. With good care it should last at least two years. It may well last longer than that, but it is good practice to replace it after two years.

The use of the diaphragm requires continuous motivation and

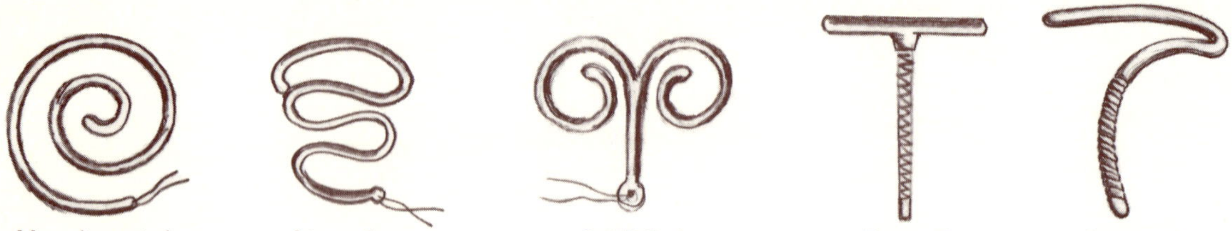

FIGURE 13.7 IUD: some typical forms

memory (this may break down when sexual activity becomes spontaneous). Once quite popular it is used today by less than 10 percent of couples. Nor is its effectiveness too great. Out of one hundred women using it for one full year, about nine are likely to become pregnant.

Intrauterine Device (IUD) The principle of the IUD has been used for centuries. Though it has been known since ancient times that a foreign object placed in the uterus prevents pregnancy, not until recently have materials been developed that the body can easily accept.

Usually made of plastic or plastic wrapped in copper, the devices vary in shape and size (see Figure 13.7). The coil-like devices are preformed and may be inserted by being pushed through a small pencil-sized tube into the uterus, where they resume their original shape. Devices of other shapes may be inserted with the aid of anesthesia. The contraceptive efficiency of an IUD is directly proportional to the surface area of the device. A few devices are made of stainless steel.

The IUD is inserted by a physician, usually during menstruation, when the opening of the cervix is dilated (see Figure 13.8). Physicians also commonly do a Pap smear to check for uterine cancer, and a pelvic examination to determine the position and size of the uterus so the IUD can be safely inserted. Insertion often results in some immediate bleeding and menstrual-like pains for a couple of days. The physician may want to check in a month or so to be sure insertion was done correctly. Some women may cramp, spot-bleed between periods, and have backaches for several months. The first menstrual flows may be heavier and last longer. If pains are severe and persist, the IUD may need to be removed.

Once inserted, the device can remain in place for a year or more. No other contraceptive protection is necessary, and neither partner should be aware of its presence. Each device has a nylon thread attached which protrudes from the opening of the cervix. Before intercourse a woman should feel with her finger to be certain the IUD has not slipped out.

The IUD is completely "reversible." When the woman decides to

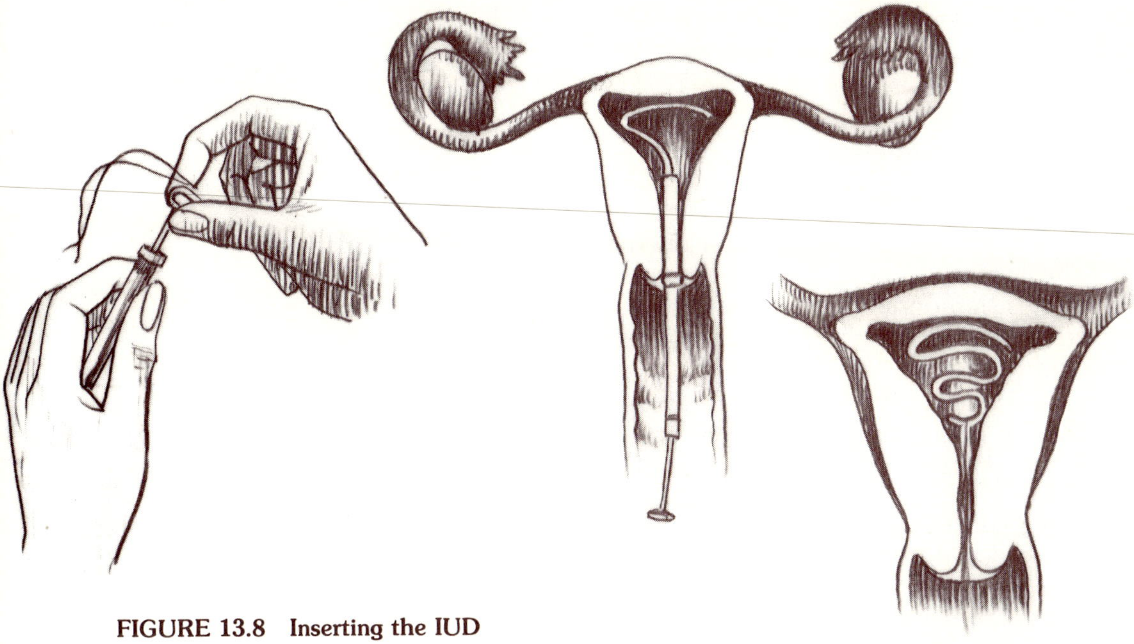

FIGURE 13.8 Inserting the IUD

become pregnant, she goes to her physician and has the IUD removed. By gently pulling on the nylon string the physician can remove the device. A woman should not do this by herself. Before long the uterus is again functioning normally and within one month to a year most women become pregnant. An occasional pregnancy may occur with the device in place. If pregnancy is confirmed, removal of the IUD is advised.

Older women and those who already have several children tend to tolerate an IUD better and have fewer expulsions than younger women and those with fewer children. Newer designs, however, are proving successful even for childless women. When bleeding and cramping are reported, they are frequently eliminated by the substitution of a smaller IUD. There are fewer expulsions from the uterus with larger IUDs, but there are also fewer pregnancies. Perforations of the uterine wall are rare and deaths from the IUD are virtually nonexistent. There is no correlation between uterine cancer and use of the IUD. Of course, the IUD offers no protection against syphilis or gonorrhea.

Out of one hundred women using the device for one year, only about three can be expected to become pregnant. The use of the IUD is unrelated to sexual intercourse, requires no daily motivation, involves no cost beyond that of initial insertion, and has no effect whatsoever on a woman's hormone levels. There is great potential for worldwide use of the IUD because of its low cost, ease of insertion, and long-term effectiveness once in place.

Chemical Contraceptives

The Douche Some people mistakenly believe that pregnancy can be prevented by washing away the semen after intercourse by douching, or washing out the vagina. Various douches have been used: hot water, cold water, vinegar, lemon juice, soap chips dissolved in water, washes available in drugstores. A large rubber syringe is filled with the fluid and emptied into the vagina.

As seen in Table 13.1, out of one-hundred women using the douche method for one year, about thirty-one become pregnant. The reason for this low effectiveness is that millions of sperm are safely inside the uterus within two minutes after ejaculation. A douche may wash out the vagina but it won't touch the uterus. Following unprotected ejaculation, regardless of the speed with which the douching is done and the preparation that is used, it's too late. Besides, leaping out of bed and making a dash for the bathroom immediately after ejaculation does detract from the enjoyment of the occasion. *Douching cannot be considered a contraceptive method.*

And a word on genital cosmetics. Drugstore shelves are cluttered with vaginal sprays, pubic hair sprays, and various kinds of "intimate" deodorants. They do nothing more than cover up odors that a good shower would wash away, they often cause irritation, they are a waste of money, and they are not particularly effective. Don't use them.

Vaginal Spermicides Various chemical preparations kill or impede the movement of sperm. These vaginal spermicides are available in the form of aerosol foams, creams, jellies, and suppositories (see Figure 13.9).

Vaginal aerosol foams are the most effective of the spermicides and the simplest to use. A pressurized container of foam is used to fill a plastic applicator, which is inserted to apply the foam high in the vagina (see Figure 13.10). It may be applied as long as one-half hour before intercourse, but it must be applied before every act of intercourse. If a woman has two sessions of intercourse in one night, she must apply double applications of foam twice. It must be left in place for at least six to eight hours after each act of intercourse. Since the foam is absorbed into the lining of the vagina, douching is not necessary. Some experts consider the foams preferable to the creams because they fill vaginal irregularities more effectively than creams and there is less vaginal leakage after intercourse.

Spermicides

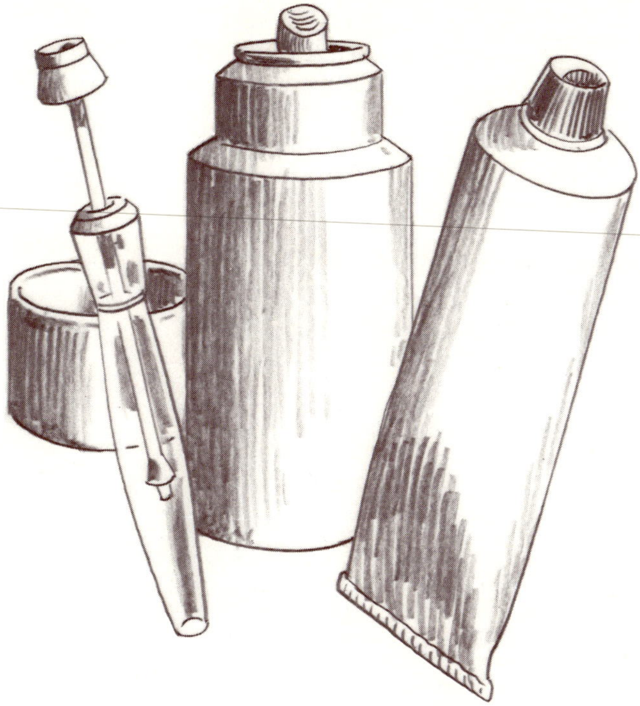

FIGURE 13.9 Spermicides

FIGURE 13.10 Application of vaginal foam

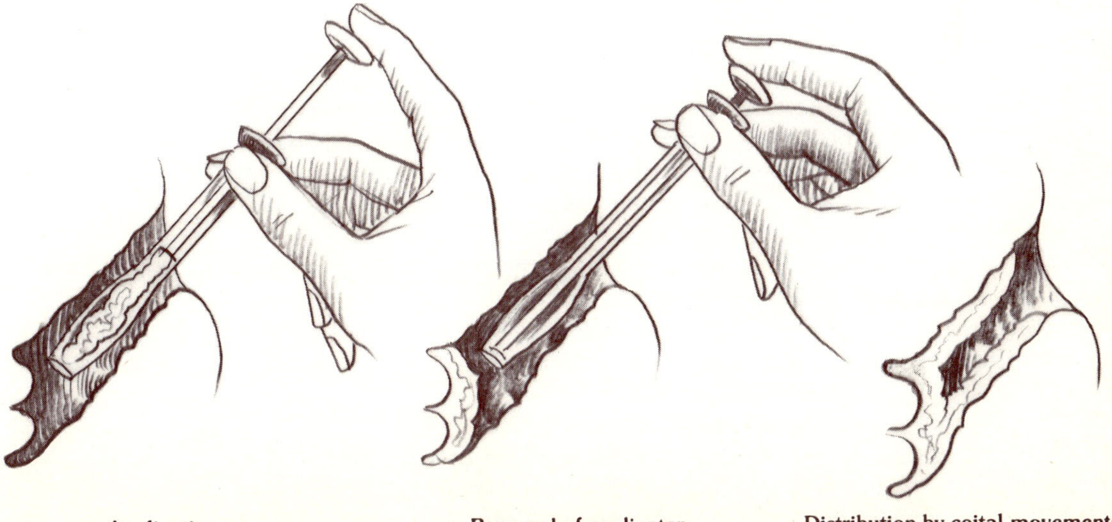

Foams can be obtained without prescription. Two popular brands of vaginal foams are Delfen and Emko. If double applications are used, these new improved vaginal foams are effective in preventing pregnancy in all but five women out of one hundred per year. If single applications are used, the effectiveness rate drops to twenty-nine per hundred woman-years. When foam and a condom are used in the same act of intercourse, the effectiveness rate is one per hundred woman-years.

Creams and jellies are designed to be used with a diaphragm, but they can be used alone. The woman selecting this method merely uses a special applicator to insert a measured amount of the spermicide into the vagina one hour or less before each act of intercourse. One application is theoretically good for only one act of intercourse. The spermicide acts to kill the sperm on contact, and the chemical base of the preparation forms a coating that keeps surviving sperm from reaching the egg. The plastic applicator deposits the preparation high in the vaginal tract at the opening into the uterus. Delfen Creme, Ortho-Creme, and Ortho-Gynol Jelly are popular brands. As with all nonprescription products, be sure to read the instructions on the label carefully. The effectiveness of jellies alone in preventing pregnancy is not good. Planned Parenthood does not recommend their use without a diaphragm.

Suppositories and foaming tablets are spermicides in solid form that melt or dissolve when placed in the vagina. A suppository is a small pencil-shaped glycerin-gelatin preparation containing a spermicide that melts at body temperature. It is inserted deep into the vagina from fifteen minutes to an hour before intercourse. Enough time must be allowed for it to melt before intercourse begins. Suppositories may be bought without a prescription and are harmless. Their reliability in preventing pregnancy is about the same as that of the creams and jellies used alone.

Foaming tablets dissolve on contact with the moisture in the vagina. They release a carbon dioxide gas to produce a foam that spreads the spermicide over the upper vaginal area. A tablet should be inserted several minutes to an hour before intercourse. They can be bought without prescription at drugstores. Their effectiveness in preventing pregnancy is considered inferior to that of creams and jellies used alone.

The action of the vaginal spermicides is completely reversible when they are discontinued. They do require insertion at some time relatively close to coitus and require memory and motivation, and even then they are less effective than a number of other contraceptives.

Hormonal Contraceptives

Most types of female oral contraceptive pills are designed to prevent ovulation. These pills, which are highly effective in preventing pregnancy, are composed of synthetic female hormones. You will recall from our earlier discussion that the pituitary gland produces the hormones FSH and LH, which are necessary for the production and release of a mature egg in the ovary. The follicles in the ovary produce both estrogen and progesterone. Among other functions, the estrogen inhibits the production of FSH, and progesterone inhibits the production of LH. When the pill is taken daily, starting on the fifth day after the beginning of menstruation, the presence of progestin (artificial progesterone) and estrogen inhibit the body's production of FSH and LH before a mature egg is produced. Ovulation does not occur and no egg is present to unite with the sperm that are released during intercourse. The woman thus fails to become pregnant. (Under the influence of *natural* estrogen and progesterone, no mature eggs are produced during pregnancy.)

The artificial hormones present in the pill also cause changes in the cervix that prevent sperm from entering the uterus, and they cause changes in the uterine lining that prevent an egg from implanting even if one were released and fertilized. Thus the combination pill, in particular, is a triple threat to pregnancy.

There are various types of pills produced today, including combination pills, sequential pills, minipills, morning-after pills, and the three-month contraceptive injection (see Figure 13.11).

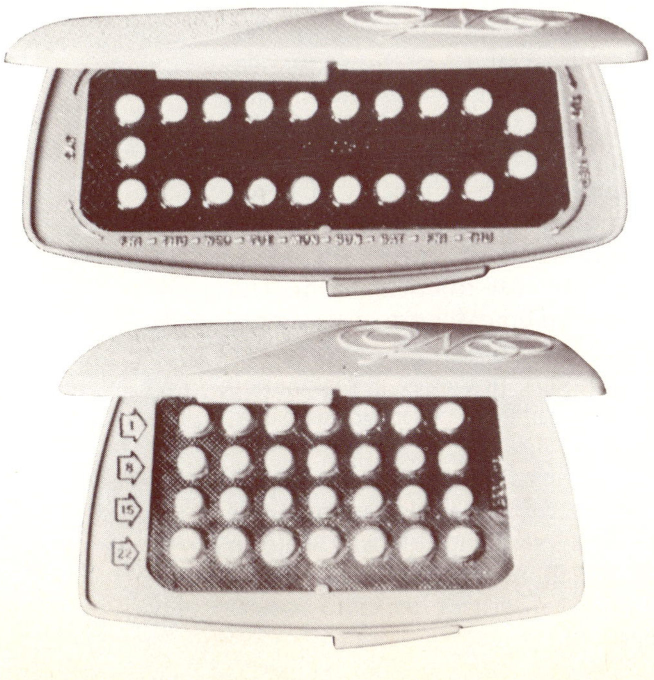

FIGURE 13.11 The pill

Combination Pills Each pill is alike and contains a combination of synthetic estrogen and progestin. These pills are designed to be taken for twenty or twenty-one days of the menstrual cycle, starting on day five and ending on day twenty-four or twenty-five. Then for seven or eight days the pill is omitted, or sugar pills or iron pills are substituted for a week. Menstruation is allowed to occur. The menstrual periods tend to become regular twenty-eight-day events, and it is common for the flow to be greatly reduced. Some women experience such side effects as nausea, headache, swelling of the breasts, and spotting, symptoms that are similar to those of early pregnancy. Commonly these symptoms diminish or disappear after the first several months.

Over the years drug producers have gradually decreased the dosage of both the estrogen and progestin components, thus decreasing the incidence of side effects for many women. Out of a thousand women using the combination pill for one year, only one is apt to become pregnant (0.1 pregnancy per 100 women for one year).

Sequential Pills Because of some complaints regarding the side effects of combination pills, sequential pills were developed. They consist of two different pills, one taken from day five through day nineteen and the other from day twenty through day twenty-four. (The days may differ for different brands.) The pills taken the first fifteen days contain estrogen only; the pills taken the last five days contain both estrogen and progestin (like the combination pill). The sequential pills are packaged so that the pills are easily taken in the right order. The action of combination and sequential pills is similar, but the effectiveness of the sequential pill is less than that of the combination pill. Of a hundred women taking the sequential pill for one year, five are apt to become pregnant.

Depending on the brand used, there are minor variations in the dosage and number of pills taken. They are packaged in sets of twenty, twenty-one, and twenty-eight pills. The sets of twenty-eight pills include placebo tablets for seven out of twenty-eight days. The major advantage of all pill methods is their effectiveness and the ease of taking them. The pill is taken once a day regularly at a convenient time. It permits lovemaking to be spontaneous. There is nothing to put on, slip in, or come off. Continued motivation and memory are required, however. If pregnancy is desired, the pill is discontinued, and the liklihood of pregnancy is at least as great as before the pill was used.

The pill is a prescription drug and requires a visit to a physician, which includes a physical examination to determine that birth control pills are relatively safe for the woman to take. The exam should include a Pap smear, a breast exam, a blood pressure check, and taking of a medical history. *Do not get pills from a physician who does not examine you.* A regular checkup twice a year is recommended.

Take only the pills for which you have a prescription—one kind of pill may affect you differently than another. If you should want to change pills after a couple of months, do not buy too large a supply. Never give them to a friend unless she is taking exactly the same pill to begin with. Keep an extra package on hand to replace pills that get lost.

Take the pill at about the same time each day. This makes it easier to remember and helps to maintain a more constant level of hormones in the blood. If you forget to take a pill, take it as soon as you remember and take the next pill at its scheduled time. If you miss two pills, take two each day for the next two days and use an additional contraceptive (foam, condom, diaphragm) for the next week.

There is no evidence that the pill produces cancer. Since most physicians require a routine Pap smear (to detect uterine cancer) and breast examination every six months, there may be fewer deaths from cancer for women on the pill. Some women with blood type A may run a somewhat higher risk of blood clots. Even so, the mortality risk for full-term pregnancy is ten to fifteen times that for pill-formed clots. *But it is most important that the pills be taken only under a physician's supervision.*

Minipills Minipills contain a low dosage of progestin with no estrogen. The mode of action remains unclear, since estrogen prevents ovulation. There is evidence that changes occur in the cervical mucus, endometrium, and tubal transport.

Their advantage is that, since they do not contain estrogen, some of the side effects associated with that hormone may be reduced or abolished. They do not impair a woman's glucose tolerance as both the combination and sequential pills may do (causing a diabetes-like condition). Their bleeding patterns and pregnancy rates are not so satisfactory as those of conventional pills. Cycles tend to be irregular in about 25 percent of patients, and some develop periodic heavy bleeding. Their effectiveness in preventing pregnancy is similar to that of the IUD.

The Morning-After Pill Accidents happen. A condom may tear. A woman may be swept away in one room while her diaphragm reposes in another. Faced with the very real possibility of pregnancy, she may take the "morning-after" pill to insure against pregnancy *after* she has had intercourse. Once an egg is fertilized, several days pass before it reaches the uterus and several more before it becomes implanted in the uterine lining, so there is no need to panic. A woman in this predicament should go to a physician, hospital, or school infirmary and ask for some DES (disethylstilbesterol). Implantation and pregnancy may be prevented if two twenty-five-milligram tablets are taken twice a day for five days, starting within twenty-four hours and no later than seventy-two hours after unprotected intercourse. DES, a synthetic estrogen, causes contraction of the uterus and the expulsion of its contents. The woman may experience severe nausea. It is not to be used as a regular birth control method, but it may be effectively used in an emergency. There is concern about the possibility that DES may cause cancer in female offspring when taken over long periods. The action of the morning-after pill suggests abortion, even though the dosage and duration of therapy are both small.

Three-Month Contraceptive Injection There is limited use in the United States of a contraceptive drug that can be given by injection. Called Depo Provero, and containing synthetic progesterone, it is taken by an injection in the hip or arm every ninety days. The only known injectable contraceptive, it can prevent pregnancy for up to three months at a time with one injection. Women using it report menstrual irregularity; sometimes they have no period for months. Pregnancy may occur within three to nine months after the injections have been terminated. There is a chance, however, that it may cause temporary or permanent sterility. In addition, it has most of the adverse side effects associated with the oral contraceptives. It is recommended for women who can't use the pill or IUD, who can't remember to take the pill, or who don't like either the pill or the IUD. The Federal Drug Administration has approved its limited use in this country.

Experimental Contraceptives

Other hormonal contraceptives are now under investigation. A long-term capsule is injected into the arm or buttock and offers sterility for as long as two years. A male birth control pill is being investigated which makes conception impossible by preventing the development of sperm. It can be administered either by injection or orally. Vaccination appears to be another possibility. The idea of making a woman immune to sperm by injecting her with antibodies that would attack and reject them is being studied. A unisex birth control pill, which can be taken by either partner, is being researched. This study has been prompted by the need for a rest period for some women on the pill.

Contraceptive Practices of Students

Contraceptive practices of unmarried university students show that many students are inadequately protected from conception. During first intercourse as many as 60 percent of men and women use no form of contraception, or use an unreliable method such as withdrawal, rhythm, or the douche. The condom is the most widely used form of contraception; it is easily available even when intercourse is unplanned, and can be easily concealed until intercourse occurs. Countless women use the pill as their preferred contraceptive method.

It appears that the availability of contraceptives has little effect on the proportion of nonvirgins on campus. Few men and women students view fear of pregnancy as a major reason for remaining virgins, even though many of them are careless about birth control. The easy availability of contraceptive devices on campus does not appear to indicate increased promiscuity or the collapse of the moral structure. Sexual behavior is regulated by other value systems, such as religion, and individual nonmarital sex codes may be maintained even with the easy availability of perfect or near-perfect contraceptive techniques.

Sterilization

Sterilization, or surgery that prevents parenthood, is a method of birth control that is common in the United States and other industrialized countries, and is an instrument of population policy in some Third World countries, most notably India. It is a method of permanent fertility control that is virtually 100 percent effective. A man or woman who has been properly sterilized can have children only if a second operation is successfully performed to undo the work of the first—and the success rate of these second operations is only 20 to 25 percent. Sterilization does not remove any of the sex organs or glands and has no effect upon sexual desire or performance.

For a woman, the operation consists of cutting the two fallopian tubes and closing off the cut ends (see Figure 13.12). It can be done as part of a cesarean delivery, by abdominal incision, by a laparoscopy, or by way of the vagina. Once the tubes have been tied, the sperm can no longer reach the egg, and the egg can no longer reach the uterus.

For a man, the operation, called a *vasectomy,* consists of cutting and tying the vas deferens, the passages through which sperm travel from the testes to the genital passages (see Figure 13.13). It requires only small cuts on both sides of the scrotum and can be safely performed in a physician's office. Following vasectomy, mature sperm may remain in the passages for up to six weeks or about twenty ejaculations. Contraceptives should be used for sexual intercourse for several weeks. Some physicians recommend the use of contraceptives for thirty days, others say until there have been fifteen to twenty ejaculations. The surest confirmation of safety is a sperm count. A man continues to produce seminal fluid as before (since much of the fluid is produced by the seminal vesi-

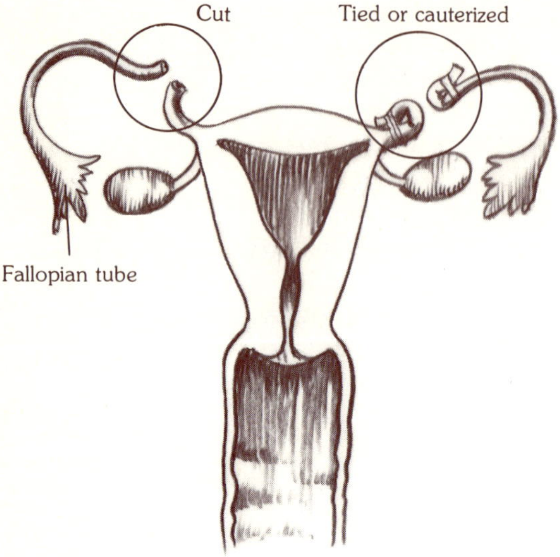

Tubal ligation, or sterilization by severing the fallopian tubes by abdominal incision.

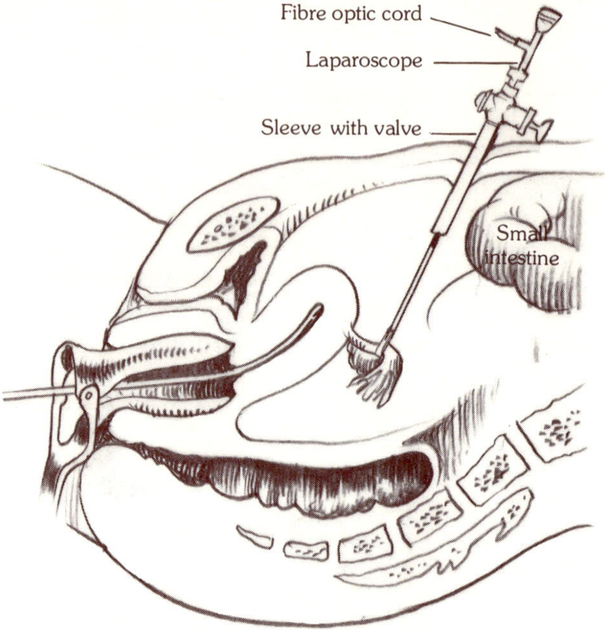

Tubal ligation by laparoscopy.

FIGURE 13.12 Sterilization of a woman

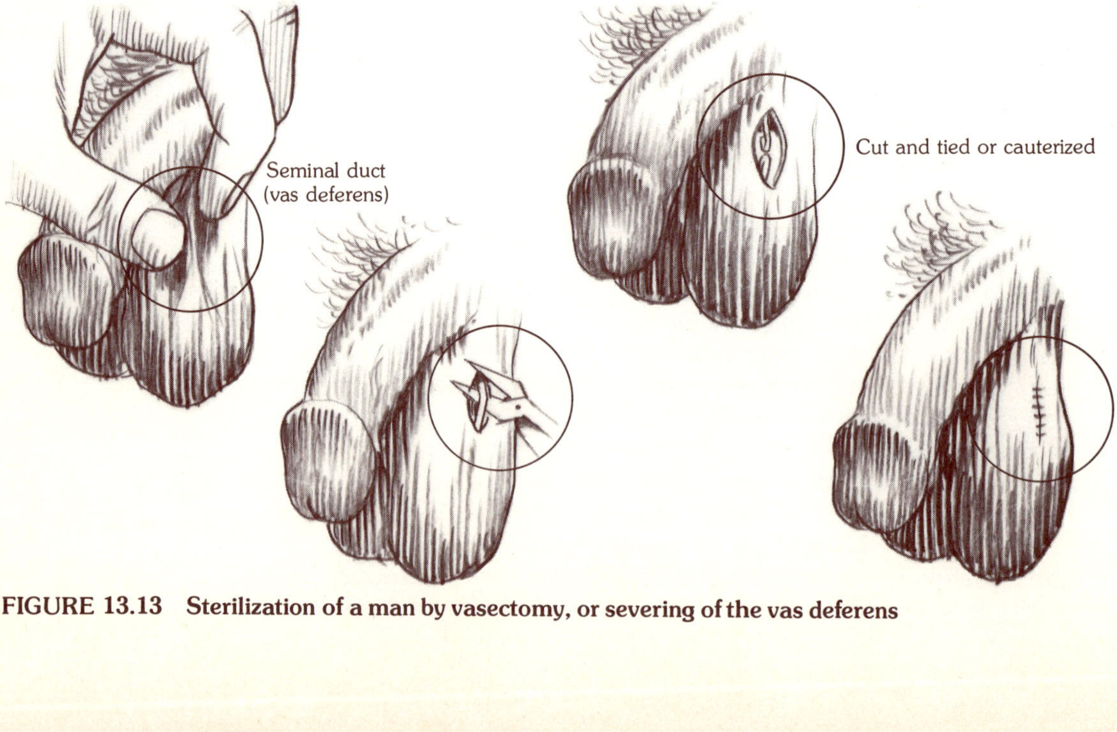

FIGURE 13.13 Sterilization of a man by vasectomy, or severing of the vas deferens

cles and prostate gland); it is still ejaculated upon orgasm, but it contains no sperm. The sperm disintegrate and are absorbed by blood vessels in the testes.

Once sterilization is performed, no further motivation or remembering is required to prevent pregnancy. The fear of pregnancy is gone. The couple can enjoy the spontaneity of intercourse any time without preparation. After the operation there is no further cost. No hormonal changes occur and ejaculatory sensations for the man are the same afterward as they were before. Sterilization in either partner interferes in *no* way with the pleasurable sensations of sexual intercourse; in fact, the libido is usually enhanced.

Yet recent surveys show a deep-rooted public fear of sterilization. Less than 10 percent of the public appear to favor surgical sterilization. More than 50 percent of the men surveyed and almost 66 percent of the women would not presently choose sterilization, even after having all of the children they wanted. A great many men needlessly fear that it will somehow rob them of sexual vigor and masculinity. Women are afraid of losing their femininity. None of this is true.

Abortion

An *abortion* can be defined medically as the removal of a growing embryo or fetus from the wall of the uterus to which it is attached. Another definition is the termination of pregnancy at any time before the fetus has attained a stage of viability. Viability may be considered as an uncertain line that ranges anywhere between 400 grams (about twenty weeks of pregnancy, approximately a 9-ounce fetus) and 1000 grams (about twenty-eight weeks of pregnancy and a fetal weight of 2 lb., 3 oz.). A fetus weighing 700 or 800 grams (1 lb., 5 oz. to 1 lb., 8 oz.) usually survives. A weight of 1000 grams (2 lb., 3 oz.) is widely used as a criterion of viability.

There are two general kinds of abortions. A *natural* abortion, commonly called a miscarriage, is the spontaneous termination of pregnancy before viability, without mechanical or medicinal intervention. It is believed that at least one out of every fifteen pregnancies ends in this manner. About 75 percent of natural abortions occur during the second and third months of pregnancy. Common causes are an abnormally developing fetus, abnormalities of the placenta, and maternal disease.

An *induced* abortion is the expulsion of an embryo or fetus by mechanical or medicinal means. It may be *therapeutic* (termination due to a physical or emotional disorder that would make continued pregnancy hazardous to the mother's health), *on demand* (termination upon request of the mother for any reason, without regard to a physical or emotional contingency), or criminal or *illegal* (termination without any medicolegal justification).

Early in 1973 the U.S. Supreme Court overruled all state laws that restricted or prohibited abortion during the first three months of pregnancy. The Court also ruled that during the next six months of pregnancy the state may "regulate the abortion procedure in ways that are reasonably related to maternal health"—for instance, by requiring hospitalization. But it is still illegal for a state to require that an abortion be approved by a panel of physicians. Only during the last trimester may any state prohibit abortions.

The Court has held that a woman's right to privacy overcomes any state interest in using abortion statutes (as some states have done) to regulate sexual conduct, even though indirectly. It also holds that a fetus is not a person under the Constitution and thus has no legal right to life. Legal abortion during the first trimester is decidedly safer than childbirth. After the first trimester, the danger to the mother increases, hence the states' authority to protect the health of the mother. The United States has now joined India, the Soviet Union, and the majority of eastern European countries in making abortion freely available. Pressure from so-called right-to-life groups, however, may still make it difficult for women to find a doctor willing to perform an abortion or a hospital that will permit its facilities to be used in some areas.

Dilatation and Curettage

The most common method of abortion is *dilatation* and *curettage* (D and C). The cervix is dilated and the inside of the uterus is scraped clean. The procedure is usually performed no sooner than the eighth week of pregnancy, by which time diagnosis of pregnancy is a certainty. It is safe through the twelfth week (from the last day of the last menstruation) when it is performed by a physician under aseptic conditions.

Suction Curettage

In suction curettage, also known as suction aspiration, a negative pressure or vacuum is used to suck out the products of conception through a suction cannula. It is recommended for use up through the twelfth week. Beyond twelve weeks the cannula tends to be obstructed by increasingly firm fetal parts. Uterine perforation may occur because of the increasing thinness of the wall. From twelve to seventeen weeks, suction curettage is sometimes performed in combination with a D and C: the suction curettage extracts the products of conception after they have been broken up by a D and C. Some suction proponents have stated that this technique takes only a minute, is simple and safe, and is so easy that a paramedic can perform it. Physicians caution that the method may be hazardous if not performed by a competent physician working under aseptic conditions.

Hypertonic Solution

The best method of aborting a fetus from sixteen to twenty-four weeks of pregnancy is through the use of a hypertonic solution such as a saline or glucose solution. Amniotic fluid is aspirated as completely as possible and an equivalent amount of either 20 percent saline or 50 percent glucose solution is introduced into the amniotic cavity. With the injection of the solution, the uterus starts to contract, and within about twenty-four to forty-eight hours the fetus and placenta are expelled. This method is not without hazard and it is not painless. If an introduced saline solution gets into a vein and reaches the brain, high fever and death may result. If glucose solution is improperly administered, serious infection can occur. A physician may perform a curettage afterward to clean out the uterus. Obviously it is preferable, whenever possible, to terminate an unwanted pregnancy earlier, through safer methods.

Abdominal Procedure

Occasionally, for a pregnancy of more than twelve weeks, an abdominal procedure may be performed to abort a fetus. If the fetus only is removed, it is known as a *hysterotomy,* but if it involves the removal of the uterus as well, it is called a hysterectomy. Although the excising of the uterus is not the usual method of inducing sterilization, the removal of a part or all of the uterus accomplishes the same end. This method of abortion may be used as late as twenty-four weeks of pregnancy or later. Much later, the chances of aborting a viable fetus become an increasing possibility.

Prostaglandins

The prostaglandins are male hormones in semen extracted from the prostate. If injected or implanted into a pregnant woman, they may induce uterine contraction resulting in expulsion of the fetus. They may be used immediately after exposure to conception up through twenty-six weeks of pregnancy.

Properly performed by a qualified physician in an aseptic setting, these methods of abortion present little hazard to a woman, often less than allowing the pregnancy to continue on to full term. While some women do suffer from emotional problems following an abortion, it is now believed that the number of women for whom abortion has a traumatic effect has been greatly exaggerated. The important thing is that a woman make up her own mind on the subject.

In countries where abortion is legally available to anyone wishing one, abortion is a common method of fertility control. There is very little danger, since the procedure can be performed at the proper time in the ideal hospital setting. In Hungary, the death rate from abortion is less than 6 per 100,000. The death rate in the United States from childbirth and its complications is almost four times as high. The earlier abortion is performed, the safer it is. In Hungary, the death rate from abortion rises from about 6 per 100,000 when performed during the first three months to 300 per 100,000 when performed during the second three months of pregnancy.

Illegal Abortion

Before abortion on demand was available in this country, physicians who studied abortion estimated that about one in every five pregnancies was terminated by means of an illegal abortion. A great many women died every year as the direct result of improperly performed illegal abortions.

Wherever legal abortions are unavailable, illegal abortions will be sought out. Even though abortion on demand is legal in the United States, some physicians and some hospitals refuse to provide it. As a result, women who live in an area where legal abortion is not available and can afford to go to another community or another state are able to have legal abortions; the poor who live in an area where legal abortion is not available must bear the children they cannot properly care for or seek out a criminal abortionist.

Illegal abortions are performed by various kinds of people. Before the Supreme Court ruling many abortionists were physicians who provided their services out of greed or compassion. Now the criminal abortionist is more apt to be a chiropractor, nurse, housewife, or some other insufficiently trained or totally untrained person.

An abortion performed by a physician outside of a qualified clinic or hospital, performed at the improper time of pregnancy, or attempted by an insufficiently trained person jeopardizes the life of the woman. Permanent damage to her reproductive organs, serious infections, even death may easily result. It is far better for her to seek out references to a well-qualified hospital that provides abortion services, even if some travel is required and at some cost to her or her family or friends, than for her to accept an illegal abortion. All claims of her friends or of the abortionist to the contrary, her life and psychological well-being are far more important.

Which Method to Choose

Fertility control is a highly individual matter that must rest upon a private decision between a man and a woman. It is plainly a matter of *which* method to choose, not *whether* or not to choose one. During a normal reproductive life, a woman may easily give birth to twelve or fifteen children. Few women would desire that many.

There are several significant criteria in selecting the method that is best in a given situation. The first and most important factor is *safety.* The ideal method should not be harmful to a person's health, nor should it reduce one's ability to have a child in the future, if one is wanted. It should be free from hazardous or unwanted side effects, both for the person using the device and for the partner. A second factor is *rate of effectiveness.* It must be effective in preventing pregnancy for the particular person using it. Its effectiveness depends on the device itself, the person using it, the method of applying the device, and the cultural, social, and economic environment surrounding its use. The device should also have use-effectiveness, or a high probability of continued use. The third factor is *ease of administration.* If it is permanently inserted (an IUD), it is expected that a professional will insert it; if it is some other mechanical device, the person using it must find it easy to use. Ideally, the device will be one that can be applied at some time other than during actual preparation for intercourse. A fourth element is *acceptability.* Acceptance must include medical factors (one's medical history, absence of side effects, physical comfort), social factors (religious attitudes, cultural hesitations), and psychological factors (personal aesthetics, one's own habits and attitudes). In some cultures, for instance, a woman is not allowed to touch her vagina with a foreign object. *Reversibility* is a fifth element. Whether a person's fertility is ever utilized or not, it is important to some people to know that pregnancy is possible, particularly for people with no children or fewer than they want. The potential of fertility is an important psychological factor in many man-woman relationships. Sixth is *expense.* Some devices (such as the IUD) require only an initial expense, while others involve a recurring cost (the pill, condom, foam). While economizing is a necessity to many couples in this country, several cents a day for a birth control device may be a prohibitive cost to couples in Third World countries. Also important is the effect the device has on a person's *libido,* or sexual feelings. In lovemaking, people should not have to be preoccupied with whether it is safe for them to give themselves to each other fully. They want to feel confident with the method of control that best suits their needs.

The method chosen must be satisfactory to both partners. A choice ought to be made in accordance with a couple's tastes and preferences, their emotional dispositions, their physical requirements, any medical limitations, and their moral standards and religious attitudes. Methods should be discussed with a physician as part of any premarital counseling. Information may also be obtained from family planning clinics or from qualified agencies. One such agency is: Planned Parenthood Federation of America, Inc., 515 Madison Avenue, New York, New York, 10022. Ask for the address of your state or area organization. The address may also be listed in a local telephone directory.

Sexually Transmitted Diseases

14

Like all other human organs, the reproductive organs are subject to a variety of infections. In addition, the reproductive organs may serve as portals of entry into the body through which some diseases, such as syphilis, may infect the entire body. For several hundred years some of these infections have been referred to as venereal diseases or VD. (The word "venereal" refers to Venus, the Roman goddess of love.) The term "venereal disease" has been applied to diseases that are mainly transmitted through sexual contact, though authorities have often differed on whether certain genital infections, such as herpes simplex, should be classified as venereal diseases. Partly because of this problem in classification and, more importantly, to allow a more straightforward approach to the control of these diseases, scientists from all over the world recently (see *World Health,* May 1975) agreed to refer to these infections as "sexually transmitted diseases" or "STD." Changing the name does not, of course, change the problem in any way, but scientists hope the new term will lead to more open and realistic attitudes toward these diseases. Such attitudes would contribute greatly to their control.

Other than their similar methods of transmission, the sexually transmitted diseases are all distinctly different from each other. What they do have in common is an affinity for the mucous membranes, such as those lining the reproductive organs, as well as a relatively weak resistance to such adverse environmental conditions as dryness and chilling. Transmission of these diseases generally requires the direct contact of warm, moist body surfaces. Sexual contact is ideal for this purpose.

No other animal is known to commonly carry any of the human STDs; the pathogens apparently evolved from harmless inhabitants of the human body, or perhaps even from soil or water inhabitants. STD should not be viewed as punishment for "sin." Too many "innocent" people, such as newborn babies and spouses of unfaithful mates, are infected to make this idea palatable.

It is best to think of these diseases an dangerous infections that happen to be commonly transmitted through sexual contact and that should receive prompt treatment before others are infected or permanent damage is inflicted upon oneself.

History of STD

The early history of the sexually transmitted diseases is obscured by the confusion and lack of knowledge that surrounded diseases in general until fairly recently. Diseases fitting the descriptions of STD, however, can be traced back for 3000 years. Hippocrates wrote of gonorrhea in 460 B.C. and several chapters of the Bible describe diseases that accurately correspond to the various stages of syphilis. The first recorded epidemic of syphilis swept through Europe in the late fifteenth century. There was widespread death and disfigurement throughout much of Europe.

Syphilis received its present name in 1530 in a poem by a physician named Fracastoro about an afflicted Greek shepherd boy named Syphilus, who had offended the sun god.

At one time gonorrhea and syphilis were thought to be the same disease. This misapprehension was corrected in 1879 by the German bacteriologist Albert Neisser, who identified the bacteria that cause gonorrhea.

Both syphilis and gonorrhea have had a variety of names. Syphilis has been called scab, pox, French pox, Gallic disease, Spanish sickness, German pox, Persian fire, lues, and syph. Gonorrhea has been called clap, dose, strain, and G.C.

Today's Incidence of STD

Both gonorrhea and syphilis are currently at epidemic proportions in the United States. The yearly number of cases of gonorrhea and syphilis together exceeds the number of cases each year of strep throat, scarlet fever, mumps, measles, hepatitis, and tuberculosis combined. There are now well over 600,000 new cases of gonorrhea officially reported each year, but it is estimated that only one case out of every four actual infections is reported. For this reason, the actual incidence is probably more than 2.5 million per year, or one case out of every 100 people in the population. An estimated half-million people in the United States suffer from untreated syphilis, and over 90,000 new cases are being added each year.

Other studies indicate that even these estimates may be too conservative. For example, during the twelve-month period ending June 30, 1973, gonorrhea screening programs cultured specimens from almost 5 million women in the United States, of which 4.9 percent were positive for gonorrhea (Center for Disease Control, *Morbidity and Mortality Report* for October 12, 1973). Although, predictably, the highest gonorrhea rates (18.9 percent) were found in visitors to STD clinics, only 12 percent of the tests were performed in such clinics. The remaining 88 percent were in other settings, where typical gonorrhea rates included 2.3 percent of women visiting private physicians for all causes, 4 percent of women hospitalized for all causes, and 7.6 percent of women enrolling in vocational training programs. Few of these women were aware of their infection, as gonorrhea is symptomless in 80 to 90 percent of infected females.

Why the Increase in STD?

The treatment of the sexually transmitted diseases was changed dramatically in the 1940s by the discovery of prontosil, the first of the sulfonamides, quickly followed by other sulfa drugs and the advent of penicillin. Syphilis and gonorrhea were among the previously obstinate and dangerous infections that suddenly became readily treatable. Before that time there was little to be done about gonorrhea. The course of the disease may or may not have been influenced by such tedious and unpleasant treatments as the irrigation of the urethra by various antiseptic fluids. Syphilis could be cured by a prolonged course of intravenous injections of the arsenical drug salvarsan or one of its variants. But the treatment of both diseases was so prolonged and difficult that many patients simply lived (and often died) with their afflictions. Before penicillin, syphilis killed half the people who caught it (and it still kills half of its untreated victims).

The introduction of sulfa drugs and penicillin in the 1940s provided a cure for both gonorrhea and syphilis in a matter of days and with often no more than a single office visit. The amount of STD in the United States dropped steadily until, in the 1950s, a very low level was reached. Then a blanket of complacency settled down over government agencies, the medical profession, and the public. Funds for STD control diminished, and STD began its spectacular resurgence (see Figure 14.1). Patients were not even being interviewed for information on sexual contacts from or to whom the infection may have passed. Medical schools underemphasized its importance and the general public became largely apathetic. Research on STD came to a halt, and there was little attempt to produce an appropriate vaccine or to develop an improved method of diagnosing gonorrhea. The incidence of both gonorrhea and syphilis soared.

According to some authorities, an important factor in the current STD epidemic is the birth control pill. "The pill" has reduced the use of condoms, the only birth control method of value in preventing the transmission of STD. In addition, the pill increases the alkalinity and moisture of the female genital tract, thus encouraging the rapid growth of gonorrhea organisms. Other contraceptive aids for women, such as vaginal jelly and foam, are acidic and thus provide an environment antagonistic to the growth of infectious organisms. The estimated risk of contracting gonorrhea for a woman engaging in a single act of unprotected intercourse with an infected partner is 40 percent; for a woman taking the pill it is almost 100 percent.

The life styles of young people have incorported increased sexual freedom and personal mobility, both of which are favorable to the spread of STD.

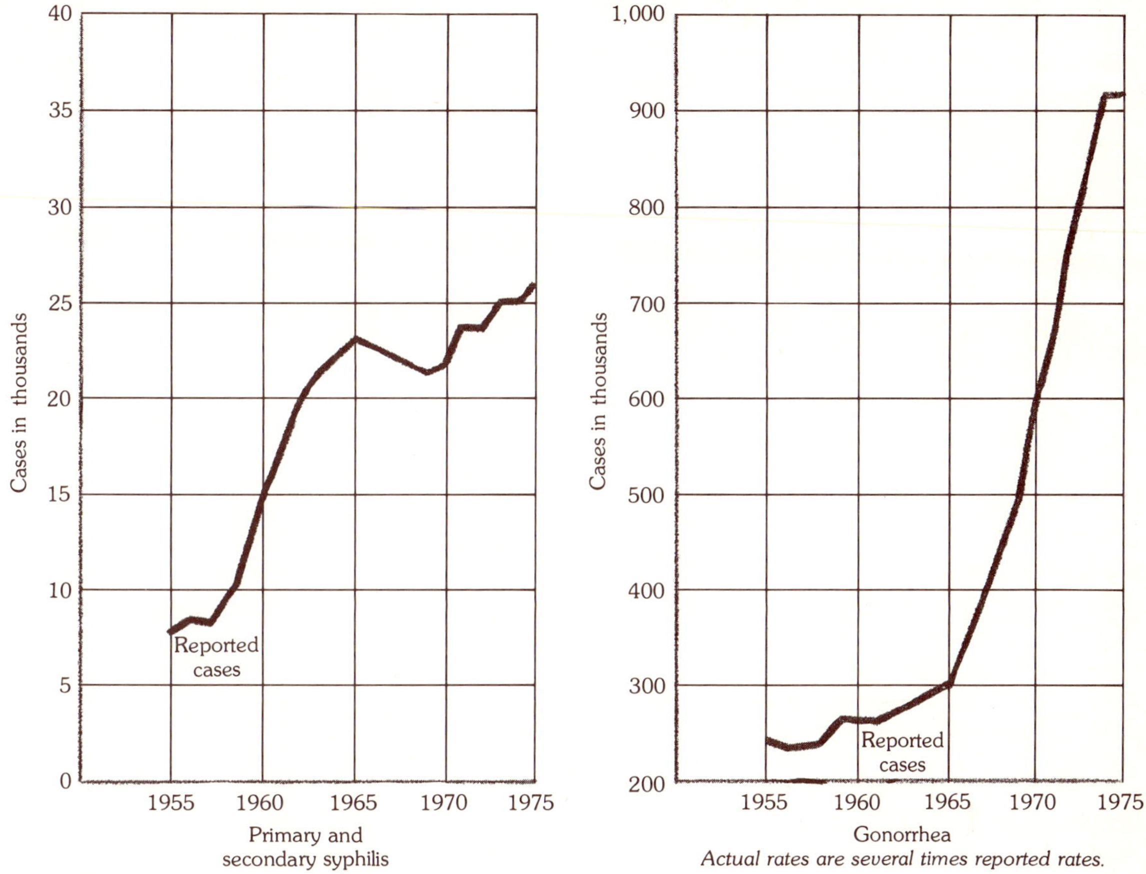

FIGURE 14.1 Reported cases of syphilis and gonorrhea (in thousands)

Gonorrhea

Gonorrhea is the *most common sexually transmitted disease* in the United States today. It is the most common communicable disease in the United States next to the common cold. Although less lethal than syphilis, gonorrhea is far more widespread and harder to control.

Gonorrhea is caused by bacteria called *Neisseria gonorrhoeae* (see Figure 14.2). This organism is often called the gonococcus, and it or the disease is sometimes simply referred to as "G.C." Common street names for gonorrhea include "the clap," "dose," "strain," and "morning drop."

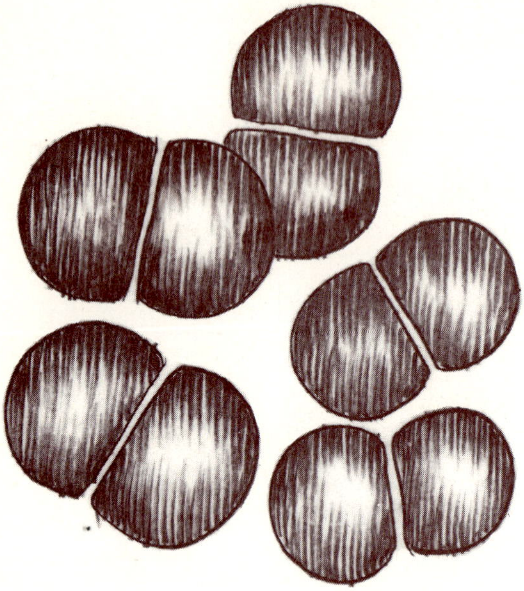

FIGURE 14.2 ***Neisseria gonorrhoeae,*** **the organism that causes gonorrhea**

Neisseria gonorrhoeae is extremely selective about where it grows, requiring just the right temperature, humidity, and nutrients. It dies or is inactivated when exposed to chill or dryness. For this reason, the transmission of gonorrhea requires contact between warm, moist body surfaces. Such inanimate objects as toilet seats are of little importance in transmitting gonorrhea.

Source and Transmission

Humans are the only natural reservoir of gonorrhea. The organism is present in the moist exudates from mucous membranes of infected persons. The gonococcus may be transmitted through various kinds of sexual activity, heterosexual and homosexual, including genital, oral-genital, and anal-genital contact.

Nature of the Disease

The gonococcus has an affinity for membranes. It most commonly infects the mucous membranes of the genitals (urogenital organs in males), throat, anus, and eye. If this organism enters the blood, it may infect the membranes lining the heart or the joints.

Course of the Disease

Once the gonococcus gains a foothold, its symptoms in a man will be entirely different from those in a woman. In most men, infection is

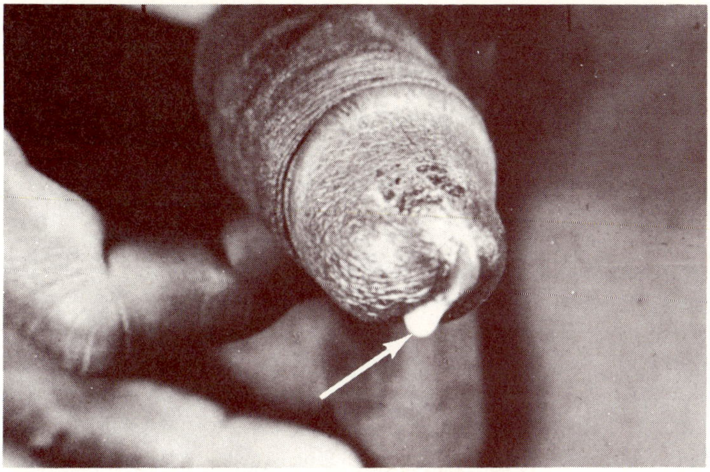

FIGURE 14.3 "Drip" from the penis of a male infected with gonorrhea

apparent from two days to a week after exposure; many, however, remain symptomless.

Gonorrhea in the Male The disease begins with a painful inflammation of the urethral canal in the penis. This causes a scalding pain upon urination. The inflammation begins at the tip of the penis and works up the urethra. The result is a "drip" of pus from the penis (see Figure 14.3). In early acute infection the discharge tends to be watery or milky. Later it becomes thick greenish-yellow, often tinged with blood.

The burning sensation that accompanies urination may subside after two or three weeks. By this time the infection may have reached the prostate gland and testicles, as well as the bladder and kidneys. Permanent damage can include urinary obstruction, chordee (downward, painful curvature of the penis on erection), inflammation and abscesses of the prostate, and sterility due to blockage of the vas deferens and epididymis. Infection of the throat occasionally occurs following oral-genital contact. Rectal gonorrhea may follow anal-genital intercourse.

In either sex, gonorrheal infection of the throat is characterized by a sore throat. Infection of the membranes of the eye (conjunctivitis) results in considerable redness and painful inflammation. Anal infection is not likely to result in any symptoms.

Gonorrhea in the Female Gonorrhea may produce no painful symptoms in women. In fact, about 80 percent of women infected do not realize they have the disease until their male partners discover their own infections. The prevalence of asymptomatic carriers is an important part of the history of the gonorrhea epidemic. Public Health Service studies show that up to 5 percent of all women in the United States may be asymptomatic carriers of the gonococcus. Although in the past it was thought that only women could have the disease without symptoms, investigators are now reporting frequent discovery of gonococci in the urethras of men who reveal no symptoms.

The symptoms of gonorrhea in the female (when they exist) are different from those in the male. The usual symptom of a woman is irritation or "smarting" of the vagina accompanied by discharge. Unfortunately, such a discharge is a most unreliable sign in the female, since she ordinarily experiences vaginal discharges quite unrelated to gonorrhea. The gonococcus prefers the cervix and fallopian tubes. In about 10 percent of cases the infection is found wholly in the rectum.

A gonorrhea infection generally moves methodically up the genital tract. In the vagina its effects are usually asymptomatic, or at least unclear. As it reaches the upper tract—the uterus, fallopian tubes, and ovaries—a pus discharge occurs and complications begin to set in.

Complications do not usually appear until after at least one menstrual cycle. If the woman is on the pill, however, complications may show up as quickly as three to five days after exposure. Birth control pills, while protecting a woman against pregnancy, have been found actually to promote gonorrhea. The pill causes an increase in the moisture content of the vagina and provides an alkaline environment that is ideally suited to the gonococcus. A woman taking contraceptive pills who has intercourse with an infected man has virtually no chance of escaping infection, and she may suffer complications much sooner than if she were not taking the pill.

Gonorrhea in Newborn Children Untreated gonorrhea in pregnant women may be responsible for conjunctivitis (an inflammation of the conjunctiva of the eye) in newborn children. This condition, which could lead to blindness, is prevented by drops of either penicillin or silver nitrate, required by law to be placed in the eyes of every newborn infant. Infection may also invade the infant's external genitalia, especially in breech deliveries. In addition to the child, physicians have become infected when gonococcal-contaminated amniotic fluid has splashed into their eyes during a delivery.

Complications One study has shown that at least 12 percent of all women with gonorrhea suffer from some degree of invasion of the fallopian tubes. This can result in sterility or ectopic pregnancy (a fertilized egg implanting itself in the fallopian tube rather than in the uterine wall) because of scar tissue that may block the free passage of the egg. Pus material may also collect into an abscess, which may rupture painfully. Gonorrhea-produced sterility is increasing and is presently the leading cause of sterility in the female.

The infection may pass from the fallopian tube into the abdominal cavity, causing a massive infection called pelvic inflammatory disease (PID).

Gonorrhea occasionally progresses into a systemic (blood-borne) infection. When this occurs, the results may be very serious, even fatal. Systemic gonorrhea may attack the joints (arthritis), heart lining (endocarditis), heart muscle, brain, membranes covering the brain (meningitis), lungs, kidneys, veins, and skin. Common symptoms of systemic gonorrhea include fever, arthritis, and sores on the skin. Even though the gonococcus is fragile outside the human body, its potential for tissue destruction and widespread complications within humans is great.

Diagnosis of Gonorrhea

A blood test is now available for the detection of gonorrhea. Other diagnostic methods involve demonstrating the presence of *Neisseria gonorrhoeae* organisms in stained microscope slides and in cultures of special growth media. For either slides or cultures, the sources of bacteria include the urethra of the male, the cervix of the female, the anus, and the throat.

Since women usually notice no symptoms of gonorrhea, periodic laboratory tests for gonorrhea are advisable even in the absence of symptoms, if there is any chance of exposure to the disease.

Very often a patient may be infected with both syphilis and gonorrhea at the same time. While examining for gonorrhea, a physician should also be alert for symptoms of syphilis.

Treatment of Gonorrhea

The gonococcus has a long history of developing resistance to everything that has been used for its treatment. Drugs that were highly effective when they were first used have gradually lost their effectiveness—potassium salts, silver compounds, sulfa drugs, and, most recently, penicillin. Penicillin is still the drug most commonly used against gonorrhea, though much larger doses are now required than when the drug was first available. A typical dosage is now 4.8 million units. Even at this high level, penicillin often fails to cure gonorrhea completely. Fortunately, there are other drugs that may be used when penicillin fails or when the patient is hypersensitive (allergic) to penicillin.

There is no effective home remedy for gonorrhea. Nothing can be mixed up or bought from a drugstore or by mail that will cure this or any other sexually transmitted disease. The infected person must see a private physician or a local public health department for effective treatment. It is most important that gonorrhea be treated promptly, before any permanent damage can occur.

Immunity to Gonorrhea

There is no vaccine being marketed at this time that will prevent gonorrhea, though experimental vaccines are being produced. No immunity results from a case of gonorrhea. After a penicillin treatment wears off in a few days, reinfection can occur.

Syphilis

Syphilis is the most serious sexually transmitted disease. Other names for syphilis include "siff," "pox," "lues," and "bad blood." Syphilis is entirely different from gonorrhea. While gonorrhea is usually confined to the urogenital system in males and the reproductive organs in females, syphilis enters the bloodstream and is thus a systemic (bodywide) infection. The main similarity between these two diseases is that both are transmitted primarily by sexual contact.

The organism that causes syphilis is a spirochete (spiral bacterium) called *Treponema pallidum* (see Figure 14.4). This germ is very frail and cannot survive drying or chilling. It is killed within a few seconds after exposure to air. Since the germ is so easily killed by air, it is easy to see why syphilis must be transmitted by sexual intercourse, kissing, or other intimate body contacts. The germ requires warm, moist skin or mucous membrane surfaces for its penetration into the body. After the spirochetes burrow through the skin or mucous membrane and enter the blood, they are carried throughout the body. Because its symptoms are so varied that they can resemble any one of many other diseases, syphilis has been called the "great imitator."

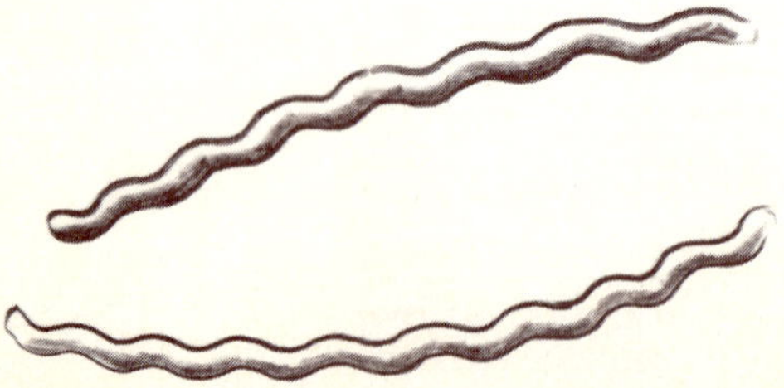

FIGURE 14.4 ***Treponema pallidum,*** **the organism that causes syphilis**

Primary Syphilis

After infection with syphilis, there may be a symptomless incubation period of ten to ninety days, although the usual period is three to four weeks. During this time the spirochetes multiply in the body.

The first symptom that appears is the primary lesion or chancre (pronounced "shanker"). This is a sore that appears at the exact spot where infection took place. The typical chancre (see Figure 14.5) is pink to red in color, raised, firm, and painless. It is usually the size of a dime, but it may be so small that it resembles a pimple. The chancre is swarming with spirochetes. Any contact with it is likely to result in a syphilitic infection.

The usual location of the chancre is on or near the sex organs, but it can be on the lip, finger, or any part of the body. In women the chancre is often within the vagina, and since it is painless, it may go unnoticed.

Even if the primary syphilis is not treated (which it definitely should be), the chancre will disappear spontaneously in three to six weeks. But this disappearance of the chancre does not mean that the disease is cured. It is just progressing to the next stage. At about the time the chancre disappears, blood tests for syphilis become positive.

FIGURE 14.5 Chancres are painless lesions, pink, raised, ulcerated, and firm. The chancre may occur anywhere on the body.

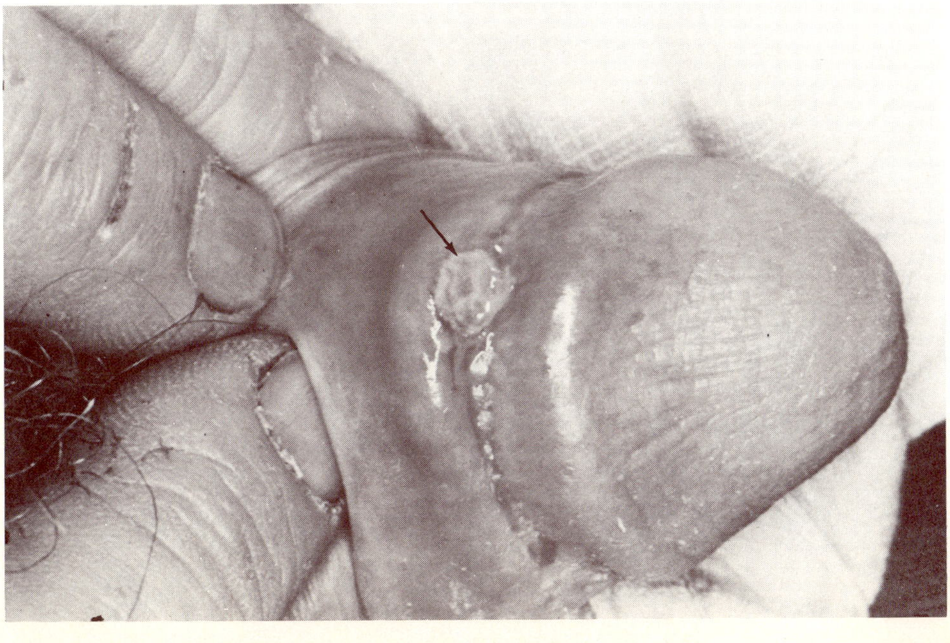

Secondary Syphilis

In secondary syphilis, the true systemic nature of syphilis becomes obvious. Symptoms may appear throughout the body, starting one to six months after the appearance of the chancre, though in many cases this stage is skipped over. The most common symptom of secondary syphilis is a rash (see Figure 14.6) that does not itch. This rash is quite variable in appearance; it may cover the entire body or any part of it. A common site of the rash is the palms of the hands or the soles of the feet. Large, moist

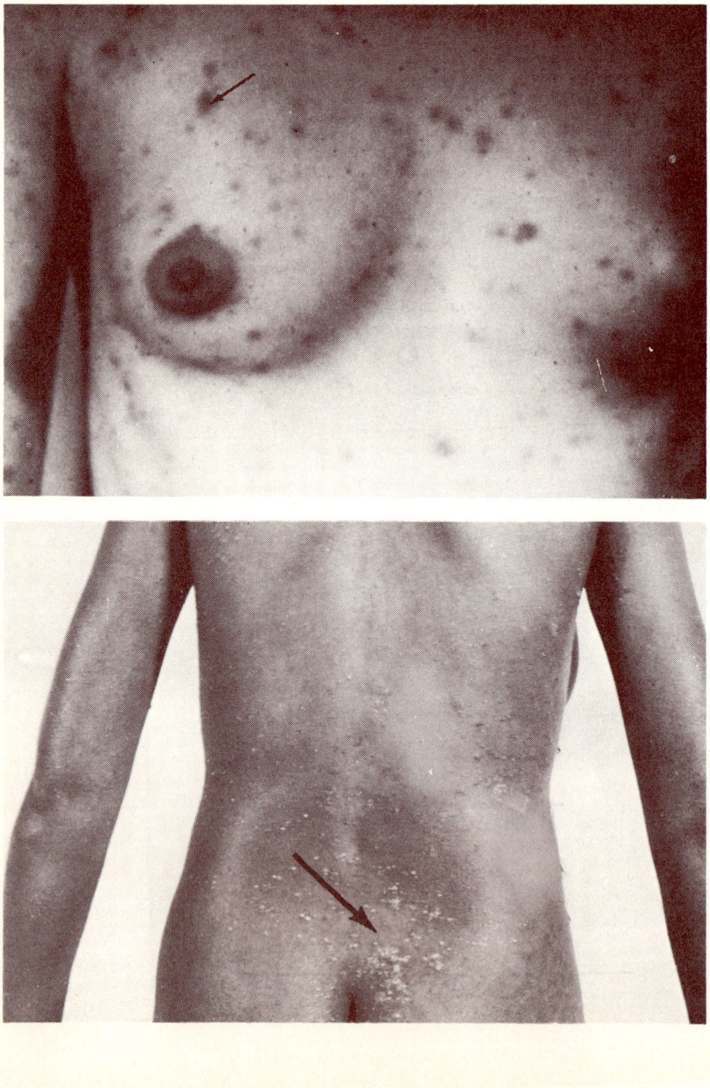

FIGURE 14.6 Rash of secondary syphilis on breast and back

sores may develop on or around the sex organs or in the mouth. These moist sores are loaded with syphilitic germs. Contact with them may cause syphilitic infection. Secondary syphilis is extremely contagious.

Other symptoms that may occur in secondary syphilis include sore throat, headache, slight fever, red eyes, pain in the joints, and patches of hair that fall out. Anyone who has these symptoms and might have been exposed to syphilis should explain this fact to a physician. Because syphilis can easily be mistaken for many other diseases, it is difficult to diagnose. Without an accurate diagnosis, it may not be properly treated. Syphilis at this secondary stage is best diagnosed by means of specific blood tests for the disease.

The symptoms of secondary syphilis last from several days to several months. Then, like the chancre of primary syphilis, they disappear even without treatment. Syphilis has then entered the latent stage.

Latent Syphilis

Latency begins with the disappearance of untreated secondary symptoms; it may extend for a few months or for a lifetime. Latency may be divided into two stages: a potentially infectious stage, early latent syphilis, and a noninfectious later stage, late latent syphilis.

These phases, commonly called "hidden syphilis," are usually not recognizable by visible signs or symptoms. They are detected only by blood tests. Latent syphilis is usually discovered during routine blood examinations.

Early Latent Syphilis If the disease remains untreated there may be a series of recurring infectious lesions of the skin or mucous membranes similar to those of secondary syphilis for the first two to four years. Whenever these lesions are present, the disease may be transmitted through contact. During the long latent period the disease loses some of its infectiousness, and after the first two years a person can rarely transmit syphilis through sexual intercourse, although a syphilitic pregnant woman can still transmit it to her unborn child (congenital syphilis) for an additional two years.

Late Latent Syphilis When the victim has lost all ability to infect, the disease has entered the late latent period, lasting anywhere from several months to a lifetime. During this period there are no discernible signs of illness. A routine blood test will reveal the presence of syphilis but the victim will have no obvious symptoms. In this latent stage, progressive degeneration of the brain, spinal cord, hearing, sight, or bones may be occurring unnoticed. If and when the symptoms of this degeneration appear, the victim then slips into the last and most destructive stage.

Late Syphilis

Many people who have contracted syphilis and allowed it to progress untreated may develop a late stage that will incapacitate or kill them. Although almost any part of the body may be affected, only the most common manifestations will be discussed here.

Cardiovascular Syphilis The lesions in most cases of cardiovascular syphilis are located in the thoracic aorta. The elastic tissue is destroyed and the aorta bulges, producing an aneurysm. The infection may also involve the aortic value, causing an insufficient flow of blood. The symptoms of cardiovascular syphilis differ in no unique way from those of other heart and vascular disorders.

Neurosyphilis The symptoms of neurosyphilis arise from a widespread destruction of tissues of the brain and spinal cord by large numbers of *Treponema pallidum.* The brain damage of late syphilis is called paresis or *dementia paralytica.* The mental changes vary but most commonly become manifest in gradual changes of personality, decreased ability to work, and impairment of concentration and judgment. These changes produce abnormal behavior, including delusions, loss of memory, lack of insight, apathy or violent rages, convulsions, and disorientation. Neurosyphilis is responsible for many deaths, as well as for many chronic cases in mental institutions.

Paralysis Paralysis is the most common outcome of the progressive destruction of the spinal cord by large numbers of spirochetes. In treated cases life can be prolonged, but permanent care may be necessary because extreme degeneration may have taken place before treatment.

Loss of Vision Syphilis involves degeneration of the optic nerve; it is usually first noticed as a loss of peripheral vision. Central vision may be lost in advanced cases, leaving the victim completely blind.

Syphilis in Pregnancy

If a woman is infected with syphilis at the time of conception or shortly thereafter, the primary chancre appearing on her may be very mild or completely suppressed. Secondary symptoms in her skin are likely to be absent, and if she has not had blood tests during her pregnancy she may have no indication that she has syphilis until the birth of her child. Infection of a fetus takes place when the spirochetes of syphilis cross the placental membranes within the womb. Such infection of the fetus apparently does not occur before the fifth month of fetal life. Consequently, adequate treatment of a previously syphilitic pregnant woman before the fifth fetal month should ensure the child's safety. Treatment given a mother after the fifth month may also cure the syphilitic fetus. Because of these conditions and because syphilis can also be acquired during pregnancy, blood tests during the first half of pregnancy and during the seventh month are considered adequate for detecting syphilis.

In a majority of cases the fetus becomes infected quite late in pregnancy, and the more recent the mother's syphilitic infection, the greater the probability that the child will be born with syphilis. A severe infection is very likely to lead to death of the fetus before birth, and syphilis is a common cause of stillbirth. Among the infants born alive to untreated syphilitic mothers, approximately 50 percent have syphilis at birth. Syphilis obtained in this manner is termed congenital syphilis.

Congenital Syphilis

A syphilitic infant may show secondary lesions at birth, may appear normal at birth and develop lesions within a few months, or may remain without symptoms until adolescence, when the symptoms of late syphilis may appear. As a rule, the earlier the symptoms appear, the more severe the infection. Syphilis is capable of producing many types of lesions, but never do all of them occur in one infant.

Of the various secondary symptoms appearing at birth, *snuffles*—an inflammation of the nose with a discharge of *Treponema pallidum* spirochetes—is most frequent. This discharge may interfere with breathing, is extremely infectious, and accounts for many infections of people who handle such children. During fetal development the growth of the nasal bones may be disturbed, resulting in the deformity known as "saddle nose" (see Figure 14.7). Skin lesions at birth are frequent and are often

FIGURE 14.7 Saddle nose (destruction of the septum in congenital syphilis)

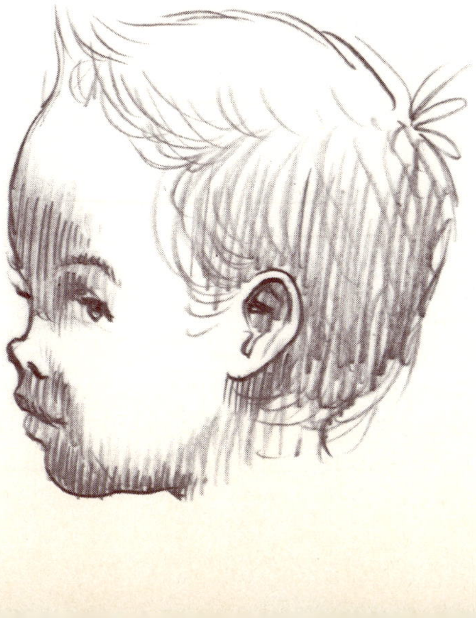

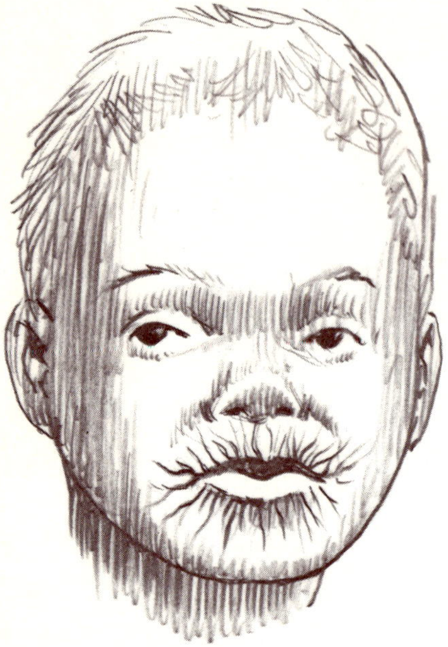

FIGURE 14.8 Congenital syphilis, showing rhagades (scars around the mouth)

similar to the rash seen in secondary stages of venereal syphilis. In a high proportion of children, the palms of hands, soles of feet, or skin about the mouth may be reddened, inflamed, and thickened at birth or shortly after birth. When this condition occurs around the mouth, fissures may radiate in all directions. After healing, these lesions leave radiating scars about the mouth known as *rhagades* (see Figure 14.8).

Following the secondary lesions, the course of untreated congenital syphilis is similar to that of venereal syphilis. These late symptoms may appear in a few months, at six or seven years of age, or in the late teens. Some of the more common are "Hutchinson's teeth" (see Figure 14.9), which are notched or screwdriver-like permanent central incisors; *keratitis,* a condition of the eyes uncommon in young children but very common in older children and capable of causing permanent blindness; and various injuries to bones and body joints.

Diagnosis of Syphilis

Early diagnosis followed by prompt and adequate treatment can completely cure syphilis.

Microscopic Examination The lesions of early syphilis are rich in *Treponema pallidum;* this fact provides the best means for conclusive

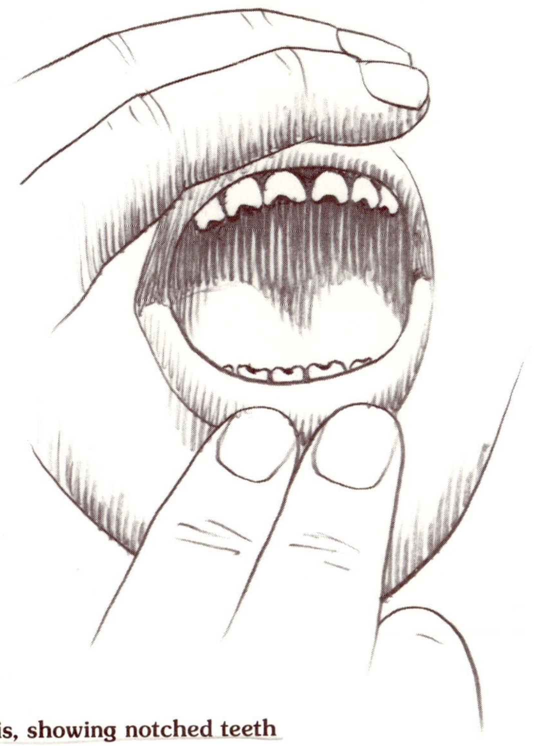

FIGURE 14.9 Congenital syphilis, showing notched teeth

diagnosis of the disease. *Treponema pallidum* taken from a chancre of primary syphilis or from skin lesions of secondary syphilis can readily be seen under a microscope by what is termed "dark-field illumination."

Blood Tests for Syphilis Blood tests become positive only after a general invasion of the body by spirochetes. After syphilis infection (and occasionally following some other conditions) the blood contains an antibody-like substance called *reagin.* All of the blood tests for syphilis based on reagin in the blood are modifications of the original Wassermann test (an old test for determining blood reagin which was much less sensitive than present tests).

Besides the reagin tests, there are others for *Treponema pallidum* spirochetes and specific antibodies produced by the body in response to syphilis infection. They are positive for syphilis only, are quite expensive, and involve complicated procedures that cannot be used as easily as the reagin tests for screening large numbers of individuals.

Syphilis Therapy

The purposes of treatment are to destroy all spirochetes, to initiate the healing of existing lesions, and to prevent further damage to the body. Treatment of syphilis also serves to prevent the spread of the disease to others. The earlier this treatment is begun, the more effective it is in accomplishing these purposes.

In the mid-1940s penicillin began to replace the lengthy, expensive, and difficult treatment of syphilis with arsenic products and bismuth preparations. Since that time penicillin alone has been used to treat syphilis around the world.

The primary consideration in treatment is maintenance of a high penicillin level in the blood and tissues for a period of time sufficient to destroy all spirochetes present in the body. Consequently, treatment varies with progressive stages of the disease. Unfortunately, the widespread use of penicillin for treatment of a variety of other disorders has frequently added some difficulties to the diagnosis of syphilis. Syphilitic infection may be masked completely or its course altered by smaller doses of penicillin than are necessary to eliminate all the spirochetes. Larger doses of penicillin are required to treat syphilis than for most other diseases. When a patient's allergy to penicillin precludes the use of this preferred drug, Erythromycin and Tetracycline are good alternatives. No matter what drug is used, inadequate therapy may lead to a relapse. There is no home remedy, mail-order cure, or nonprescription product available from the drugstore that will cure syphilis; it must have professional treatment by a physician.

Research is going forward on development of a vaccine against syphilis and prospects are now very encouraging.

Genital Herpes Virus Infections

Some of the most common, troublesome, and persistent genital infections are caused by viruses from the *herpes simplex* group (see Figure 14.10). Herpes simplex viruses are apparently carried by most people at all times, though usually in a state of latency (dormancy). Some 70 to 90 percent of adults carry antibodies against herpes simplex, but these antibodies do not prevent occasional activation of the virus. In addition to genital sores, herpes viruses are associated with cold sores, fever blisters, eczema, corneal infection, meningitis, encephalitis, and possibly uterine and other cancers. Two types of herpes viruses, type 1 and type 2, have been identified to date. Type 1 typically attacks the upper parts of the body while type 2 typically attacks below the waist, but there are many exceptions to these generalizations.

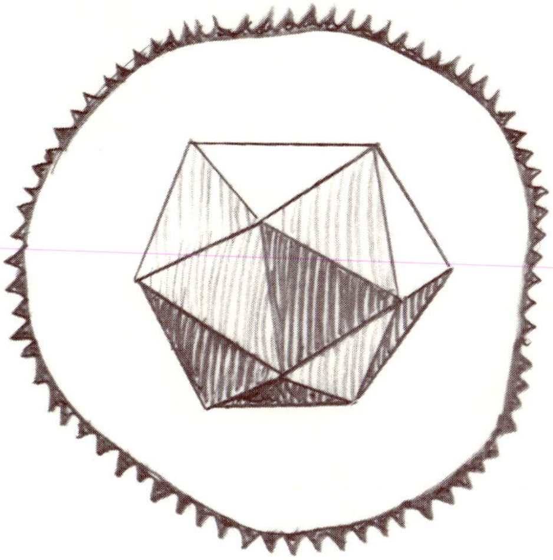

FIGURE 14.10 A herpes simplex virus particle, only several billionths of a meter in diameter

Most people receive their initial infection with herpes virus during childhood. The antibodies carried by most adults are transferred across the placenta to the fetus during pregnancy so most infants are protected from infection during the first few months after birth. If the mother acquires her first infection during pregnancy, however, and the child is born before sufficient maternal antibodies can be transferred across the placenta, severe infection of the newborn may occur, often with fatal consequences. The virus may be widely distributed in infant tissues, producing severe lesions in skin, mucous membranes, liver, and brain.

Much more typically, infection occurs during childhood and without serious complications. Children are usually infected through contact with the virus in the saliva of other children or adults or through contact with the eczema or other lesions of infected persons. About 90 percent of initial childhood infections are symptomless; about 10 percent of children suffer a mild fever and general discomfort lasting only a few days. Following initial infection, the herpes virus usually is carried in the body cells in a latent state, and is periodically reactivated by various stimuli such as fever, mechanical irritation, and certain foods.

Genital herpes simplex sores in adults may result from either the reactivation of latent herpes infections or from newly acquired virus transmitted through genital or orogenital sexual contact. These sores may occur on the labia or within the vagina in women and on the penis or within the urethra in men.

In someone not already carrying the virus, the symptoms of genital herpes usually appear about six days after sexual contact with an infected person. Subsequent attacks are caused by reactivation of the virus, which apparently stays in the nerve endings between attacks. The average person may have four or five recurrences in the first year and two or three in subsequent years. The infection is contagious whenever there is a recurrence of lesions.

Genital herpes usually starts with some minor itching or a slight rash. Then a cluster of small blisters forms. These then break open to form one more more red, eroded lesions that are exquisitely painful, especially during sexual intercourse. In a few cases the pain may radiate into the legs, and there may be severe swelling that makes urination difficult. In a first attack, the sores usually disappear in two to four weeks, while subsequent attacks usually clear up in one or two weeks.

Unlike gonorrhea and syphilis, there is no specific treatment for herpes simplex. Viruses in general are not susceptible to control by antibiotics or other drugs. Various treatments have been tried, but none is universally effective or accepted as safe. The fact that genital herpes lesions clear up with the passage of time even if they go untreated tends to make any form of treatment appear to work at least part of the time. One of the more common treatments has been painting the lesions with a red dye and then exposing the area to light, which appears to shorten the duration of the outbreak. In experiments with animals, however, this treatment has appeared to increase the cancer-causing tendencies of the herpes viruses. Many authorities thus discourage its use. Some doctors feel they are able to prevent recurrent genital herpes attacks with repeated small pox or tuberculosis vaccinations, but other doctors doubt the effectiveness of this approach. What is really needed is a specific herpes vaccine. Several laboratories are working on the problem, but a successful vaccine appears to be several years in the future.

Uterine Cancer: A Sexually Transmitted Disease?

A possible though still unproven association has been suggested between a herpes simplex virus (type 2) and cancer of the cervix or uterus. The virus is often found within cancerous cells, but no cause-and-effect relationship has been established. Preliminary studies do indicate that women who suffer herpes type 2 infections are eight times more likely to develop cervical cancer than those who are free of the disease.

Some cancer researchers suspect that cervical cancer may be positively correlated with early and promiscuous sexual activity. According to those who accept this association, the incidence of cervical cancer is higher among women who begin sexual intercourse young and among those with a history of many sex partners. Conversely, the incidence of uterine cancer has been reported to be low among virgins, women whose sexual activity started late, and women with histories of few sex partners. Such a relationship, if it indeed exists, would be compatible with the role of a sexually transmitted herpes simplex virus as a causal agent for cervical cancer, since the herpes viruses are noted for their ability to lie dormant for many years. The incidence of uterine cancer increases with age, although it is of course possible that the cells of some particular younger women might be more susceptible to infection by a virus.

Other factors might also account for an association between early intercourse or multiple sex partners and cervical cancer, again assuming that such an association exists. Genetic mutation of the cervical cells is one such possibility. The cause of such mutation might be repeated mechanical trauma during coitus or perhaps some carcinogenic (cancer-causing) chemical in semen, although this seems extremely unlikely. Still another possibility is that the stimulus for cancer production might be irritation and weakening of the cervical tissues by chronic infection with one or more of the many sexually transmitted pathogens.

Three Uncommon Sexually Transmitted Diseases

The following three diseases occur throughout the world, but are uncommon in most parts of the United States. Each is almost totally preventable by merely washing with soap and water immediately after exposure. Together they amount to about 1600 reported cases per year in the United States, mainly in the southern states.

Chancroid

Chancroid, also known as "soft chancre" or "soft sore," is a localized infection usually acquired by sexual contact and caused by a bacillus called *Hemophilus ducreyi.* About three to five days after exposure to the bacillus a small red area appears at the site of infection. This enlarges into a pimple-like growth that soon breaks down, forming an ulcer (open sore) with ragged edges and exuding pus (see Figure 14.11). If a cut or abrasion of the skin exists at the time of exposure, the lesion may appear within twenty-four hours. The ulcers bleed easily and are soft and very painful.

In roughly half of all cases the disease is self-limiting and heals by itself. In the other half, in about a week the lymph glands near the ulcer may swell, accumulate large amounts of pus, and rupture spontaneously. Also, if a lesion is located in a body area that is hard to keep clean, is hidden, or does not receive prompt treatment, rapidly destructive ulcerations can destroy much of the local tissue. The bacillus can be spread to surrounding areas of the body, causing multiple lesions to develop. Systemic reactions are rare, pain is the most frequent complaint, and extreme tissue destruction is the most severe complication.

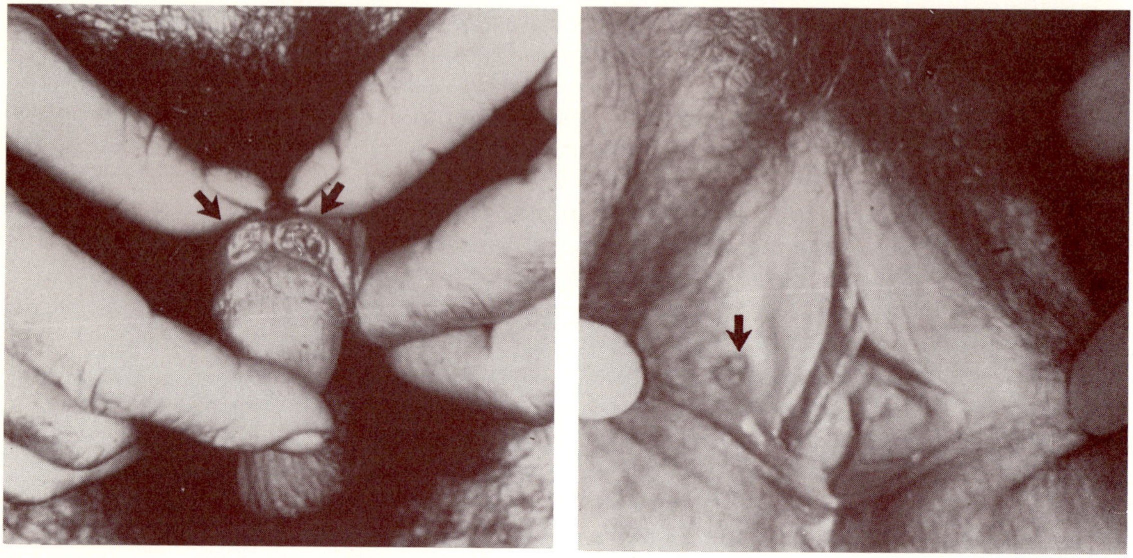

FIGURE 14.11 Chancroid ulcers

Chancroid has been confused with the chancre stage of syphilis. Chancroid can be readily distinguished because its lesions are usually multiple and tender (instead of firm or hard) with a slightly grayish base.

Various antibiotics are used to treat chancroid. Chancroid is mainly a disease of people who do not use soap and water frequently enough to keep the genital areas clean. The key to prevention of chancroid is cleanliness; the use of soap and water immediately after sexual exposure is a reliable preventive measure. As with many other STDs, symptomless carriers are an important source of infection.

Granuloma Inguinale

Granuloma inguinale causes small rounded, fleshy masses of pus-filled ulcerations on the skin covering the external genitals and groin (inguinal) region of the body. It occasionally spreads to the lymph nodes in the area. It is a chronic and progressive disease, caused by a bacillus called *Calymmatobacterium granulomatis.*

This disease is not necessarily transmitted by sexual contact only; it may be spread by contaminated objects as well. It is a disease of those who do not or cannot maintain standards of cleanliness.

The incubation period of granuloma inguinale is apparently quite variable, ranging from eight to over a hundred days. If untreated, the infection spreads peripherally and may involve a large area of skin and mucous membrane of the genital region. It may be successfully treated with antibiotics.

Lymphogranuloma Venereum

Lymphogranuloma venereum is a sexually acquired infection of the lymph channels and lymph glands near the genital organs. It is caused by a very small bacterium of the *Chlamydia* group.

The disease starts as a small, painless primary lesion (sore) at the site of entry of the bacteria, usually on the genitals. This lesion appears about seven to twelve days after infection has taken place and disappears soon thereafter. It is often of such short duration that it escapes notice. About ten to thirty days after exposure the lymph nodes in the groin region enlarge, fill with pus, and may rupture and drain continuously. Fever, chills, headache, and joint pains may be present. Chronic infection of the pelvic lymphatic ducts may block drainage of fluid from this region, causing swelling of genital tissues. Lymphogranuloma venereum may be successfully treated with sulfa drugs or antibiotics.

Other Infections of the Reproductive and Urinary Organs

In addition to the true STDs, the reproductive organs are susceptible to several other kinds of infections that are not usually classified as STDs because they are very commonly transmitted through nonsexual means, although each of these infections may also be contracted through sexual contact.

In recent years there has been a great increase in these infections. This may be related to an increase in casual sexual contacts and definitely is related to modern birth control methods. Birth control pills change the vaginal environment, creating a moist, alkaline condition, favoring infection by *Candida, Trichomonas,* and herpes viruses, as well as gonorrhea. At the same time, pills and IUDs have somewhat replaced such birth control methods as condoms and vaginal foams, which actively help prevent the transmission of infections.

Candida

One of the more troublesome infections of the sexual organs, and especially the vagina, is caused by a yeastlike organism called *Candida albicans* (see Figure 14.12). This organism is a normal inhabitant of the mouth, digestive tract, and vagina, but it is usually held in check by the other organisms present and by the body's natural defenses.

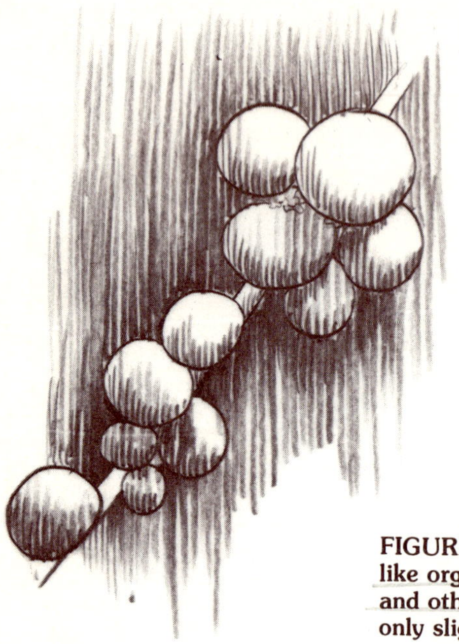

FIGURE 14.12 ***Candida albicans.*** **This yeast-like organism is a common cause of vaginitis and other infections. The cells are microscopic, only slightly larger than bacteria.**

Various factors can act to reduce normal defenses against *Candida* (also called a "yeast" infection), allowing it to erupt into a serious infection. One of these factors is intensive antibiotic therapy for some other infection. During such therapy the normal bacterial flora of the intestine and vagina may be reduced in numbers, allowing *Candida* to flourish instead. Poor nutrition may also lead to *Candida* eruption, as may any general weakening of one's health. Diabetes, which impairs the body defenses against most kinds of infections, is frequently associated with severe Candida infections. Hormone therapy, including use of birth control pills, as well as pregnancy may alter the vaginal environment to favor growth of *Candida*. A moist environment also encourages the organism; spending many hours in a wet swimsuit or in clothing that does not "breathe" freely, such as nylon underwear or panty hose, sometimes leads to severe *Candida* infections of the vagina and labia.

Vaginal candidiasis (the medical name for *Candida* infection) is the most troublesome of the *Candida* infections. The characteristic symptoms of vaginal candidiasis include burning and itching and a whitish discharge, which can be quite abundant. There may be patches of white *pseudomembrane* (false membrane) on the vaginal lining. Treatment of vaginal candidiasis involves several considerations. First is keeping the vaginal area dry and correcting any contributing conditions such as poor nutrition. A variety of effective oral and vaginal medications are available by prescription. It is important that male sex partners use condoms during the period of infection to avoid "ping-pong" infections in which the male is infected and later reinfects the female.

Other sites of *Candida* infection include the penis, vulva, and mouth cavity. Infection of the mouth cavity is called "thrush" and occurs most commonly among infants, elderly persons, and patients on intensive antibiotic therapy over long periods of time. *Candida* rarely enters the blood, but if it does it may cause serious or even fatal kidney or heart damage if not treated.

Trichomonas

Another common cause of vaginitis is infection by the protozoan (or one-celled animal) *Trichomonas vaginalis* (see Figure 14.13). *Trichomonas* lives in the vaginas of many women without producing noticeable symptoms. Symptomless infections of the male prostate gland, urethra, and seminal vessels are also common. Under certain conditions, however, *Trichomonas* can multiply enormously in either male or female reproductive organs. Symptoms in the female can include intense itching and burning of the vagina, small rashlike spots on its lining, and a profuse thin, foamy, yellowish discharge that may have a foul odor. Symptoms in the male are rare, and include urethritis or, even more rarely, inflammation of the prostate or seminal vesicles.

FIGURE 14.13 ***Trichomonas vaginalis*, a microscopic one-celled animal common in the vaginas of women throughout the world**

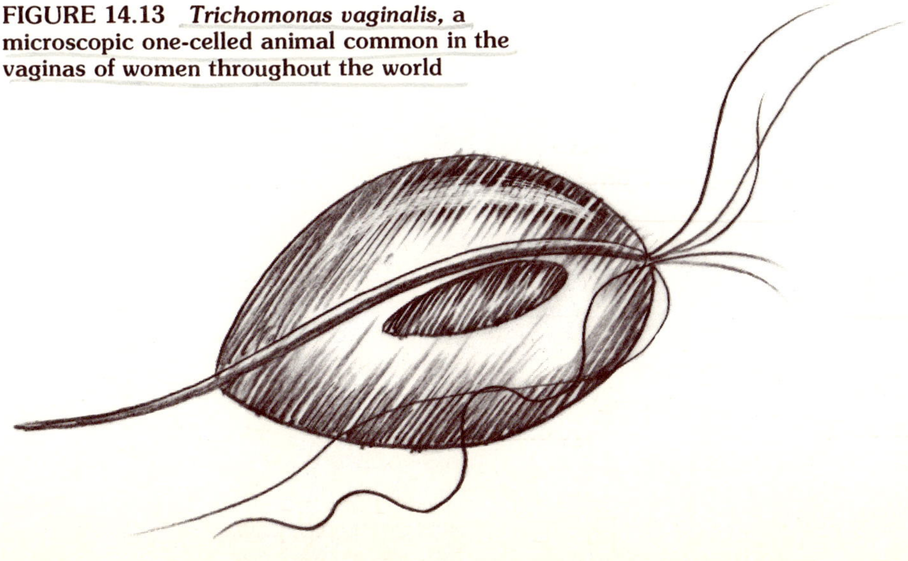

Trichomonas is a common infection among adult females throughout the world. The organism is transmitted from person to person by contact with vaginal and urethral discharges of infected persons during sexual contact, during birth, and possibly by contact with infected articles. Symptomless vaginal infections are often converted into troublesome vaginitis through modification of the vaginal environment produced by the hormonal changes associated with birth control pills or pregnancy.

Trichomoniasis can be successfully treated by medically prescribed oral or vaginal medications. Simultaneous treatment of sex partners is important in preventing reinfection. Even though a partner may be symptomless, he may well carry the organism.

Urethritis and Cystitis

Urethritis is any infection or inflammation of the male or female urethra. Cystitis is any infection or inflammation of the urinary bladder. These conditions may exist independently of each other or simultaneously. Either may result from a variety of causes. Both are extremely common.

Urethritis is more often a problem in males than in females, owing to the greater length of the male urethra. In either sex its symptoms may include a burning or stinging sensation during urination. In severe cases urination may be quite painful and may also become difficult, as swelling of the urethral lining restricts the flow of urine. More advanced cases may be complicated by the formation of scar tissue and adhesions that may require catheterization (insertion of a tube) to permit the drainage of urine. In addition, if urethritis is not promptly treated, the infection may spread via the urethra to the bladder, with a resulting cystitis.

Numerous infectious agents have been associated with urethritis. The catch-all terms "nonspecific urethritis" (NSU) and "nongonorrheal urethritis" (NGU) are often used to describe cases in which gonorrhea has been ruled out but the specific pathogen has not been identified. Many cases are believed to involve several extremely minute forms of bacteria called mycoplasma and chlamydia. The chlamydia that causes the eye infection trachoma has recently been implicated as a frequent cause of urethritis.[1]

Urethritis is sometimes associated with a period of increased sexual activity during which irritation of the urethra increases its susceptibility to infection. The urethritis may be the result of a pathogen newly acquired through sexual contact or of a pathogen that has already been present but which only later establishes infection of the irritated urethra. Many cases occur in the absence of any change in sexual habits or partners.

[1]"Most Common U.S. Venereal Disease: Would You Believe Trachoma?" *Medical World News,* vol. 15, no. 36 (October 4, 1974), pp. 16–17.

Most cases of urethritis respond well to antibiotics and sulfa drugs. In addition to the medication, treatment usually includes increased fluid intake, avoidance of alcohol and caffeine, and moderation in sexual activity until the infection is healed.

Symptoms of cystitis may include frequent urination and burning during urination. In severe cases, there may be a continual urge to urinate, there may be pain in the lower abdomen, and blood may appear in the urine.

Cystitis rarely is a primary condition; it usually is secondary to an infection of the kidney, prostate, or urethra. It may result from any condition, such as an enlarged prostate or urethral stricture, which interferes with the complete emptying of the bladder. The incidence is quite high among poorly controlled cases of diabetes and among people (especially women) who increase the level of their sexual activity. This latter is the so-called honeymoon cystitis and is the result of bacteria's being massaged up through the urethra into the bladder during sexual intercourse. (The female urethra is quite short.) Acute cystitis related to intercourse usually manifests itself about thirty-six hours after the sexual encounter. The most effective prevention is postcoital urination to flush the bacteria from the urethra and bladder. If necessary, urine flow may be stimulated by drinking several glasses of fluid soon after coitus.

Cystitis is usually treated with antibacterial drugs (sulfa drugs or antibiotics). Increased fluid intake is important, as is the frequent and complete drainage of urine from the bladder. Alcoholic beverages should be avoided until the infection is cured.

Pubic Lice

Pubic lice, commonly called "crab lice" or "crabs" because of their crablike appearance (see Figure 14.14), are small, gray insects (1/16 inch long) that live as external parasites on the body. They live in body hair, holding onto the shaft of the hair with their crablike pincers. They prefer pubic hair but will also live in the hair under arms and in eyebrows and beards, but never scalp hair (which is too fine in texture). Crab lice do not really pinch with their claws, but they do feed on human blood, causing an intense itching and discoloration of the skin. They often remain attached for days, with their sucking mouth parts inserted into the skin of an unfortunate host. Female lice attach eggs, called nits, to the body hair. These eggs hatch in six to eight days. Since sexual maturity is reached in only fourteen to twenty-one days and each female lays up to fifty eggs, a crab louse infection can grow to alarming proportions in just a short time. Heavy infestations may result in fever and other disorders caused by toxins injected by the feeding lice.

Pubic lice may be transmitted through sexual intercourse, but they can also be spread through less intimate physical contact with infested

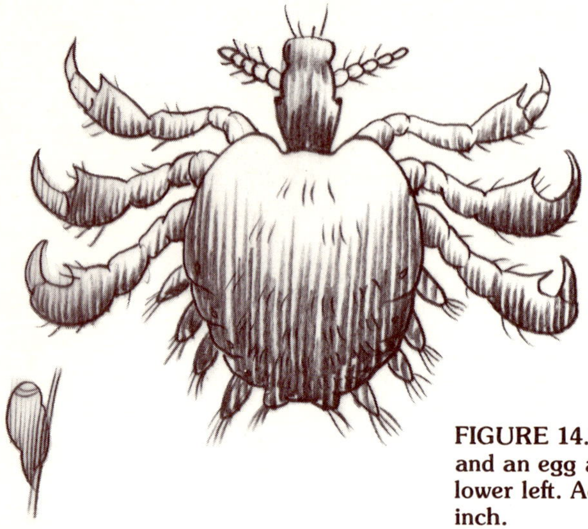

FIGURE 14.14 Pubic louse (crab louse) and an egg attached to human hair, lower left. Actual size of louse is 1/16 inch.

people or by use of contaminated clothing, toilet seats, bedding, or other materials.

Crabs can usually be killed by washing the affected body parts with a special lotion, such as Kwell, available at most pharmacies. Several applications are required. Contrary to popular belief, infested hair need *not* be shaved, and exposed clothing need not be thrown away. However, it should not be worn until it is cleaned or thoroughly washed in hot water.

Scabies (Itch or Seven-Year Itch)

Scabies is a highly contagious skin disease caused by microscopic spider-like mites that burrow into the skin. The mites (see Figure 14.15), ranging from about one-fourth to one-half millimeter in length, are "caught" by sexual or other close contact with an infested person. Their burrows appear as slightly discolored lines on the skin, ranging from several millimeters to several centimeters in length. Other symptoms are small blisters and a rash in the area of the burrows and intense itching. The itching may be severe enough to interfere with sleep, and scratching tends to favor the spread of the mites. The mites multiply prolifically through mating and laying eggs in their tunnels.

Areas of the body commonly attacked include the thin skin between the fingers, the inside bends of the knees and elbows, the wrists, the genitals, the thighs, the skin beneath the breasts, the shoulder blades, and the buttocks, though any part of the body may be infested. Newly infested persons usually do not experience any itching for about a month, so an infestation may progress considerably before a person is aware of it.

In treating scabies, the skin first must be softened thoroughly with a prolonged hot bath or shower and thorough scrubbing to allow the medication to reach the mites, which are protected in their tunnels. Then a 25 percent solution of benzyl benzoate is applied to the entire body except the eyes, nose, and mouth. A second application is made the following day. All members of a living group should be treated at one time to prevent reinfestation. Clothing and bedding need not be sterilized.

Preventing the Sexually Transmitted Diseases

So far, our discussion of STDs has centered upon recognition of their symptoms and the importance of obtaining prompt treatment if infection occurs. But from both personal and public health standpoints, it is much more desirable to prevent any disease than to treat it. The prevention of these diseases requires action by both the individual and public health personnel.

Personal Prevention

As with most other diseases, the ultimate responsibility for the prevention of the sexually transmitted diseases lies with the individual. The

FIGURE 14.15 The itch mite, *Sarcoptes scabiei*

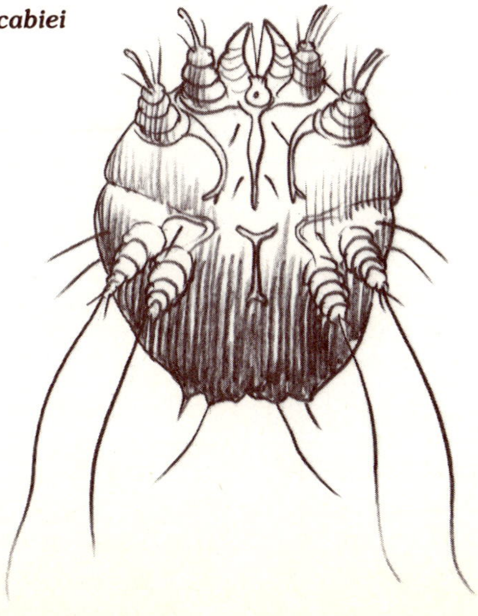

most important personal preventative measure is the avoidance of sexual contact with anyone who is likely to be infected. In view of today's high incidence of STD, that would include anyone who has sexual contact with a variety of partners or who has sexual contact with a single partner who in turn has a variety of sex partners. Remember that diseases can be transmitted through either heterosexual or homosexual contact and through either genital-genital, oral-genital, or anal-genital sex, and even through certain petting practices.

The prime mechanism for prevention of the sexually transmitted diseases, then, is selective sexual behavior. Unfortunately, for the public as a whole, this mechanism has failed because it has never been widely practiced; the current STD epidemic is glaring evidence of this failure. Thus, for the person who chooses to be somewhat less discriminate in the choice of sex partners, it becomes important to make maximum use of other personal preventive (prophylactic) methods to reduce the chances of infection. Note that we use the word "reduce" rather than "eliminate," since even the best of the currently available prophylactic methods are far from totally effective.

The single most important personal preventive method is probably the liberal use of soap and water immediately after sexual contact. The pathogens of the diseases that enter the body through the skin can often be killed or removed in this manner. The three less common diseases, chancroid, lymphogranuloma venereum, and granuloma inguinale, can be almost entirely eliminated by this simple technique.

Urination by a man immediately after sexual contact and prompt douching by a woman may help reduce the chance of infection with gonorrhea. (But remember that douching is not effective as a birth control measure and that frequent douching often results in vaginal irritations and infections. Thus douching should be reserved for disease prevention or for special situations upon the recommendation of a physician.)

The use of a condom over the penis will help prevent the transmission of STD, especially gonorrhea, in either direction—from male to female or from female to male. To be effective, the condom must be applied onto the erect penis at the very start of any sexual activity, before any sexual contact is made. Even though a condom is used, it is still important to wash with soap and water immediately after contact because the condom covers only the penis, and several of the diseases, especially syphilis, can enter the body through the skin at any point whatsoever. The condom thus affords limited protection against syphilis. In its favor, however, it should be noted that the condom is the only commonly used device that is effective both as a prophylactic against gonorrhea and as a contraceptive. Carefully and consistently used, it can be reasonably effective for both purposes. Although it has traditionally been a man's responsibility to make sure of its availability for coitus, an enlightened woman might want to keep a supply of condoms available to protect herself against STD and, if not otherwise protected, against pregnancy.

Antibiotics have been used on a prophylactic basis, administered either before or after possible exposure to STD, but this practice cannot be recommended for routine use because it tends to breed antibiotic-resistant strains of pathogens, including but not limited to those that cause the sexually transmitted diseases, and because it tends to build allergies to the antibiotics in those who receive them.

The ideal personal preventive would, of course, be a vaccine for each disease. Few communicable diseases have ever really been controlled until effective vaccines have been developed against them.

Public Health Measures

Many methods are used by public health agencies in their fight against the sexually transmitted diseases, and while STD is still rampant, it seems certain that the incidence would be even greater than it is without the efforts of dedicated public health workers.

Most public health departments carry out programs of education concerned with prevention and symptoms of sexually transmitted diseases and the importance of prompt treatment. The media used often include newspapers, billboards, radio, TV, and posters in public places. Some public health departments assist local schools in their STD education programs, providing classroom materials and teacher training for effective STD instruction.

Clinics for the diagnosis and treatment of STD are also common functions of public health departments. The services of clinics are usually offered at little or no cost to the individual. Laws in most states have been revised to allow the treatment of minors, often as young as twelve years of age, without obtaining permission from their parents or otherwise notifying them. It has been found that when parental permission must be obtained as a condition of treatment, many young people avoid treatment out of fear of reprisal from parents, thus tragically risking permanent damage from infection.

Another important public health function in STD control is case finding. In many localities, each patient treated for a sexually transmitted disease, especially for syphilis, is interviewed to determine from whom the disease may have been caught and to whom it may have been transmitted. These people can then be contacted, notified that they may be infected, and asked to visit the public health department or their private physicians for STD testing. Since so many cases of STD are symptomless, this is the only way in which many infected people can learn of their disease before serious damage is done.

One of the real barriers to effective case finding is that while by law every case of STD a physician treats must be reported to the local health department, in reality the majority of cases are not reported. The reporting rate for privately treated gonorrhea is especially low, even though gonorrhea reports are essentially for statistical purposes rather than for case finding. Many public health departments lack adequate funds for thorough case finding even for deadly syphilis.

While it may seem obvious, the STD patient should be warned to refrain from sexual contact with previous partners until they have been tested and, if necessary, treated. It is common (and frustrating) in STD clinics to find that a newly cured patient has gone back to the same partner and become reinfected again and again.

A technique that has revealed thousands of cases of syphilis is compulsory blood testing for certain people, such as applicants for marriage licenses, pregnant women, military personnel, hospital patients, and new employees of many corporations. Most of the cases detected in this way are in the symptomless latent period, and without detection and treatment many would progress into late syphilis, with its irreversible damage to vital organs and death.

It is an excellent idea for anyone who has a variety of sexual partners to obtain *an annual blood test for syphilis.* Many cases progress directly into the latent and eventually the late stages without ever exhibiting any noticeable symptoms. Yearly blood tests can reliably detect such cases, and the cost of the tests is minimal or even free if they are obtained through public health departments or free clinics.

In summary, while public health departments are making great efforts to control STD, syphilis, gonorrhea, and genital herpes remain as epidemic diseases. It is imperative for the individual to take reasonable precautions against infection, to know the symptoms of these diseases, and to seek prompt treatment if these symptoms develop.

Sex and the Law

15

Many of the greatest social problems in American history have been produced by laws designed to regulate morality, attitudes, and sexual behavior. Most people agree that we need laws to protect the institution of the family and to protect an individual from coercion, the young from deviant adults, and the public from flagrant displays of sexual acts. But the law seldom stops there. Throughout American history, laws have been used to try to determine or enforce standards of morality. From state to state the laws designed to regulate sexual expression vary widely and are frequently archaic.

Many of the current laws governing sexual expression in the United States can be traced either directly or indirectly to Anthony Comstock (1844–1915), a self-styled moralist from New York State. He helped form the Committee for the Suppression of Vice, and in 1873 Comstock and his committee were instrumental in having Congress pass the Comstock Act (March 3, 1873), which prohibited the mailing of obscene materials and set forth severe penalties. The Comstock Act made the Post Office Department a special agent that defined what was obscene, and could legally open any mail to look for obscene materials. Anything that could have the slightest connection with sex was considered obscene.

The Comstock Act indirectly banned the importation and shipment of contraceptive materials or devices through the mail as obscene materials. By 1905 Congress had amended the law to punish both the sender and the receiver of such "obscene materials." Following the lead of the federal government, every state except New Mexico enacted its own antiobscenity law, patterned after the Comstock Act. During this period many of the laws relating to sexual matters were first enacted.

Sexual statutes can be divided into two broad areas. First are the laws that have been enacted to guide the physical health of individuals and society. Laws regulating contraception, sterilization, artificial insemination, abortion, sexually transmitted disease, and educational requirements of paramedical personnel are examples of such legislation. The second area includes legal restraints on sexual behavior. These are the laws that try to dictate social morality: laws controlling marriage and divorce, bigamy, adultery, prostitution, obscenity, rape, child molestation, deviant sexual behavior, and "crimes against nature."

In 1955 the American Law Institute, while preparing a model penal code, formulated a legal code governing sexual behavior. It was recommended that states should legislate a uniform set of laws that would protect individuals and society adequately and realistically. In 1962 Illinois became the first state to revise its sexual laws according to the suggestions in the Model Penal Code. Since then a few other states have fully or partially enacted the recommendations. In 1967 the President's Crime

Commission again recommended removing from criminal law many of the sexual acts between consenting adults now considered illegal in most states, contending that these matters are private, or at most social ills, and are not proper matters for legislation.

Nearly all U.S. laws pertaining to sex have their beginnings in the Judeo-Christian tradition of sexual ethics. The basis of most laws concerning sexual behavior depends upon the ethical and religious backgrounds of legislators, which greatly influence decisions concerning such legislation. Any act against procreation, children, and family still tends to be considered a sin and to be prohibited. In the past, few politicians were even willing to raise the issues openly because of the risk to their reputations and careers.

Contraception Laws

Legally, contraception is the intentional prevention of fertilization of the human ovum. Contraception is achieved through the use of contraceptive drugs, devices, and methods, and by sterilization. In law, contraception is often referred to as "birth control" or "family planning."

The Comstock Act greatly limited the distribution of contraceptives in the United States during the past century. In 1965 the United States Supreme Court overturned the last law restricting the use of contraceptives (*Massachusetts v. Griswold*). This decision held that a Massachusetts law prohibiting the use of birth control devices by married couples was unconstitutional because it infringed upon the right of marital privacy. In 1970 Congress passed the Family Planning Services and Population Research Act, making contraceptive services available to all desiring them. This act and subsequent modifications have greatly increased the availability of contraceptive information and devices in all states.

Contraceptives are legally available to adults in all states. Also, many states have laws similar to the California law giving minors legal access to contraceptives that can be bought without a prescription, such as condoms (prophylactics) and contraceptive foam.

Sterilization

Sterilization, which is "any procedure by which an individual is made incapable of reproduction" without impairing potential for sexual activity, is a form of contraception.

Legally sterilization is classified as either compulsory or voluntary. The first sterilization laws passed in the United States provided for compulsory sterilization of individuals for eugenic reasons—where the possibility existed that a child might inherit an abnormal condition.

The first compulsory sterilization law was enacted in Indiana in 1907. It called for the compulsory sterilization of certain mental patients for eugenic reasons. From 1907 to 1966 most states passed compulsory sterilization legislation.

Relaxation of laws governing voluntary sterilization for socioeconomic reasons came during the late 1960s. The last law prohibiting voluntary sterilization (in Utah) was removed in 1972. Voluntary sterilization of adults is legal when consent has been given. Most states possess a law similar to a California law that prohibits clinics, physicians, and hospitals from requiring individuals who want to be sterilized to meet any nonmedical qualifications, such as age or previous number of children. There is no law that requires the consent of a spouse when an individual requests sterilization. Nevertheless, some physicians will not perform such operations for fear of possible malpractice suits. However, there has been no successful malpractice suit against any physician based upon the nonnegligent performance of a voluntary sterilization operation when the informed consent of the patient has been obtained.

Minors cannot legally give consent for most medical care without parental consent, except when the person is considered an "emancipated minor"—anyone fifteen years of age and older who lives away from home, who is married, or who is in the armed forces. Consequently, a nonemancipated minor may not be sterilized without prior parental consent.

Abortion Law

Abortion has always been practiced in spite of restrictive taboos or laws (including the death penalty). Although the general impression today is that abortion has always been illegal, it was not until well into the nineteenth century that abortion was legally prohibited in the United States. Before 1803, abortion was regarded as an offense against the church and was punishable by religious penalties. In 1803 Connecticut passed the first anti-abortion law in the United States. The reason for this restrictive legislation was the recognized dangers to the patient inherent in an operative procedure performed outside of a hospital.

Beginning in 1821, each of the states enacted its own abortion laws. These laws varied considerably. In January 1973 the U.S. Supreme Court ruled that the decision to have an abortion in the first trimester (twelve weeks) of pregnancy is a personal decision to be made by the pregnant woman and her physician, without interference from any state. This very controversial ruling invalidated almost all existing state abortion laws. But this ruling had come more than ten years after the American

Law Institute (in 1962) had passed a model law governing abortion which recommended that an abortion be permitted when the mother's physical or mental health would be impaired by the birth, when there was likelihood that the child would be born with serious mental or physical defects, and when the pregnancy was the result of rape or incest. The American Medical Association endorsed these recommendations in 1967. By the time of the Supreme Court ruling in 1973, only seventeen states and the District of Columbia had passed legislation based upon these recommendations.

Today physicians may perform abortions in the first trimester on any or no grounds. The abortion need not be performed in a hospital; it may be an office procedure. From the twelfth week on, control of abortion has been left mainly to the states. During the second trimester of pregnancy (up to twenty-six weeks), states may impose only those restrictions that are reasonably related to the health of the mother. These abortions must be performed in a licensed hospital. During the last three months of pregnancy most states permit an abortion only in order to preserve the life and health (including the mental health) of a woman.

Artificial Insemination

Artificial insemination is the mechanical deposition of living sperm into the cervical opening of a woman to achieve conception. This method of achieving conception was used as early as the fourteenth century with horses. The first human artificial insemination in the United States was accomplished by a physician named Marion Sims in 1866. In 1909 another American physician reported the first use of a donor's sperm rather than that of the woman's husband.

The child conceived by artificial insemination has had an uncertain legal status in the past. Jurists in some states have ruled that these children are illegitimate, while other states feel the procedure is completely legal and that all children conceived by artificial insemination are legitimate. Three states (California, Georgia, and Oklahoma) have been instrumental in providing legal status to children produced by artificial insemination from a donor other than the mother's husband. In 1969 California enacted a statute that provided that a child artificially conceived is legitimate if the husband of the woman has consented in writing to the insemination. Few states require written consent for artificial insemination, but most physicians and attorneys advise couples to sign a document of consent to protect the parents, the child, and the doctor.

Semen or sperm banks provide other legal problems. There are no laws controlling standards for such banks, or for liability to any malformed children conceived owing to improper processing or storage of sperm. New York City has local regulations protecting confidentiality and legal conditions for sperm donors.

Sexually Transmitted Diseases

There are scores of state laws outlining the responsibility for control of sexually transmitted diseases. Most states require testing for syphilis of couples before marriage and of women during pregnancy. Failure to report a case of any sexually transmitted disease or refusal to accept treatment is a misdemeanor in most states. These laws are highly variable from state to state.

Paramedical Personnel

The legal status of physicians is well established, but the services of paramedical personnel—those professions who render specific services indirectly related to the practice of medicine—come under a wide range of legislation. The paramedical personnel most directly related to sexual health are midwives, physicians' assistants, and nurse practitioners.

A *midwife* is a woman who provides prenatal and postnatal care to a mother and her child, and attends normal childbirth. Midwives have practiced their profession throughout the history of the United States. Many states legalized the practice of midwifery around the time of World War I, but many repealed these laws later. A unique example is California. California licensed midwives in 1917 and repealed the certification in 1949. This legislation prevented any new certificates from being issued, but allowed previously licensed midwives to continue to practice. In 1973 there were only three women (all over seventy years old) who held certificates authorizing them to practice midwifery in California. California, along with many other states, is currently reviewing the concept of expanding the duties of physicians' assistants or registered nurses to include midwifery. Other states, such as New York, have continued to license midwifery as a paramedical profession.

A *physician's assistant* is a graduate of a state-approved program and is licensed to perform medical services under the supervision of a physician. Many states have approved the use of such assistants by general practitioners, but their use by specialists, such as gynecologists, is legal in only a few states. Expansion of this program has led to an expansion of the responsibilities and services of registered nurses into a role called *nurse practitioner*. With specified advanced training, qualified nurse practitioners perform in a manner similar to physicians' assistants.

Legal Restraints on Sexual Behavior

There are three categories of sexual behavior that are subject to legislation. First are the laws affecting sexual behavior between *consenting adults*. The second group of offenses involves *force* or *violence*, or *crimes against children*. Third are laws regulating *commercial exploitation of sex*.

Sexual Behavior Between Consenting Adults

In many states the constitutionality of laws regulating sexual behavior between consenting adults in private is coming under attack by many segments of society. The changes began in 1967, when the United States Supreme Court struck down all state laws banning interracial marriage. Today the controversy has moved toward freedom of sexual behavior of consenting adults in private when the behavior is heterosexual. But in many states today a married couple, theoretically, can be arrested for most sexual acts conducted in the privacy of their bedrooms. The following is an overview of some of these laws.

Marriage, Divorce, and Annulment The legal definition of marriage is "a personal relationship arising out of a civil contract to which the consent of the parties in maintaining the contract is necessary." Divorce is the legal dissolution of a marriage, releasing both individuals to remarry. Annulment is a legal pronouncement declaring a marriage invalid. The difference between divorce and annulment is that a divorce terminates a valid marriage, while annulment declares that the marriage was never valid.

All states have their own statutes regulating marriage, divorce, and annulment. Thirteen states and the District of Columbia still recognize *common-law marriage*, in which a couple is considered married even though a legal ceremony has not been performed, if they have lived together as husband and wife for a specified number of years. All other states require a legal ceremony before a marriage is recognized. States also place restrictions upon individuals who wish to marry (testing for disease, minimum age, and so on). Some people evade these regulations by marrying in another state with more lenient laws and returning home, because all states recognize a marriage as valid as long as it conforms to the laws of the state in which it was performed.

A divorce is more difficult to obtain than a marriage. Most states require proof of a crime against the marriage as grounds for a divorce. These grounds (adultery, insanity, conviction of a felony, general cruelty, physical cruelty, mental cruelty, and so on) are used to find one individual "guilty" of an offense, which can result in an uneven awarding of property to the "innocent" party. On January 1, 1970, California enacted the Family Law Act, in which the word for termination of a marriage was changed from "divorce" to "dissolution." The law provides for dissolution of a marriage on the basis of "irreconcilable differences." There are no guilty or innocent parties, and the property must be divided evenly. Colorado, Connecticut, Iowa, Michigan, North Dakota, Flordia, New Jersey, and Texas have also adopted divorce laws removing fault from the procedure.

Seduction In legal terms, seduction is sexual intercourse submitted to because of the promise of marriage or a fraudulent representation of being married. A man can usually escape prosecution for seduction by marrying the woman. If the girl is under the *age of consent* (the age at which a girl can legally consent to sexual intercourse) the man can be prosecuted for statutory rape instead of seduction.

Bigamy Bigamy (or polygamy) is the criminal offense of entering into a marriage with one person while still legally married to another. All states permit a second or subsequent marriage to take place only if the spouse is dead or has been absent for five or more successive years and is believed dead, or if a former marriage has been legally dissolved or annulled. If someone willingly and knowingly marries while not meeting these qualifications, he or she has committed bigamy. Bigamy statutes apply to persons who marry within or outside of a state as long as they cohabit (live together) within the state.

The term *polygyny* is used when a man has more than one wife, and *polyandry* when a woman has more than one husband. Early English common law classified bigamy as an offense against the church, and it was punishable by religious penalties. It was not until 1604 that bigamy was made a criminal offense. The Puritans brought this legal concept with them to America and bigamy has been a crime in all states since then.

Adultery, Fornication, and Cohabitation Adultery is voluntary sexual intercourse by a married person with someone other than his or her spouse. Fornication is the act of sexual intercourse between consenting unmarried adults. Cohabitation is living together as husband and wife.

The concept of adultery goes back to the beginnings of history. The English Puritans brought the adultery laws of England with them to America. In Massachusetts the Puritans first made adultery a crime punishable by death; then in 1694 the death penalty was replaced by public whipping and the wearing of the letter "A" for "adulterer" or "adulteress." Later Connecticut required the letter "A" be branded on the foreheads of those found guilty of adultery. The penalties for adultery have diminished until today in most states it is a misdemeanor punishable only by a fine.

Sexual intercourse, or the act of *fornication,* between consenting unmarried adults is prohibited in thirty-one states. Fornication, whether adulterous or not, is not illegal in nineteen states; however, adulterous cohabitation is illegal. If one or both individuals who live together are married to other persons, they are guilty of adulterous cohabitation. A person may be convicted of adulterous cohabitation even though he or she is also cohabiting with a legal spouse at the same time.

Illegitimacy A child conceived and born to a woman who is not married is termed an *illegitimate child.* If the woman marries, either before or after the child's birth, the marriage and the father's acknowledgment of responsibility for the child legitimizes the child. Children born after annulled, voided, or dissolved marriages are considered legitimate. Any child born to parents who are married and living together is presumed to be legitimate, unless the man is impotent at the time of conception of the child.

Illegitimate children often face legal difficulties involving identity, determination of paternity, child support, and inheritance rights. In many states the birth certificate still contains the information that such a child is illegitimate. In all states illegitimate children have the right to inherit from their mothers. In forty-four states they have no right to inherit from their fathers. (A father may, of course, bequeath property or money to such a child if he wishes.) Only in two states (Arizona and North Dakota) are all children considered legitimate and entitled to equal rights. Forty-six states require the father to support the illegitimate child.

Incest Incest is the marriage or act of sexual intercourse between individuals who are biological (blood) relatives. The degree of relationship beyond which a sexual relationship is not bigamous varies from state to state. Most state laws stipulate that marriage or sexual intercourse is incestuous if it takes place between parent and child, grandparent and grandchild, brother and sister, uncle and niece, or aunt and nephew. California statutes on incest apply equally to illegitimate, legitimate, and half relatives; they do not apply to adoptive or step-relatives.

Private Consensual Sexual Acts (oral sex, anal sex, bestiality). Many states still prohibit sexual acts that do not have the potential to result in conception. In these states kissing, caressing, and vaginal intercourse are the only legal sexual acts. The illegal sexual acts usually are oral-genital acts, anal intercourse, and intercourse with animals. Some states also include mutual masturbation and sexual acts with dead bodies. These acts are often referred to as "unnatural" sexual acts, or "crimes against nature."

In 1962 Illinois became the first state to revise its sexual laws along the lines suggested by the Model Penal Code of 1955. Thus Illinois removed all laws against any sexual act between consenting adults in private. Connecticut, Colorado, Oregon, Hawaii, Delaware, and Ohio changed their laws along the same lines in the following years. California joined the group in 1975. Some states (Kansas, New York, Minnesota, Utah) have reduced penalties for these sexual acts to misdemeanors.

Homosexuality No state has any law requiring punishment for homosexuality, but homosexuals may nevertheless be arrested and brought to trial for their acts. State laws against "unnatural" acts (oral-genital sex, anal intercourse, mutual masturbation) do not specify the sexes of the participants, so homosexuals of both sexes may be arrested if they are apprehended performing these acts with persons of the same sex as they. Very few homosexuals are arrested for such acts unless they occur in public (a restroom, a threater, a park, an automobile), or unless an individual is solicited for such acts. When this happens, the homosexual is usually arrested for "a lewd or lascivious act" ("a willful, wrongful act which seriously injures the person or property of another or seriously disturbs or endangers the public peace or health, or openly outrages public decency") or for "disorderly conduct" (loitering in a public place to engage in or solicit anyone to engage in "lewd, dissolute, lascivious, or unlawful acts"). Only rarely is the solicited person prosecuted for participation in the act.

Sexual Crimes of Force or Violence, or Against Children

Offenses of force or violence or involving children are considered the most serious of all sexual offenses. The treatment of persons charged with these crimes is often subject to serious charges of racism, sexism, and inconsistency of prosecution. They are difficult to prosecute because usually the victim is the only witness and is often unable to provide the reliable, consistent evidence necessary for conviction. In some of these crimes, "implied consent" (failure to resist) can change the whole legal picture. There are serious disagreements among jurists as to the appropriate penalties for many of these crimes. Consequently, the penalties issued by judges vary widely.

Rape Rape has historically been defined as the act of forcing a woman to submit to sexual intercourse against her will. The crime is legally termed *forcible rape*. *Statutory rape* is any act of intercourse with a female under the age of consent, as defined by the statutes of the state in which the crime is committed. The age of consent varies widely from state to state, but most often it is eighteen years. The Model Penal Code recommends that the age for statutory rape be less than ten years and that a male who has intercourse with a consenting female under sixteen be guilty of "corruption of a minor" if he is at least four years older than the girl. Such a law would alleviate many of the problems associated with consenting teenage sexual acts.

California law defines forcible rape as an act of genital contact with any penetration, however slight, which is forced upon a female against her will (by physical violence, constraint, or threat of violence), if she is unable to give her informed consent (because she is mentally retarded, mentally ill, intoxicated, or unconscious), or if she believes that the man is her husband. The California law, as cumbersome as it is, is less vaguely worded than those of most states. Consequently the most difficult problem in obtaining a conviction for rape is often establishing that a rape has taken place. This alone often protects the male from prosecution.

Technically, under other paragraphs of California law and the laws of most states, a man cannot rape his own wife, and a boy under the age of fourteen cannot be charged with rape. But if either compels the woman to submit to intercourse, or attempted intercourse, he may be charged with assault.

Child Molestation Sexual molestation of minors usually involve rape, forcible oral and anal sex acts, or manipulation of a child's external genital organs. The legal definition of a minor or minor child varies from state to state. These laws are designed to protect children from sexual exploitation by others, since they are presumed to be incapable of giving informed consent. The statutes do not differentiate between sex acts forced upon children by adults and sexual experimentation among young people with each other. Most laws apply to all persons above a specified age (fourteen years under California law), although minors are tried in juvenile court.

Commercial Exploitation of Sex

The commercial exploitation of sex involves prostitution and obscenity or pornography. Very little public sentiment has been raised in recent years for or against the regulation of prostitution, although many women at the International Woman's Year Conference in Mexico City (1975) advocated the international legalization of prostitution. But public concern about obscenity laws is widespread.

Prostitution Prostitution is indiscriminate sexual intercourse for pay. It is illegal in most states. Prostitution is usually defined as a voluntary sexual act between two consenting adults for money, but some states include crimes involving force in their prostitution statutes.

Prostitution has existed in all civilizations and has usually been tolerated and regulated by law or social custom. The first major legislation outlawing prostitution in the United States was the Mann Act of 1910. Known as the White Slave Traffic Act, it prohibited interstate transportation of women for immoral purposes. By 1925 every state had passed legislation against commercialized prostitution. These laws were reinforced by the May Act of 1941, which allowed the federal government to assume police authority over eradication of prostitution in communities that failed to do it themselves.

Prostitution laws take many forms. In California it is not illegal to be a prostitute, but if a woman is apprehended either soliciting or engaging in prostitution she may be prosecuted under the "lewd and lascivious acts" and "disorderly conduct" statutes. A male prostitute is dealt with as a homosexual and prosecuted by the "unnatural sex acts" laws of the state or the "disorderly conduct" statutes.

Most prosecutions involve specific laws associated with prostitution, such as pimping, pandering, running a house of prostitution, or sending a minor to a house of prostitution. Although the terms "pimp" and "pander" are often used interchangeably, the law differentiates between the two. A pimp is any person (male or female) who derives any earnings or support from a prostitute. A panderer is any person who procures (assists, induces, persuades, or encourages) some one into prostitution or to work in a house of prostitution. A house of prostitution, "house of ill fame," or "disorderly house," is any place used for prostitution. It may be in a hotel, an apartment, a motel, or a bar—any room that is knowingly rented for the purposes of prostitution.

Obscenity The first major obscenity law was the Comstock Act of 1873. Under this act it is a felony to knowingly place into the U.S. mails any obscene, lewd, or lascivious book, pamphlet, picture, or other indecent publication. The U.S. Postal Service has the responsibility of enforcing the Comstock Act in its present form. Since 1873 most states passed "little Comstock laws" of their own.

In 1957 the U.S. Supreme Court settled a landmark case (*Roth* v. *U.S. Supreme Court*) by ruling that obscenity is not within the constitutional protection of freedom of speech or press. Especially important in this decision was the concept that sex and obscenity are not synonymous. Obscene material is only that which deals with sex in a lewd and lascivious manner. And the standard for judging obscenity is whether, to the *average person,* applying *contemporary community standards,* the "total content" of the material is lewd and lascivious.

Between 1957 and 1968 the Supreme Court wrote fifty-five separate opinions in thirteen cases in attempts to formulate a definition of obscenity.

The laws of most states define obscene matter as any written material, pictorial representation, motion picture, chemical, mechanical, or electrical reproduction, machine, or material that, taken as a whole, by contemporary standards, (1) is lewd or lascivious to the average person; (2) goes beyond customary limits of representation of such matters; (3) is utterly without redeeming social value.

In 1972 another major Supreme Court decision upheld the California State Alcoholic Beverage Control Board regulation that prohibits the sale of alcoholic beverages in an establishment that offers live or filmed explicit sexual entertainment. Such "live sex acts" are within the law because of the difficulty of proving that the performances are indeed obscene according to the three criteria mentioned.

The Sex Offender

Many states require that convicted sex offenders register with local law-enforcement officials. Registration must take place upon release from the penal institution where the offender has been confined, and the person remains a "registered sex offender" until legally released from this registration. All registered sex offenders are subject to questioning whenever a sex offense is committed in the community. Persons required to register are those convicted of the majority of sex crimes listed in this chapter within the state or in another state. Persons judged to be *mentally disordered* sex offenders (sexual psychopaths), regardless of the nature of crime, are also registered in many states.

The purpose of registration of sexual offenders is to deter the commission of future crimes, to facilitate arrest of repeat offenders, and, in the case of mentally disordered sex offenders, to protect society and to rehabilitate them.

Many federal, state, and local sex laws commit an individual to a penal institution so that the person can be materially benefited by its reformatory and education discipline. Many feel that rehabilitation is not possible until two specific recommendations of the Model Penal Code have been put into practice:

1. Sex offenders should be offered help and understanding, rather than contempt and punishment.

2. If a preventive approach to sex offenses is to be effective, there must be wider dissemination of accurate sex information; through such education, children will gain a more scientific and objective understanding of human sexuality.

Sexual Myths and Fallacies

16

There is no other area so shrouded in myth, fallacy, and superstition as that of human sexuality. While myths are beliefs that have no basis in reality, they arise for a variety of reasons, serve many purposes, and have existed for millenniums. One of the primary factors contributing to the emergence and acceptance of myths has been lack of adequate anatomical and physiological knowledge. It must be remembered that most of our current sophisticated understanding of human functioning is still relatively new. For instance, it wasn't until the middle 1700s, when the English anatomist and surgeon John Hunter did pertinent research in human sexual anatomy and physiology, that all the reproductive organs were identified and objectively studied. It wasn't realized until the nineteenth century that the union of sperm and egg are essential to create a baby. For that matter, to this day some primitive peoples still don't make the association between intercourse and conception. It wasn't until the early 1960s that the union of human sperm and ova was observed. Although people lacked scientific data to explain sexual functions accurately, the need for explanation and order still existed. Thus when gaps could not be filled with truth, misconceptions fitted just as nicely.

Many fallacies have gained acceptance because they are partially true. Many misconceptions have arisen from the observation of animals, their sexual habits, or their relationship to the physical environment. What was true of animals was believed to be true of humans as well. While similarities do exist, there are many differences. As a result, some gross misapprehensions have resulted from such comparisons.

Finally, religion has provided fertile soil for the generation of fallacies, and those that can be traced back to religious origins are frequently the ones that do the most psychological damage. These myths are closer to what would be called taboos. Not only do they distort facts; they are also likely to instill in the believer fear of retribution if the religious code is transgressed. Moreover, religious fallacies carry strong moralistic overtones that contribute to attitude formation, making acceptance of one's own sexuality difficult, or making it impossible to derive pleasure from sex except under special conditions, such as when reproduction is desired.

In spite of recent and widely disseminated results of significant scientific sexual research, myths of all sorts are still prevalent and persistent. Even with the more relaxed societal attitudes, many people continue to feel so uncomfortable about sex that they are not motivated to acquire the education necessary to dispel misconceptions.

Sexual myths and fallacies are contagious; they spread from one person to another, and from generation to generation. Quite frequently sex education is obtained from well-intentioned but misinformed parents or from members of a peer group who are quite unqualified to provide factual information. In any event, people continue to pass on whatever information they possess when the situation presents itself, and thus myths may go unchallenged for many more years. Unfortunate as it may be, it is not only the uneducated or ignorant who pass on misconceptions, but professional people as well, people who are in positions of influence, such as physicians, marriage counselors, clergymen, and college professors. Just because these people are highly educated in one particular field, they are not necessarily experts qualified to give instruction or even advice in sexual matters. They are subject to the same misconceptions and negative attitudes that distort other people's understanding of sex. It is therefore imperative that each individual exercise discretion when it comes to choosing sources of sexual information. Accuracy must be verified before accepting any dictum as indisputable truth, and dubious information must not be offered to others until it has been examined for its validity.

While many myths are benign and have no ill effect on a person's sexual functioning, others are so seriously circumscribing that men and women may actually become sexual cripples because of them. The kinds of fallacy that lead to tragic consequences usually conjure up intense feelings of inferiority or guilt. Once guilt and inferiority are internalized, even when the truth is made evident, it may be impossible to rectify the psychological damage. Myths also have considerable influence on sex roles and have helped to maintain the double standard. Sometimes there is a basic fallacy in both male and female versions. Instead of fostering close relationships and mutual understanding between the sexes, people come to feel there is no common ground for communication between them and members of the opposite sex. Another reason that myths may be destructive relates to the period when women were not held in very high regard by men, and at times were tolerated only as cheap labor and reproductive machines. Only recently have American women begun to realize the degree to which they have been sexually repressed.

Entire books have been written on sexual myths. The following items have been selected because they are still commonly accepted by many people.

Myths Based on Sexual Functions

The following myths are based on misunderstandings of the structures or functions of sexual apparatus. As noted earlier, the physiological basis of sexual response has only recently been understood. It is understandable that the average person could have some strange ideas when so little was known until recently about the precise response of male and female reproductive systems to sexual stimulation. If a woman believed orgasm a physiological impossibility, then of course she wouldn't be likely to achieve an orgasm. And if a man equated penis size with sexual adequacy, then his penis size would surely affect his performance or lack of it.

Myth: A large penis is sexually more satisfying to a woman than a small one, and a man with a small penis is less sexually potent than a man with a large one.

Fact: The length and diameter of the penis has absolutely nothing to do with a man's sexual ability as long as the penis is long enough to reach the vagina and maintain contact with it.* When the vagina is not distended it is only about three and one-half inches long, and of these inches only about the first is supplied with nerve endings involved in sexual stimulation. The vaginal walls are composed of muscular tissue that grips the penis and expands to accommodate the penis, whatever size it may be. A normal penis ranges anywhere from two to ten inches, and is perfectly functional at either end of the range. The size of the penis could have nothing but a psychological effect on a woman's satisfaction. If she believed that a large penis caused greater satisfaction, then it would. This, of course, works the other way also. In fact, one of the authors once knew a woman who believed the only good sex partner was one with a small penis because "they know what to do with it." So while a man could very well be impotent because of penile size, it would not be because of the penis itself but rather because of psychological anxieties stemming from feelings of inadequacy. Remember, if you don't think you can, then you certainly can't, and nowhere is this more true than in sexual functioning.

It should also be mentioned that there is no correlation between the size of a man's body and the size of his penis. Heredity is the determinant of penis size. A very tall, large man may have a smaller penis than a short, thin man. In addition, a penis that is long in the flaccid state does not necessarily increase to greater dimensions than a smaller flaccid penis. For example, the penises of black males are generally longer than the penises of white males when they are flaccid; however, when they are erect there is little size variance between the races, and both are within standard population norms.

Myth: There is a difference between clitoral and vaginal orgasm.

Fact: An orgasm is an orgasm, whether it is brought about by strictly clitoral stimulation or vaginal stimulation. There is only one kind of orgasm. Even if the clitoris hasn't been directly or intentionally stimulated, it has been indirectly stimulated by the man's penile thrusting and by the pubic contact of the bodies. Often women experience or-

*See *Medical Aspects of Human Sexuality,* August 1975, p. 67.

gasms of greater intensity when clitoral stimulation has been direct, but the physiological response is the same. The clitoris participates in all orgasms, for as the pelvic movements of the man press against the vaginal walls, they stimulate nerves extending down from the clitoris.*

Myth: Intercourse is dangerous during the menstrual period.

Fact: Menstruation has been the subject of numerous misconceptions for centuries. Women have actually been considered "unclean" during this time, and among some religious groups they still are. Sometimes they were even compelled to leave their homes during the menstrual period. Blood often evokes negative feelings associated with injury and violence. While many people feel uncomfortable having intercourse during menstruation because of the possibility of staining the sheets or fear of infection, in reality menstrual blood is not harmful to either man or woman. In fact, many women have heightened sexual desire during these days, and both partners may therefore find coitus particularly rewarding. As for stains, an old towel should eliminate any concern in this regard.

Myth: Women don't experience nocturnal orgasms like those experienced by men ("wet dreams").

Fact: According to Kinsey's *Sexual Behavior in the Human Female,* 70 percent of the female subjects reported having dreams of a truly sexual nature, and of these about half said that their dreams resulted in orgasm. Men may have been reluctant to accept the validity of these findings because women leave no visible evidence of orgasm such as the ejaculate of men. Examination of the vulval region after the nocturnal orgasmic occurrence, however, reveals vaginal secretions just as though sexual stimulation had been of a real physical nature.

Myth: Sexual intercourse is not safe during pregnancy.

Fact: While physicians are almost unanimous in permitting coitus up until the last four to six weeks before delivery, many now say that it is permissible up until the time that labor pains actually begin, provided that pregnancy is normal and that no adverse conditions exist that might threaten the fetus. The general conditions for continuing intercourse during pregnancy would include an absence of pain for the woman during coitus, an absence of bleeding, and no indication of rupture of the fetal membranes. Of course, every woman should consult her physician concerning the advisability of intercourse during each of her pregnancies, and her own feelings about it should be respected. During the last weeks she becomes increasingly uncomfortable and may not feel enthusiastic about intercourse. Remember too that during a woman's orgasm the uterus contracts much as it does

*For further information, see *Medical Aspects of Human Sexuality,* August 1975, p. 29.

during labor. During the last three weeks of pregnancy, such orgasmic contractions could bring on premature labor.

Myth: A woman can't get pregnant while she is lactating (nursing a child).

Fact: While menstruation is often suppressed for several months following delivery when a woman nurses her child, it is possible for conception to occur. Pregnancy is somewhat less likely, but about 20 percent of women who nurse without using any birth control measure do get pregnant. Even though there may be no menstrual flow for several months, ovulation precedes menstruation and thus conception is possible.

Myth: There is an absolutely safe period during the menstrual cycle when there is no possibility of conception.

Fact: *Usually* a woman will ovulate about the middle of the menstrual cycle (fourteenth day) and *normally* this would be the only time that conception could occur. Even women with exceptionally regular and predictable ovulation times, however, may not always ovulate on schedule. Also, ovulation sometimes occurs more than once a month. This is the reason that the rhythm method of birth control is so unreliable. Humans are not machines, never varying in their performance. Therefore, if partners are serious about contraception, they should never assume certain days to be safe, and a more reliable method of birth control should be used at *all* times of the month.

Myth: Simultaneous orgasms are more satisfying than those experienced separately by each partner.

Fact: Again we say that an orgasm is an orgasm, no matter when it happens. Many couples continuously strive to achieve simultaneous orgasm because of the psychological rewards they associate with it. Physiologically speaking, however, there are many valid arguments in favor of separate orgasms. For instance, the movements of the man and woman are quite different at the time of orgasm and are not compatible. The man's tendency is to thrust deeply into the vagina and to hold that position for a period of time, whereas the woman's tendency near orgasm is to have the same stroking movements continued without interruption, and perhaps with a little acceleration in pace. These two patterns cannot be accommodated at the same time. In addition, orgasm is a time of maximum personal awareness and reduced awareness of the external environment. Many people experience great pleasure in the perception of their partners' orgasms, and this perception is reduced during their own orgasms. In any case, the object of sexual activity is not to follow unrealistic rules, but rather that both partners be as satisfied as possible and that it be an enjoyable, nonfrustrating experience.

Myth: Castration always causes a man to completely lose his sex drive and potency.

Fact: Castration is the removal of either the testicles or ovaries. Most women don't feel that their sexuality is completely lost when their ovaries are removed, but men tend to feel more threatened by loss of the testicles. When the testicles are removed, because of either injury or disease, there is a drastic decrease in the male sex hormone testosterone, but the testicles are not the only structures that produce male hormones. The adrenal glands just above the kidneys also produce them.

The effects of castration are variable, especially in relation to the age at which castration occurs. When a sexually immature boy loses his testicles, further sexual development is halted. He will never develop the secondary sex characteristics of an adult male. When castration occurs after a man is sexually mature, however, and especially if he has had considerable satisfactory sexual experience, impotence is not the inevitable outcome. Supplemental injections of testosterone are often used to supply a man's body with the amount that he can no longer produce, if he feels he needs them. While sexual drive may decrease, and erections may not be quite so frequent or strong, it is the psychological trauma rather than the physical fact of castration that results in impotence. Reassurance and encouragement from the sexual partner and an informed and healthy attitude on the part of the man are the most crucial factors in the successful continuity of intercourse following castration.

Myth: After menopause or panhysterectomy (including ovary removal) a woman's sexual desire gradually disappears.

Fact: After the ovaries stop producing ova or when the ovaries are removed, there is a decrease in the hormones (estrogen and progesterone) produced by the ovaries. However, this is no reason for a woman to lose her sexual desire. In fact, many women experience increased sex drive because they no longer fear pregnancy. On the other hand, some women do go through periods of mental depression or physical discomfort due to the sudden change in hormone balance. When this hormone deficiency is severe, the physician can prescribe medication to replace the estrogens no longer being produced.*

Myth: All men go through a climateric similar to female menopause, after which they can no longer father a child.

Fact: In the female, the climateric consists of actual physical and sometimes mental changes that signal the end of reproductive ability. Most

*For further discussion, see *Medical Aspects of Human Sexuality,* August 1975, pp. 104–110.

men do not experience a climateric in the sense that fertility is lost. As men age, testicular functioning does decrease and fertility is thus reduced, but the production of sperm is seldom completely lost. There is much controversy over whether men experience a true physiological climateric or whether it is more psychosexual in nature.* Recent scientific research indicates that some men do experience a true physical climateric associated with diminished sexual vigor, but in the majority, erection, intercourse, and fatherhood are possible into old age. In both sexes, emotional stability and acceptance of the gradual changes accompanying aging have considerable influence on sexual desire.

Myth: There is a bone in the penis that is responsible for getting and maintaining an erection.

Fact: This fallacy probably relates to the presence of a bone in the penis of some animals, such as the dog. The human penis, however, contains no bone, and erection is due to blood pouring into dilated arteries in the erectile tissue. Erection is maintained because the veins in the erectile tissue constrict, thus preventing escape of blood from the penis.

Myth: Humans can get "hung up" during intercourse (*penis captivus*).

Fact: While many people will swear this has happened to someone they know, there are no factual data to support such a contention. It can happen in animals having bones in the penis, because glands on the sides of the penis swell after entry into the vagina at the same time that the vagina constricts, preventing withdrawal before ejaculation. There is no corresponding phenomenon in humans. If the vagina goes into spasm (*vaginisimus*), however, withdrawal may be difficult, but it is never impossible. The discomfort of the spasm or fear of being hung up causes the man to lose his erection, facilitating easy withdrawal.

Myth: Absence of a hymen is proof that virginity is lost.

Fact: In most girls, the hymen is a thin membrane that partially closes off the entrance to the vagina. While the hymen may survive to be ruptured during first intercourse, girls today are so much more active than their grandmothers were that this thin membrane is likely to have been ruptured before intercourse. There are a few girls whose hymens are so flexible that they can have several sexual experiences and still have intact hymens. The presence or absence of the hymen is no proof of virginity. Even a physician may not be able to tell unless coitus has just occurred or unless sexual experience is very frequent.

Myth: Atheletes should not have intercourse the night before performing because it drains them of their strength or makes them too relaxed.

Fact: There are no scientific data to substantiate this old belief. Never-

*See *Medical Aspects of Human Sexuality*, April 1975, pp. 109–113.

theless, many coaches continue to instruct their players to abstain from intercourse or masturbation the night before playing. They may say that the increased tension improves performance. The truth is that tension interferes with body control.

Myth: Girls living in warmer or tropical climates begin menstruation earlier.

Fact: The menarche has nothing to do with climate, but rather is a matter of heredity. Girls usually begin menstruating at about the same age as their mothers did. However, physical conditions of the girl or the environment do influence the age of menarche. For example, anemia or malnutrition causes a delay, and so do hormonal or emotional disturbances.

Myth: There is no such thing as a multiorgasmic woman.

Fact: Many people still find it difficult to accept the fact that many women, in fact about 50 percent, are capable of experiencing many orgasms during one session of lovemaking. While it sometimes takes women longer to reach orgasm, once they get there, with continued stimulation it is very possible for them to have several—three, five, or even more. Frequently women say that the second or third is more intensive than the first. In men it is usually just the opposite. If a man is capable of having a second or third orgasm during one session of lovemaking, the first orgasm is likely to be the most intense and satisfying.

Myth: When men wake up with an erection, this is due to their having a full bladder.

Fact: Such erections are the result of dreams just before waking and have nothing to do with a distended bladder, although the bladder is probably full at this time. When the penis is tumescent it is impossible to urinate, as the prostate gland shuts off the flow of urine from the bladder into the urethra. The presence of morning erection can be very significant when a potency problem exists. Such erection indicates that the problem is not of an organic nature but rather is psychological in origin. This may be a good time to attempt intercourse, for if the attempt is successful, the man's confidence in his ability to function can greatly improve matters.

Misconceptions Dealing with Sex Drive and Activity

The sex drive is comparable to such other drives as hunger and thirst in that it initiates certain behavior patterns that are expected to satisfy it. Many restraints, however, have been imposed upon the behavior available to satisfy the sex drive. Often these restraints take the form of attitudes developed through the acceptance of misconceptions. The sex drive is more likely to be a reflection of what an individual perceives it should be rather than a strictly physiological reaction. For instance, some older people believe that sexual activity is not appropriate to their age group, and thus sexual expression may be completely obviated even though the body's sexual capacity remains intact. Other people may strive to experience sex primarily with partners who have particular racial or physical characteristics, because they believe that the sex drive is greater among such persons, when actually other partners may be just as satisfactory. While the reasoning behind such myths is invalid, the fact remains that sex drives will usually be dealt with and satisfied in accordance with what is felt to be expected or acceptable.

Myth: There are substances, such as particular foods or drugs (aphrodisiacs), that are capable of increasing sexual desire.

Fact: People have been trying for centuries to find an effective aphrodisiac. The fact remains, however, that to date no substance has been found that possesses this quality and still is safe. Innumerable food items have been valued for their effectiveness in increasing sexual activity or desire, but their effectiveness is attributable to the power of suggestion rather than to the actual constituents of the food or drink. The most famous aphrodisiac perhaps is "Spanish fly," derived from dried beetles. This substance produces an irritation of the urinary tract, causing increased blood congestion in the reproductive organs. The penile erection produced by this drug is uncomfortable or downright painful, and it is not accompanied by sexual desire. In addition, it is a poison, and just one drop too much can be lethal.

Recently two drugs have accidently been discovered to have aphrodisiac effects in addition to those for which they were developed. One is PCPA, an experimental drug being used in the treatment of schizophrenia. The other is the widely publicized drug L-dopa, currently being prescribed for persons with Parkinson's disease. Both of these drugs have many side effects that do not warrant their use as sexual stimulants. The time may soon be at hand, though, when a safe and effective drug will be available to help the dragging libido.

Myth: Alcohol acts as a sexual stimulant.

Fact: Despite alcohol's reputation as a sexual stimulant, it is just the opposite. Alcohol acts as a depressant and reduces sexual sensitivity. Moderate amounts sometime appear to stimulate sexuality by reducing inhibitions, but excessive quantities produce temporary impotence in men and impaired orgasmic response in women.

Myth: The intensity of sexual desire varies with ethnic group.

Fact: Sexual desire and degree of sexual activeness appears to be evenly distributed among peoples throughout the world, despite the many myths to the contrary. Certain groups may appear to be more passionate than others, but this is related to their cultural attitudes toward sex and lack of inhibitions in regard to sexual expression.

In America, black people have often been credited with an unusually high level of sexual activity. Sociological studies reveal a correspondence between sexual activity and economic-educational status. People who come from depressed economic and educational environments do exhibit higher levels of sexual activity, but this is as true of white, yellow, red, and brown people as of black. The myth has been persistent because, unfortunately, blacks constitute a large portion of the socioeconomically deprived.

Myth: Masturbation is bad or morally wrong, and can cause many problems.

Fact: This is perhaps one of the best-known and most damaging of all myths. Most parents at one time or another try to prevent their children from masturbating by the use of threats, moral condemnation, or physical punishment. Despite parental objections, masturbation almost always continues, but is accompanied by guilt feelings or fear of punishment. It is certainly hoped that by the time you have read this much of the book, you realize that masturbation is not abnormal, and that nearly 100 percent of the population do masturbate, although some are reluctant to admit it. Masturbation serves as a natural outlet for sexual tensions under many circumstances when other sexual gratification is impossible. It does no harm whatsoever unless you think it does. In one form or another, masturbation actually begins in infancy, and it is really a learning experience that should help prepare the individual for the role of a normal sexually functioning adult.

Many sexual maladjustments in adults can be traced back to parental attitudes toward masturbation. Once a child associates the genitals with shame, guilt, sin, punishment, and fear, sexual expression at any level becomes increasingly difficult. While children may have to be taught when and where masturbation is appropriate, this can be done without prohibiting it altogether, or making it out to be nasty, dirty behavior. One of the greatest responsibilities of parents is helping a child to grow up without guilt feelings, to have a good self-image, and to learn how to express love for others. If an individual never learns self-love and self-respect, it is impossible for such a person to feel these things for others.

Myth: Men have a much stronger sex drive than women do.

Fact: While there is no way to determine objectively which sex has the stronger sex drive, if either, the supposedly great variation between the sexes cannot be demonstrated. Men have traditionally played the role of aggressor and women have been expected to be passive or merely submissive. The double standard is disappearing, and women are proving themselves to be as potentially aggressive as men—often causing insecure men to feel that their masculinity is threatened. Increasingly women are demanding a broad range of sexual experience, including diversity of partners, and they have increased expectations of performance from their partners. There is one factor that cannot be overlooked in considering sexual cravings versus gender, and it has probably contributed greatly to the male's overestimation of his sex drive. Specifically, the penis is more quickly excited and the result of such excitement is the obvious erection. Some women, on the other hand, may respond more slowly, and of course they can offer no obvious evidence corresponding to the tumescent penis. Does this mean that women desire sex less than men? Consider, for example, the large number of women who complain that their husbands can't meet their sexual demands.

Myth: Physical activity greatly reduces sexual desire.

Fact: Physical activity to the point of exhaustion does reduce the sex urge, but when physical activity is designed specifically as a means of getting the mind off sexual needs, it will not achieve its purpose for any appreciable length of time. When people try to divert their attention from sexual cravings by expending energy in some other way, this in itself can increase sexual desire. That which we deliberately try to forget is also that which is most likely not to be forgotten. As for cold showers, they will reduce sex drive for about as long as it takes to dry off the body. But if a person ardently believes in the effectiveness of cold showers, or anything else, they may in fact be psychologically effective.

Myth: Women with unusually great sexual appetites are nymphomanics, and the equivalent condition in the male, satyriasis, is quite common also.

Fact: There are extremely few true nymphomaniacs in the commonly accepted meaning of the term, and even fewer satyrs, if there are any at all. The currently accepted phrase to describe such behavior is "compulsive sexuality." The sexually compulsive person differs greatly from a person with a very good sex drive. For example, the sexually compulsive person is unable to control sexual behavior, and true sexual satisfaction is never experienced. In contrast to the sexual compulsive, even promiscuous persons have the ability to control their actions, and while their choice of sexual partners may be very liberal, such choices are self-determined and sexual gratification is attained. The women most frequently labeled as nymphomanics are those whose sexual appetites just happen to be greater than their mates'. The use of such a term implies that her behavior is abnormal while his is normal, and it is a defense mechanism used to mask male feelings of inadequacy. Many men are not aware that a great many women are capable of multiple orgasms, and there are still many men who believe that women are just not supposed to enjoy sex as much as men. When given a choice between the unresponsive and the responsive woman, most men would prefer a woman who participates in and delights in lovemaking, and consider themselves fortunate when they have found such a partner.

Myth: People are allocated just so many sexual experiences, and when they are used up, sexual activity stops.

Fact: There is absolutely no evidence to support this myth. In fact, just the opposite is true. The length of time that a person can expect to be sexually functional is directly related to frequency and regularity of sexual activity, and regularity supports rather than suppresses both sexual desire and sexual performance. Like any other part of the body when it is not used, the sex organs may atrophy and lose their ability to function when they are not used. (This is the reason that members of religious orders and others dedicated to some "unworldly" ideal are able to remain celibate for a lifetime.) Some men erroneously believe that they have just a certain amount of sperm, and when it is used up, so are their sex lives. Men continue to produce sperm continuously throughout their lives, and ejaculated sperm are efficiently and easily replenished. Also, orgasm cannot occur so often that another can never again be experienced. There is a refractory period after each male orgasm during which another is physiologically impossible, but within a period of time (variable according to age and individual) sexual desire and orgasmic ability always return.

Myth: Sterilization of either sex diminishes sexual drive.

Fact: Unlike castration, which involves removal of the sex glands (ovaries or testicles), which can interfere with sex drive, sterilization neither removes these glands nor suppresses the production of sex hormones. The only thing that sterilization does is prevent the union of sperm and egg. In men the vas deferens is cut, and in women the fallopian tubes are cut and tied. If pregnancy is not desired, then sterilization may actually increase the sex drive because there is no longer fear of an unwanted pregnancy. There are people who say their sex drive has decreased following sterilization, but this decrease is psychological and definitely not physiological in origin.

Myth: Sexual desire and ability are lost in the middle years, and the psychological need for sex is not so great in older couples as it was during their youth.

Fact: Unfortunately, for many years people closely associated the appropriateness of intercourse with reproductive ability. Thus people often believed that sex after the reproductive years was not only unnecessary but actually undignified. This idea appears now to be current only among the young; their elders know better. According to statistics, marital coitus remains part of the relationship of most couples until they reach their middle seventies, and for only a little less than half of couples in their eighties and nineties. Sex, love, and romance are not limited to the young. Sex is a very positive psychological support to the aging person whose role in life is changing, who is unsure about the meaning of his or her life, and who may very well feel like a burden. Continued sexual activity assures each partner of feeling loved, of still being attractive; it supports continuing high self-esteem. This is a time during a couple's life when communication with each other is likely to be more important than it was when they were preoccupied by work and parental responsibilities, and what more beautiful way is there to say "I still love and need you" than to enjoy each other sexually?

Myths and Reproductive Processes

Conception, pregnancy, birth, fertility, and contraception have always had special significance for all peoples, and rightly so, because the very existence of humans depends upon these interrelated processes. Because of lack of understanding of the functioning of the reproductive system, however, such processes were often viewed as magical, mystical, or otherwise supernatural, and beyond human intervention. Consequently myths have arisen regarding almost every aspect of reproduction, and many are still clung to tenaciously because ignorance is pentrated so very slowly.

Myth: Mating between closely related individuals produces defective genes.

Fact: Mating between closely related individuals does not produce defective genes, but it does increase the probability that both members of such a couple will be carrying one or more of the same recessive genes. A recessive gene is one that is a part of a person's genetic make-up but which is not evident because it will visibly manifest itself only when it is paired with another recessive gene like itself. Recessive genes may or may not be harmful. It is known that all us carry many recessive genes that we are not even aware of. Thus the more ancestors a man and woman have in common, the more likely it is that they are carrying identical recessive genes. This means that the odds that identical beneficial genes will unite are increased, as well as the risk that harmful combinations will occur. So while some couples will produce defective offspring, others will encounter no congenital problems in their offspring. While marriages between first cousins or people more closely related do dramatically increase the chances of congenital defects in offspring, marriages between second cousins involve little greater risk than random unions.

Myth: If women urinate immediately following intercourse, pregnancy will be prevented.

Fact: Urination, no matter how immediately it follows intercourse, is of absolutely no contraceptive value. In the first place, the vaginal canal, in which semen is deposited, is completely separate from the urethra, through which urine passes. Therefore, urine could not come in contact with the semen ejaculated into the vagina. Some people also believe that the semen will flow out of the vagina when a woman assumes a sitting position, and that this will help prevent conception. While a small amount of seminal fluid may escape from the vagina, by this time thousands of sperm have already entered the cervical opening. Finally, even if urine were somehow to be introduced into the vagina after intercourse, it has little power to kill sperm.

Myth: Pregnancy can't occur unless intercourse has taken place.

Fact: Of course intercourse is the normal method of conception, but artificial insemination is a successful and not uncommon method of inducing conception without the act of intercourse. Many couples also believe that pregnancy can't occur as long as the penis does not enter the vagina. It is quite possible for conception to occur if sperm are deposited in the genital area, even though the vagina has not been penetrated, or if fingers that have semen on them are introduced into the vagina. In any event, it is possible for a woman to conceive and bear a child without penile penetration. There have been cases in which a physician has had to cut the hymen to permit the birth of a child.

Myth: If a couple engages in oral sex and the woman swallows some semen, pregnancy can occur.

Fact: Absolutely not. The semen that is swallowed would be digested like any other liquid that is ingested. Semen is composed of the same basic nutrients as other foods: protein, carbohydrate, and fat. The average ejaculation has been reported to contain about 36 calories.

Myth: In order for pregnancy to occur, a woman must have an orgasm.

Fact: The female orgasm has no functional value as far as the union of sperm and ovum are concerned. Pregnancy following rape is an excellent example of this point. Since intercourse is necessary for the propagation of the species, however, the pleasure of orgasm is very functional.

Myth: After the menopausal period (change of life) has begun, and no menstrual periods have occurred for a few months, contraceptive measures are no longer necessary.

Fact: Women don't just suddenly stop ovulating forever even when they definitely have begun going through menopause. Contraceptive measures should continue to be used for at least one year following the last menstrual period. Should a period occur during these twelve months, another year must go by before the woman can consider herself safe. Even after a year there are no iron-clad guarantees; it may take several years to be positive that pregnancy is no longer possible. There are plenty of change-of-life babies to prove the point.

Myth: A prematurely born seventh-month fetus has a better survival chance than an eighth-month fetus.

Fact: This is a common belief but it is not true. The longer a fetus remains within the uterus, as long as it does not go much beyond term, the better are its chances of survival. Weight, for instance, is a very important factor in determining the survival chances of a fetus, and a seven-month fetus weighs about two pounds less than an eight-month fetus. Other factors influencing survival chances are the degree of development of the respiratory and digestive systems, both of which are more fully developed in the eight-month fetus. The amount of subcutaneous fat is also greater in the eight-month fetus, and this is significant because a newborn, even a full-term baby, is not able to withstand temperature fluctuations very well, and fat helps to regulate temperature. Also, antibodies are transferred from the mother to the fetus through the placenta, and such transference doesn't occur until late in pregnancy. These antibodies are important in protecting the infant from several diseases for the first few months following birth. Statistically, the seven-month fetus has a 50 percent survival chance, the eight-month fetus 90 percent, and the full-term baby 99 percent. In addition, low birth weight is associated with increased incidence of neurological defects.

Myth: An unborn child can be marked by events or emotions that the mother has experienced during pregnancy.

Fact: This is untrue in almost every instance; however, there is some truth to the belief that the emotional state of the mother can have an effect on the unborn child. Birthmarks or discolorations on the infant's body bear no relationship to the events of pregnancy, but were genetically determined at conception. Some women still believe that reading good literature or listening to Beethoven will have some influence on the child; this too is absolutely untrue. There is no direct connection between the circulatory and nervous systems of the mother and those of the fetus. The only things that can affect the fetus are certain chemicals and organisms that are allowed to pass the placental barrier from the mother's blood into that of the fetus. These substances include some poisons, antibodies, viruses, and bacteria. If the mother undergoes great emotional stress during pregnancy, the stress does affect the levels of hormones in her body, such as epinephrine, and these hormones influence the developing fetus to some extent. Social experiences, however, have no effect on the unborn child.

Myth: The semen of a previous mate can have an effect on children fathered by a woman's new mate.

Fact: There is no scientific evidence to support this idea, which is known as "telegony." It is quite impossible for a child to be genetically influenced by anyone other than the woman who contributed the egg and the man whose sperm penetrated that egg. This myth probably arose from the observation that animals often produce litters of offspring that bear little or no resemblance to each other. Female dogs, for instance, release ova over a period of several days, and it is likely that she would mate with more than one male. Consequently, the littermates may not share the same sire, but each offspring receives only the genes of the male that sired it and is never influenced by the genes of any other male. No matter how many sexual partners a woman has had, her child will have only the genetic characteristics of the man whose sperm penetrated that particular ovum. There is an outside possibility that a woman may conceive a child by a particular mate and then ovulate again within a few days. If the woman has more than one sex partner, it would be possible for the second ovum to be fertilized by another man. This would result in the birth of twins who would be related to each other only as half-siblings.

Myth: It is possible for humans to reproduce by unfertilized eggs (*parthenogenesis*) the way lower animals sometimes do.

Fact: To begin with, parthenogenesis occurs when an egg is in some manner stimulated so that it starts developing without being fertilized by a sperm. This is a rather common occurrence among the lower animals, especially among insects. Experimentally, various stimuli have been used to induce parthenogenesis in mammals such as rabbits. It has been done to human ova, but development didn't proceed very far and there is no record of the actual birth of a child from an ovum that was induced to develop in this way. If a method of human parthenogenesis were ever developed, all offspring produced in this manner would be female, because the only sex chromosome carried by the ovum is the X chromosome. If the practice became common, it would lead to a very unusual population distribution.

Myth: If either mate has any black ancestry, however little and however remote, the couple may have a child who is very black, even though both parents appear white.

Fact: The mechanism of color inheritance dictates that a child cannot be darker than the sum of the darkness of both parents, and it is more likely that the offspring would be lighter than this. So if both parents had light skin color and a child "they" produced was decidely darker, than it would not be a matter of throwback but rather a case of deception.

Myth: One testicle contains only male-producing sperm (Y), whereas the other contains only female-producing sperm (X).

Fact: The male definitely does determine a child's sex, but the testicles are not differential in the production of X-bearing and Y-bearing sperm. When germ cells go through spermatogenesis, they produce an equal number of X- and Y-bearing gametes. Therefore, it would be impossible for either testicle to produce only one kind of sperm. Females, in contrast, produce only one kind of gamete, X-bearing ova, and therefore have no influence in the determination of the child's sex.

Myth: Humans are capable of cross-breeding with infrahuman animals.

Fact: It is impossible for a human to sire or conceive an offspring by any other animal. It is not possible for any different genera to cross-breed. It is sometimes possible, however, for different species within the same genus to mate and produce offspring. The mating of horse and donkey produces a mule; the mating of lions and tigers produces offspring called ligers. All such offspring of related species are sterile and cannot reproduce themselves. Humans can and do have coitus with infrahuman animals, but offspring never result.

Myth: Masturbation can make a man sterile or impotent.

Fact: Masturbation in no way affects a man's ability to get an erection unless it should occur so closely before actual intercourse that he would still be in the refractory period during which erection would be impossible for a limited period of time. Masturbation in no way causes sterility, but it may affect the fertility level. Frequent masturbation or intercourse (several ejaculations a day) does temporarily lower the sperm content of the semen, thereby reducing the chance of fertility during any one ejaculation, but definitely not to the point of rendering him sterile. Sperm are easily and readily replenished.

Myth: Birth control pills often cause cancer.

Fact: Birth control pills rarely cause cancer; however, if cancer is present, it may develop and spread faster because the estrogen contained in the pill has a catalytic effect on cancer. This is one of the primary reasons that women should have yearly exams while they are taking the pill. These examinations have detected many cancers that would probably not have been found otherwise. This is particularly true of breast and cervical cancers. Among problems that do occur more frequently among pill users than among other women are an increased incidence of blood clots and disturbances in blood-sugar level. When these risks are weighed against the risks involved in pregnancy, however, pregnancy turns out to be the more dangerous of the two.

Myth: Contraceptives can cause sterility.

Fact: The only contraceptive measure that causes permanent sterility is actual sterilization by cutting and tying the vas deferens in males and the fallopian tubes in females. If a couple is unable to have children after contraception has been discontinued, the problem most likely existed before the use of the contraceptive measure and is not a consequence of it.

Myths and Homosexuality

Homosexuality has been known throughout recorded history. In some cultures, such as that of the ancient Greeks, it was considered a more pure and beautiful expression of love than heterosexual union. The fact remains, however, that within our own cultural climate homosexuality is not generally considered acceptable behavior, and in some places such activity is criminal. For the most part, scientific research on human sexuality has centered on the heterosexual relationship, and much less attention has been devoted to exploring the dimensions of homosexuality. This is not to say that no factual data are available, but there still exists no clear or comprehensive understanding of this phenomenon. To complicate the situation, there is still much controversy among behavioral specialists as to whether homosexuality is deviant behavior or merely a variation in normal sexual expression. We are still asking what its causes are, whether it should be treated, and if so how. In the meantime, the average individual, straight or gay, is too often left to deal with the homosexual subculture solely on the basis of personal feelings and a variety of misconceptions. While certain myths can be dispelled with ease, it is difficult to counter some beliefs about homosexuality because of lack of sufficient data, or because the rapidly expanding pool of information may well disprove what today is considered true.

Myth: Homosexuality is due to hereditary or hormonal defects.

Fact: To date heredity has not been proved to be directly responsible for homosexuality. Neither has it been proved to have no influence on homosexuality. In fact, there is no single factor that can be demonstrated to be the cause. It appears that a series of events leads or predisposes an individual toward homosexuality. The primary causative factor—at least the one most widely cited—is emotional disturbance related to unstable home environment during childhood development. Within the framework of family influence, the psychosocial maladjustments are very diverse and difficult to isolate, for adverse parental influences may or may not lead a person to assume a homosexual orientation. There is mixed evidence on the question of hormone imbalance as a causal factor in homosexuality. Chemical analysis of urine from both homosexual and heterosexual individuals has in some studies indicated a slight variance in hormone balance—that is, the ratio of one hormone to another. Exactly what significance these findings hold may not be known for years; research is still in progress. To date genetic and hormonal influences are believed to be minimal, if they exist at all, but no one really knows.

Myth: Homosexuals are more creative than heterosexuals.

Fact: It does appear that many homosexuals are found in professions that demand a rather high degree of creativity, such as the arts, dress designing, interior decorating, hair styling, and so on. It is a mistake to associate occupation with homosexuality, however. In the first place, only a small percentage of homosexuals can actually be identified by their mannerisms or style of dress or interests. The artistic professions tend to be more tolerant of the overt (obvious) homosexual because the individualistic, innovative person is valuable, and the overt homosexual certainly is not a conformist. Homosexuals may also be drawn into these professions because of the social segregation they often experience. The person who is "different" is excluded from most peer groups in adolescence. Therefore, activities must be undertaken that can be done on an individual rather than a group basis. Thus creativity is encouraged.

Myth: Homosexuals are a threat to society, and represent a special threat to children.

Fact: Actually, the reverse is more often true—society represents a threat to the homosexual. Since they are so often ridiculed or rejected, homosexuals tend to segregate themselves from the "straight" segment of society. They constitute a subculture that has its own language, its own areas of residence, its own business and pleasure establishments. The threat felt by the straight population, however invalid it may be, is due to the fact that homosexuality contradicts the values of marriage and the family. Society increasingly accepts changes in values involving heterosexuals; for example, divorce, transitory nonmarital cohabitation, serial monogomy, and increasing voluntary childlessness. When it comes to the homosexual, however, society is less tolerant because the homosexual life style is unconventional; it is hard on the Hell's Angels and the Hari Krishna people too. As for the threat that homosexuals may represent to children, it is not typical for homosexuals to force their attentions upon children, and even when they do become involved in sexual acts with minors, the child is more likely to be harmed by the reactions of the adults who learn about it than by the experience itself. The highest incidence of forced attentions upon unwilling heterosexuals occurs within prisons, which are certainly not comparable with the outside community.

Myth: Most prostitutes are also lesbians.

Fact: Most prostitutes are not lesbians. Whether or not a prostitute is homosexual depends upon the reason she chose prostitution as a profession. When a woman becomes a prostitute because of intense dislike for men and uses prostitution as a means of getting back at them, then she is likely to be a homosexual. For many prostitutes, however, their profession is merely a means of livelihood. Such a woman usually has a sexual relationship with a special man in her life. There are no statistics available as to the exact incidence of homosexuality among prostitutes, but certainly most prostitutes are not lesbians.

Myth: If a person has a homosexual experience during youth, that person is likely to become strictly homosexual later on in life.

Fact: It is not unusual at all for adolescents or preadolescents to have one or more homosexual experiences. There is a period of adjustment during which children must transfer their interest and affection from friends of the same sex to those of the opposite sex. This is a period when children have "best friends" with whom they are close, and sexual inquisitiveness is common. It is very normal for both boys and girls to explore each other, and perhaps even go beyond exploration. It is also common for an adolescent to have what used to be called a "crush" on an older person of the same sex, usually a teacher or camp counselor. This intense interest in a person of the same sex is a normal stage that gradually leads to a higher level of maturity, which permits acceptance of and curiosity about the opposite sex. There are very few people who have never had some sort of homosexual experience, and the preadolescent or adolescent homosexual experience in no way indicates that the individual will be homosexual as an adult. The only lasting damage that these encounters can have is an unwarranted feeling of guilt or an equally unwarranted fear or assumption that one must be basically homosexual.

Myths About Sexual Norms and Sex Offenders

Sexual behavior cannot be arbitrarily defined as normal, abnormal, perverse, or even criminal. Ultimately, standards lie only within the perception and consequent interpretation of the individual. What legally constitutes abnormal or criminal sexual behavior is therefore subject to considerable variation from state to state and even among communities. Misconceptions that erroneously categorize a particular behavior as abnormal frequently result in the unjustified labeling of persons as perverted when in fact they are merely expressing their sexuality in a less inhibited way than some other people. The myths about the "typical" sex offender—whose behavior, incidentally, rarely constitutes a physical threat to anyone—have instilled excessive and unwarranted fear in a major segment of the public.

Myth: Transvestites and transsexuals are the same, and both are homosexual.

Fact: Although it is possible for elements of all three conditions to exist in one person, each is a separate type of behavior. The transvestite is one who gets sexual stimulation from dressing up in clothes of the opposite sex. Most transvestites are neither homosexual nor transsexual, and the majority of them are married. There is no denial of gender, but transvestites often view themselves as having two personalities, one male and one female. The transsexual, on the other hand, totally rejects the biological sex with which he or she was born. While occasionally there is an abnormality in the sex chromosomes or sex hormones, the problem is usually extremely difficult to trace to its origins. Some transsexuals report that they have always felt that they belonged to the opposite sex, from the time of their earliest memories, though no biological abnormality can be found. Transsexuals are never homosexual. They feel that they are trapped in the wrong body, and the sexual attention they desire from persons of the same sex is based upon their conviction that they actually belong to the opposite sex. It is now possible for transsexuals to have sex-change operations, which have proved to be very successful from the psychological standpoint.

Myth: All sex offenders are dangerous to society.

Fact: Under the penal codes of many states, any act of intercourse outside the confines of marriage is a crime, and so are many sex acts commonly performed by married couples. Under laws of this kind, most of the population could be found guilty of some sex offense, but few persons would define such behavior as deviant, and in fact it would be extremely unusual for such people to be arrested for their "crimes." The sex acts for which people are most commonly arrested are exhibitionism, voyeurism, forcible and statutory rape, and various homosexual acts. The only one of these sex offenders who is dangerous to society is the forcible rapist. The behavior of exhibitionists, voyeurs, and homosexuals is not characteristically forceful or aggressive, but is more indicative of insecurity, fear of the opposite sex, shyness, or, in the case of statutory rape, unwise choice of sex partner. Exhibitionists alone account for almost one-third of all sex-associated arrests. While these offenders are certainly neurotic, they are seldom psychotic. The belief that the typical sex offender is a homicidal maniac is a myth. Homicidal maniacs do exist, of course, and their crimes are widely publicized. But they can in no way be related to the typical—or more accurately the most often arrested and convicted—sex offender. Once a person has established a sexual behavior pattern, such as exhibitionism, there is virtually no way for him to commit a more serious crime, because the personality dynamics that make for exhibitionism militate against the performance of aggressive, forceful acts.

Myth: Sex offenders of any kind are seldom cured.

Fact: Sometimes the cure is effected when the offender is arrested; that's what usually happens when men are charged with statutory rape. Exhibitionism, voyeurism, and other nonforceful deviant acts are evidence of neuroses. Typically, neurotic behavior responds well to psychotherapy; however, since these offenders are rarely given an opportunity for therapy, repeated arrests and convictions are common. The pedophile or child molester is frequently arrested and convicted for his crime only once. Most child molesters are not strangers to the children they molest, and their acts frequently do not involve coitus. If they do, then the charge is rape. The rapist and rapist-murderer are the sex offenders who must not be allowed to repeat their crimes. The others deserve our pity and our help more than our wrath.

Myth: Child molesters are usually old men who are likely to rape and kill children.

Fact: The Kinsey reports have disproved the idea that old men (over sixty-five) are most likely to be child molesters. As a group, they are the least likely to be guilty of any kind of sexual offense. The average age of the child molester is about thirty-five; men over fifty account for only about one-sixth of child molestation arrests. Again it should be pointed out that the pedophile is most often a family member or at least a familar person to the child, that such acts are not necessarily forceful, and that violence is not common even when the child doesn't cooperate. If parents and other adults can keep their heads, the child is quite likely to suffer no psychological damage.

Myth: Pornography leads people to sexual excesses, and even to commit sex crimes.

Fact: Pornography is a very loose term used to refer to just about any kind of erotic material. Most research to date indicates that erotic material of any description has no effect on the rate of sex crimes committed by either the young or the old, and that persons arrested for sex crimes are most inclined to have backgrounds of little sexual permissiveness. Sexual repression is found to be a leading factor in the development of unacceptable sexual behavior. As far as sexual acting out is concerned, pornography's influence is related to the individual's capacity for imagination. Sexual activity may increase for a short period following exposure to erotic material, but very seldom affects degree of sexual aggressiveness, and moral codes are not likely to be altered.

Bibliography

Arey, Leslie. *Developmental Anatomy,* 7th ed. Philadelphia: Saunders, 1974.
Beserra, Sarah S., Nancy M. Jewel, and Melody W. Mathews. *Sex Code of California.* Sausalito: Public Education and Research Committee, 1973.
Brown, Norman O. *Love's Body.* New York: Random House, 1966.
Chesser, Eustace. Strange Loves: The Human Aspects of Sexual Deviation. New York: Morrow, 1971.
Cohn, Frederick. *Understanding Human Sexuality.* Englewood Cliffs, N.J.: Hall, 1974.
Comfort, Alex. *The Joy of Sex.* New York: Fireside Books, Simon & Schuster, 1972.
Conn, Howard F. *Current Therapy, 1974.* Philadelphia: Saunders, 1974.
Deutsch, Ronald M. *The Key to Feminine Response in Marriage.* New York: Random House, 1968.
Ford, Clellan S., and Frank A. Beach. *Patterns of Sexual Behavior.* New York: Harper & Row, 1951.
Fulton, Gere B. *Sexual Awareness.* Boston: Holbrook Press, 1974.
Hamilton, W. J., and H. W. Mossman. *Human Embryology: Prenatal Development of Form and Function,* 4th ed. Baltimore: Williams & Wilkins, 1972.
Hellman, Louis M., and Jack A. Prichard. *Williams Obstetrics,* 16th ed. New York: Appleton-Century-Crofts, 1971.
Hettlinger, Richrd F. *Human Sexuality: A Psychosocial Perspective.* Belmont, Calif.: Wadsworth, 1975.
Johnson, Warren R., and Edwin G. Belzer, Jr. *Human Sexual Behavior and Sex Education,* 3rd ed. Philadelphia: Lea & Febiger, 1973.
Kaplan, Helen S., and Clifford J. Sage. "Sexual Patterns at Different Ages." *Medical Aspects of Human Sexuality* 15, no. 6 (June 1971): 11.
Katchadourian, Herant A., and Donald T. Lunde. *Fundamentals of Human Sexuality,* 2nd ed. New York: Holt, Rinehard & Winston, 1975.
Kupperman, Herbert S. "Male Climacteric." *Medical World News* 15, no. 24 (June 28, 1974): pg. 32–44.
Lederer, William J., and Don D. Jackson. *The Mirages of Marriage.* New York: Norton, 1968.
Lewinsohn, Richard. *A History of Sexual Customs.* New York: Harper & Row, 1958.
MagaBack, Human Sexuality: An Age of Ambiguity. Boston: Little, Brown, 1975. Bruce Henderson, Writer.
Masters, William H., and Virginia E. Johnson. *Human Sexual Response.* Boston: Little, Brown, 1966.
——— and ———. *Human Sexual Inadequacy.* Boston: Little, Brown, 1970.
McCown, Chester C. *Man, Morals, and History.* New York: Harper & Row, 1958.
Maxwell, Roland. *Management of the Infertile Couple.* Springfield, Ill.: Charles C Thomas, 1968.

Money, J., and Anke A. Ehrhardt. *Man and Woman, Boy and Girl: The Differentiation and Dimorphism of Gender Identity from Conception to Maturity.* Baltimore: Johns Hopkins University Press, 1972.

Moore, Keith L. *The Developing Human.* Philadelphia: Saunders, 1973.

National Institute of Mental Health. *Biological Rhythms in Psychiatry and Medicine.* U.S. Public Health Service publication no. 2008. Washington, D.C.: U.S. Government Printing Office, 1970.

Oster, Gerald. "Conception and Contraception." *Natural History* 91, no. 7 (August–September 1972).

Pengelley, Eric T. *Sex and Human Life.* Reading, Mass.: Addison-Wesley, 1974.

Pierson, Elaine C., and William V. D'Antonio. *Female and Male Dimensions of Human Sexuality.* Philadelphia: Lippincott, 1974.

Racy, John. "Marital Partners Who Misuse Sex." *Medical Aspects of Human Sexuality* 8, no. 11 (November 1974): 67–68.

Reuben, David. *Everything You Always Wanted to Know About Sex.* New York: McKay, 1969.

Rhodin, Johannes A. G. *Histology.* New York: Oxford University Press, 1974.

Saghir, M. T., and E. Robins. *Male and Female Homosexuality.* Baltimore: Williams & Wilkins, 1973.

Shope, David F. *Interpersonal Sexuality.* Englewood Cliffs, N.J.: Prentice-Hall, 1974.

Thommen, George S. *Is This Your Day?* New York: Crown, 1973.

Turner, C. D. *General Endocrinology,* 5th ed. Philadelphia: Saunders, 1971.

Vander, Arthur J., James H. Sherman, and Dorothy S. Luciano. *Human Physiology: The Mechanisms of Body Functions,* 2nd ed. New York: McGraw-Hill, 1975.

Walker, P. A., and J. Money. "Prenatal Androgenization of Females." *Hormones* 3 (March 1972): 118–128.

Wilson, Samuel T., Richard L. Roe, and Lucy E. Autrey. *Readings in Human Sexuality.* St. Paul, Minn.: West, 1975.

Index

76 77 78 79 80 9 8 7 6 5 4 3 2 1